Commissioning Editor: Laurence Hunter
Project Development Manager: Barbara Simmons
Project Controller: Nancy Arnott
Designer: Erik Bigland

Churchill's Pocketbook of

Surgery

Andrew T. Raftery BSc MD CI Biol MI Biol FRCS (Eng) FRCS(E)

Consultant Surgeon, Sheffield Kidney Institute, Northern General Hospital NHS Trust, Sheffield, UK;
Member (formerly Chairman), Court of Examiners, Royal College of Surgeons of England;
Member of Panel of Examiners, Intercollegiate Speciality Board in General Surgery;
Honorary Clinical Lecturer in Surgery, University of Sheffield

SECOND EDITION

CHURCHILL LIVINGSTONE

EDINBURGH LONDON NEW YORK PHILADELPHIA ST LOUIS SYDNEY TORONTO 2001

CHURCHILL LIVINGSTONE
An imprint of Harcourt Publishers Limited

First published 2001

ISBN 0443 070423
International Student Edition 0443 070431

British Library Cataloguing in Publication Data
A catalogue record for this book is available from the British Library

Library of Congress Cataloging in Publication Data
A catalog record for this book is available from the Library of Congress

Medical knowledge is constantly changing. As new information becomes available, changes in treatment, procedures, equipment and the use of drugs become necessary. The editors/authors/contributors and the publishers have, as far as it is possible, taken care to ensure that the information given in this text is accurate and up to date. However, readers are strongly advised to confirm that the information, especially with regard to drug usage, complies with the latest legislation and standards of practice.

The publisher's policy is to use **paper manufactured from sustainable forests**

Printed in China

PREFACE

Second Edition

I am grateful to the publishers, Churchill Livingstone, for the invitation to produce a second edition of the 'Pocketbook of Surgery'. I am particularly pleased that, in these days of self-directed, student-centred, problem-based learning, that there is still a place for the small book offering a didactic approach to the acquisition of surgical knowledge. In the five years since the first edition appeared much has changed and therefore most chapters have been revised. Particularly the chapters on Shock and Trauma, Breast, and Transplantation have been extensively revised. A small number of X-ray images has been included to illustrate some of the more common surgical conditions. I hope that this second edition will continue to help the student to understand the basic principles involved in the practice of surgery as well as providing basic information on aetiology, diagnosis, and management of a variety of surgical conditions. I just hope it sells as well as the first edition!

Sheffield 2001 A.T.R.

PREFACE

First Edition

It is well recognized but regrettable fact that a considerable number of medical students do not possess a textbook of surgery. The provision of extensive library facilities may be one reason, although I suspect the impecunious state of the present-day medical student may be a more relevant reason.

The aim of this small volume is to provide a concise and didactic account of the essential features of the more common surgical disorders at both a size and price to suit the pocket. An effort has been made to cover basic principles, as well as to provide basic information on aetiology, diagnosis and management, including pre-operative and postoperative care. The text covers the field of general surgery but aims also to cover the basic needs of the undergraduate as far as the surgical specialities are concerned. The book is intended to fit easily in the white coat pocket and to be used on the wards. It will give the student some idea of history taking, what physical signs to elicit, the differential diagnosis, what investigations to order and how to treat the patient.

As does everyone who writes a book of this size, I will include the usual platitude '... this book is not intended to replace a more substantive medical text but to supplement it'. I hope, however, to have included the basic information which will allow most of you to pass finals (just) and to provide the basic headings which allow the more intellectually and vocationally motivated to be guided to the appropriate parts of the more substantive texts. I hope that it will also prove most satisfactory for pre-finals cramming!

Sheffield 1995 A.T.R.

ACKNOWLEDGEMENTS

I wish to gratefully acknowledge the help, advice and criticisms of the following people who kindly read the speciality chapters: Dr Peter Brown, Consultant Radiologist, Northern General Hospital, Sheffield (Investigative procedures); Mr Alan Mearns, Consultant Cardiothoracic Surgeon, Bradford Royal Infirmary, Bradford (Thorax); Mr B J Harrison, Consultant Surgeon, Northern General Hospital, Sheffield (Breast); Mr G Proud, Consultant Surgeon, Royal Victoria Infirmary, Newcastle upon Tyne (Endocrine); Mr A Wyman, Consultant Surgeon, Northern General Hospital, Sheffield (Alimentary Tract); Mr Andrew W Bradbury, Senior Lecturer and Consultant Vascular Surgeon, The University of Edinburgh, Royal Infirmary of Edinburgh (Peripheral Vascular Surgery); Mr John Anderson, Consultant Urologist, Royal Hallamshire Hospital, Sheffield (Urology); Mr G Holt, Specialist Registrar in Orthopaedic Surgery, Northern General Hospital, Sheffield (Orthopaedics); Mr R D E Battersby, Consultant Neurosurgeon, Royal Hallamshire Hospital, Sheffield (Neurosurgery); Mr R D Griffiths, Consultant in Plastic and Reconstructive Surgery, Northern General Hospital, Sheffield (Plastic Surgery); Miss J Walker, Consultant Paediatric Surgeon, Sheffield Children's Hospital, Sheffield (Paediatric Surgery). Any errors that may have crept in, however, remain my responsibility and not theirs. I would also like to thank Mr W E G Thomas, Consultant Surgeon, Royal Hallamshire Hospital, Sheffield; Dr Matthew Bull, Consultant Radiologist, Northern General Hospital, Sheffield; Dr Sam Euinton, Consultant Radiologist, Northern General Hospital, Sheffield and Dr Alan Sprigg, Consultant Radiologist, Sheffield Children's Hospital, Sheffield for providing x-rays. I would particularly like to thank my former teachers, junior staff and students who have all contributed in some way to this book. I would also like to thank my wife Anne for her patience and encouragement throughout the production of this book. Finally, I would like to thank my secretary, Louise Griffiths, for the hard work and long hours that she has put in to typing and re-typing the manuscript.

ABBREVIATIONS

ABG	arterial blood gases
ACE	angiotensin-converting enzyme
ACTH	adrenocorticotrophic hormone
ADH	antidiuretic hormone
A&E	Accident and Emergency
AF	atrial fibrillation
AFP	α-fetoprotein
AIDS	acquired immunodeficiency syndrome
ALG	antilymphocyte globulin
ALT	alanine transaminase
ANF	antinuclear factor
APTT	activated partial thromboplastin time
ARDS	adult respiratory distress syndrome
ARF	acute renal failure
ASD	atrial septal defect
AST	aspartate transaminase
ATG	antithymocyte globulin
ATN	acute tubular necrosis
AV	arteriovenous
AXR	abdominal X-ray
BBB	bundle branch block
BCG	bacille Calmette–Guérin
BP	blood pressure
BTS	Blood Transfusion Service
CABG	coronary artery bypass graft
CAPD	continuous ambulatory peritoneal dialysis
CBD	common bile duct
CCF	congestive cardiac failure
CCU	Coronary Care Unit
CDH	congenital dislocation of the hip
CEA	carcinoembryonic antigen
CML	chronic myeloid leukaemia
CMV	cytomegalovirus
CNS	central nervous system
COPD	chronic obstructive pulmonary disease
Cr	creatinine
CRF	chronic renal failure
CRP	C-reactive protein
C&S	culture and sensitivity
CSF	cerebrospinal fluid
CT	computerized tomography
CVA	cerebrovascular accident
CVP	central venous pressure

CVVH	continuous veno-venous haemofiltration
CXR	chest X-ray
DIC	disseminated intravascular coagulation
DIVA	digital intravenous angiogram
DM	diabetes mellitus
DMSA	dimercaptosuccinic acid
DSA	digital subtraction angiography
DTPA	diethylenetriaminepentacetic acid
DU	duodenal ulcer
DVT	deep venous thrombosis
ECG	electrocardiogram
EEG	electroencephalogram
EMG	electromyography
EMSU	early morning specimen of urine
ePTFE	expanded polytetrafluoroethylene
ERCP	endoscopic retrograde cholangiopancreatography
ESR	erythrocyte sedimentation rate
EUA	examination under anaesthesia
FBC	full blood count
FDPs	fibrin degradation products
FEV1	forced expiratory volume (1 second)
FFP	fresh frozen plasma
FNAC	fine needle aspiration cytology
FOBs	faecal occult bloods
GA	general anaesthetic
GCS	Glasgow coma scale
GI	gastrointestinal
GU	genitourinary
GVH	graft-versus-host disease
HBsAg	hepatitis B surface antigen
HBV	hepatitis B virus
HCG	human chorionic gonadotrophin
5HIAA	5-hydroxyindoleacetic acid
HIV	human immunodeficiency virus
HLA	human leukocyte antigen
HRT	hormone replacement therapy
HSV	highly selective vagotomy
HVA	homovanillic acid
ICP	intracranial pressure
IGTN	ingrowing toenail
IHD	ischaemic heart disease
INR	International Normalized Ratio
ITP	idiopathic thrombocytopenic purpura

ITU	Intensive Therapy Unit
IVC	inferior vena cava
IVDSA	intravenous digital subtraction angiography
IVU	intravenous urography
JVP	jugular venous pressure
KCCT	kaolin cephalin clotting time
KUB	kidney ureter bladder (plain X-ray)
LA	left atrium
LAD	left axis deviation
LBBB	left bundle branch block
LE	lupus erythematosus
LDH	lactate dehydrogenase
LFTs	liver function tests
LH	luteinizing hormone
LHRH	luteinizing hormone releasing hormone
LIF	left iliac fossa
LP	lumbar puncture
LV	left ventricle
LVF	left ventricular failure
MEN	multiple endocrine neoplasia
MI	myocardial infarction
MLC	mixed lymphocyte culture
MRI	magnetic resonance imaging
MSSU	midstream specimen of urine
MTP	metatarsophalangeal
NG	nasogastric
NMR	nuclear magnetic resonance
NSAID	non-steroidal anti-inflammatory drug
OA	osteoarthritis
OGD	oesophago-gastro-duodenoscopy
PA	pulmonary artery
PAP	prostatic acid phosphatase
PCA	patient-controlled analgesia
PCV	packed cell volume
PDA	patent ductus arteriosus
PDS	polydioxanone
PE	pulmonary embolus
PEEP	positive end-expiratory pressure
PND	paroxysmal nocturnal dyspnoea
PR	per rectum
PSA	prostate-specific antigen
PTA	percutaneous transluminal angioplasty
PTFE	polytetrafluoroethylene

PTH	parathyroid hormone
PT	prothrombin time
PTC	percutaneous transhepatic cholangiography
PTT	partial thromboplastin time
PUO	pyrexia of unknown origin
PV	per vaginam
PVD	peripheral vascular disease
RA	rheumatoid arthritis
RAD	right axis deviation
RBBB	right bundle branch block
RIF	right iliac fossa
RTA	road traffic accident
RUQ	right upper quadrant
RV	right ventricle
RVF	right ventricular failure
SBE	subacute bacterial endocarditis
SLE	systemic lupus erythematosus
SVC	superior vena cava
TB	tuberculosis
TED	thromboembolic deterrent
TENS	transcutaneous electrical nerve stimulation
TFTs	thyroid function tests
TIA	transient ischaemic attack
TNM	tumour, node, metastasis
TPN	total parenteral nutrition
TSH	thyroid stimulating hormone
TURP	transurethral resection of the prostate
U&Es	urea and electrolytes
UC	ulcerative colitis
UO	urine output
URTI	upper respiratory tract infection
USS	ultrasound scan
UTI	urinary tract infection
VDRL	venereal disease research laboratory
VF	ventricular fibrillation
VMA	vanillyl mandelic acid
V/Q	ventilation/perfusion ratio
VSD	ventricular septal defect
WCC	white cell count
WLE	wide local incision
ZN	Ziehl–Neelsen

TERMS AND DEFINITIONS

Students starting a surgical firm will be introduced to a number of terms and definitions which it is often taken for granted they will have heard before. As a useful reminder, these are listed below.

TERMS

Angio- Relating to (blood) vessels, e.g. angiogram – contrast imaging of an artery; cholangiogram – contrast imaging of the bile ducts.

Antegrade Going in the direction of flow, e.g. antegrade pyelogram – injection of contrast medium under imaging control into the renal pelvis percutaneously to delineate a distal obstruction.

Chole- Related to the biliary tree or bile, e.g. cholelithiasis – gallstones; cholecystectomy – removal of the gall bladder; choledochoscopy – examination of the bile ducts with an instrument.

-cele A cavity containing gas or fluid, e.g. hydrocele – collection of fluid between the layers of the tunica vaginalis of the testes; lymphocele – a localized collection of lymph; galactocele – a cavity containing milk in a lactating breast.

-docho- Related to ducts, e.g. choledochoscopy – examination of the bile ducts with an instrument; mammadochectomy – removal of the lactiferous ducts of the breast (for duct ectasia).

-ectasia Related to dilatation of the ducts, e.g. mammary duct ectasia – abnormal dilatation of the lactiferous ducts with periductal inflammation; sialectasia – dilatation of salivary gland ducts.

-ectomy Cutting something out, e.g. appendicectomy, gastrectomy, parotidectomy.

-gram An imaging technique using radio-opaque contrast medium, e.g. angiogram – visualization of the arterial tree; venogram – visualization of veins, e.g. to look for deep vein thrombosis; cholangiogram – to visualize the bile ducts.

Lith- Stone, e.g. pyelolithotomy – removal of a stone from the renal pelvis by opening the renal pelvis; cholelithiasis – gallstones.

-oscopy The inspection of a cavity, tube or organ with an instrument, e.g. cystoscopy – inspection of the bladder; laparoscopy – inspection of the abdominal cavity; colonoscopy – inspection of the colon; endoscopy – general term for inspection of internal organs.

-ostomy Opening something into another cavity or to the outside, e.g. colostomy – an opening of the colon onto the skin; gastroenterostomy – an opening of the stomach into the small bowel.

-otomy Making an opening in something, e.g. laparotomy – exploring the abdomen; cystotomy – opening the bladder.

Per- Going through a structure, e.g. percutaneous – going through the skin.

-plasty Refashioning something to alter function, e.g. pyloroplasty – to relieve pyloric obstruction, ileocystoplasty – to enlarge the bladder with a piece of ileum; angioplasty – to widen an obstruction in an artery.

Pyelo- Relating to the pelvis of the kidney, e.g. pyelogram – contrast imaging showing the renal pelvis; pyelonephritis – inflammation of kidney and renal pelvis.

Retrograde Going in a reverse direction against flow, e.g. endoscopic retrograde cholangiopancreatogram (ERCP) – retrograde injection of contrast medium up the common bile duct via cannulation of the papilla of Vater via a duodenoscope; retrograde pyelogram – injection of contrast medium in a reversed direction up the ureter to delineate the ureter and renal pelvis.

Trans- Going across a structure, e.g. percutaneous transluminal angioplasty – going through the skin and across an obstructed lumen in an artery to widen it and improve distal blood flow.

SOME IMPORTANT DEFINITIONS

Abscess A localized collection of pus.

Aneurysm An abnormal dilatation of an artery.

Cyst A fluid-filled cavity.

Fistula An abnormal communication between two epithelial surfaces (endothelial in the case of an arteriovenous fistula), e.g. colovesical fistula – between the sigmoid colon and the bladder, occurring usually as a complication of diverticulitis, carcinoma, or Crohn's disease.

Gangrene Death of tissue.

Sinus A blind-ending track communicating with an epithelial surface, e.g. pilonidal sinus where the 'sharp' end of hairs burrow into the skin.

Ulcer A break in the continuity of an epithelial surface.

Varix An abnormal dilatation of a vein.

CONTENTS

BIOCHEMICAL VALUES

Venous blood: adult reference values

Analyte	Reference values	
Acid phosphatase (unstable enzyme)	0.1–0.4 i.u./l	
Alanine aminotransferase (ALT) (glutamic-pyruvic transaminase (GPT)	10–40 i.u./l	
Alkaline phosphatase	40–100 i.u./l	
Amylase	50–300 i.u./l	
α_1-Antitrypsin	2–4 g/l	
Ascorbic acid—serum	23–57 μmol/l	0.4–1.0 mg/dl
—leucocytes	1420–2270 μmol/l	25–40 mg/dl
Aspartate aminotransferase (AST) (glutamic-oxaloacetic transaminase (GOT)	10–35 i.u./l	
Bilirubin (total)	2–17 μmol/l	
Caeruloplasmin	1–2.7 μmol/l	
Calcium (total)	2.12–2.62 mmol/l	
Carbon dioxide (total)	24–30 mmol/l	
Chloride	95–105 mmol/l	
Cholesterol (fasting)	3.6–6.7 mmol/l	
Copper	11–24 μmol/l	
Creatinine	55–150 μmol/l	
Creatinine clearance	90–130 ml/min	
Creatine kinase (CK)—males	30–200 i.u./l	
—females	30–150 i.u./l	
Ethanol—marked intoxiation	65–87 mmol/l	
—coma	>109 mmol/l	
Ferritin—males	6–186 μg/ml	
—females	3–162 μg/ml	
α-Fetoprotein	2–6 units/ml	
γ-Glutamyl transferase		
(γ-GT)—males	10–55 i.u./l	
—females	5–35 i.u./l	
Glucose (fasting)	3.9–5.8 mmol/l	
Immunoglobulins (Ig): IgA	0.5–4.0 g/l (40–300 i.u./l)	
IgG	5.0–13.0 g/l (60–160 i.u./l)	
IgM—males	0.3–2.2 g/l (40–270 i.u./l)	
—females	0.4–2.5 g/l (50–300 i.u./l)	
Iron—males	14–32 μmol/l	
—females	10–28 μmol/l	
Iron binding capacity (total)	45–72 μmol/l	
Iron binding capacity (saturation)	14–47%	
Lactate	0.4–1.4 mmol/l	
Lactate dehydrogenase (LDH)	100–300 i.u./l	
Lead	0.5–1/9 μmol/l	
Magnesium	0.75–1.0 mmol/l	
5' Nucleotidase	1–11 i.u./l	
Osmolality	285–295 mOsm/kg	
Phosphatase *see* acid and alkaline		
Phosphate	0.8–1.4 mmol/l	
Potassium	3.3–4.7 mmol/l	
Proteins—total	62–82 g/l	
—albumin	36–47 g/l	
—globulins	24–37 g/l	
—electrophoresis (% of total)		
albumin 52–68		
globulin α_1 4.2–7.2		
α_2 6.8–12		
β 9.3–15		
γ 13–23		
Sodium	132–144 mmol/l	
Triglyceride (fasting)	0.6–1.7 mmol/l	
Urate—males	0.12–0.42 mmol	
—females	0.12–0.36 mmol/l	
Urea	2.5–6.6 mmol/l	

HAEMATOLOGICAL VALUES

Venous blood: adult reference values

Analyte	Reference values
Bleeding time (Ivy)	Up to 11 min
Body fluid (total)	50% (obese)–70% (lean) of body weight
Intracellular	30–40% of body weight
Extracellular	20–30% of body weight
Blood volume	
Red cell mass, men	30±5 ml/kg
women	25±5 ml/kg
Plasma volume (both sexes)	45±5 ml/kg
Erythrocyte sedimentation rate (Westergren)	0–6 mm in 1 h normal 7–20 mm in 1 h doubtful >20 mm in 1 h abnormal
Fibrinogen	1.5–4.0 g/l
Folate—serum	2–20 μg/l
—red cell	>100 μg/l
Haemoglobin—men	13–18 g/dl
—women	11.5–16.5 g/dl
Haptoglobin	0.3–2.0 g/l
Leucocytes—adults	4.0–11.0 $\times 10^9$/l
Differential white cell count	
Neutrophil granulocytes	2.5–7.5 $\times 10^9$/l
Lymphocytes	1.0–3.5 $\times 10^9$/l
Monocytes	0.2–0.8 $\times 10^9$/l
Eosinophil granulocytes	0.04–0.4 $\times 10^9$/l
Basophil granulocytes	0.01–0.1 $\times 10^9$/l
Mean corpuscular haemoglobin (MCH)	27–32 pg
Mean corpuscular haemoglobin concentration (MCHC)	30–35 g/dl
Mean corpuscular volume (MCV)	78–98 ft
Packed cell volume (PCV) or haematocrit—men	0.40–0.54
—women	0.35–0.47
Platelets	150–400 $\times 10^9$/l
Prothrombin time	11–15s
Red cell count—men	4.5–6.5 $\times 10^{12}$/l
—women	3.8–5.8 $\times 10^{12}$/l
Red cell life span (mean)	120 days
Red cell life span $T_{\frac{1}{2}}$ (^{51}Cr)	25–35 days
Reticulocytes (adults)	10–100 $\times 10^9$/l
Vitamin B_{12} (in serum as cyanocobalamin)	160–925 ng/l

1

Introduction to surgery

GENERAL

APPROACHES TO THE PATIENT

Most patients are quite happy to be seen and examined by medical students. Their usual attitude is: 'Doctors have to learn, don't they?' Some patients, however, resent being seen by students; some understandably because they are shy and embarrassed by their condition, but others because they do not feel they should be treated as 'guinea-pigs'. This latter group, are almost certainly those who in subsequent years will complain that doctors have failed to make the correct diagnosis, and one wonders exactly how this group of patients consider that medical students should learn.

Bedside manner is extremely important. It is important to establish rapport with patients so that they can trust you. Before approaching any patient on the ward, always ask the nurse in charge of the ward if you can see the patient. It may be that the patient is not well enough to be seen and examined repeatedly by students. When approaching the patient, introduce yourself with a handshake and let the patient know who you are – 'My name is John Smith. I am a medical student. Would you mind if I talk to you and examine you?' Always attend the ward at a sensible time and try to avoid disturbing the patients during their rest period. Always examine the patient with a colleague or a nurse present (chaperone). Do not carry out intimate examinations such as rectal or vaginal examinations except under strict supervision.

In the outpatient clinic there will usually be notices displayed that students may be present during the consultation and patients are told that if they do not wish to see students then they should inform the nurse in charge of the outpatient clinic. It is my practice always to ask the accompanying nurse to check with the patients whether they mind seeing students before they are brought into the consultation room. Always take plenty of time to take a history from the patient. Never rush or you may miss important points in the history.

TAKING A HISTORY

Always allow yourself plenty of time to take a full history. Develop a method of taking it and try not to write and talk to the patient at the same time. Although as students you will not normally write the patient's history in the notes, you should get used to recording it so that you know exactly how to record it in the notes when you become a qualified doctor. Initially you should record the following:

- full name
- address
- sex
- age
- ethnic group
- marital status
- occupation.

Make sure that you record the date of the examination. You will need this so that you can record subsequent progress.

The reminder of the history should be taken in the following order:

1. *The presenting complaint*. Ask the patient what symptoms he or she is complaining of. If there is more than one complaint, list them in the order in which they are most troublesome to the patient.
2. *The history of the presenting complaint*. Record the full details of the main complaint or complaints. Allow the patient to give a full record of complaints relating to a particular system and then ask any remaining questions that you may have about the abnormal system. For example, if the patient complains of indigestion, nausea and vomiting, make sure that as part of the history of the presenting complaint, which clearly relates to the alimentary tract, that you ask all other questions in this section about the alimentary tract, e.g. bowel habit, abdominal distension, jaundice.
3. *Systematic enquiry*. Once you are satisfied that you have obtained the full history of the presenting complaint and have asked all pertinent questions about the abnormal system, then you should ask direct questions about other systems. These are laid out below.
   a. *Alimentary system*. Appetite. Change in diet. Change in weight. Nausea. Difficulty in swallowing. Regurgitation. Heartburn. Flatulence. Indigestion. Vomiting. Character of the vomit, e.g. coffee grounds, blood, bile, faeculent. Abdominal pain. Abdominal distension. Change in bowel habit. Characteristics of the stool. Rectal bleeding. Change of skin colour, e.g. pallor of anaemia, jaundice.
   b. *Respiratory system*. Cough. Sputum – character of sputum, e.g. purulent, haemoptysis. Dyspnoea. Wheezing. Hoarseness. Chest pain.
   c. *Cardiovascular system*. Chest pain. Dyspnoea. Paroxysmal nocturnal dyspnoea. Orthopnoea. Palpitations. Ankle swelling. Cough. Dizziness. Intermittent claudication. Rest pain. Temperature or colour changes of hands and feet. Oedema.
   d. *Nervous system*. Blackouts. Fits, loss of consciousness. Fainting attacks. Tremor. Weakness of limbs.

Paraesthesia. Disturbances of smell, vision or hearing. Headaches. Change of behaviour.

e. *Musculoskeletal system*. Pain in joints. Swelling of joints. Limitation of movement. Muscle pain. Muscle weakness. Disturbance of gait.

f. *Genitourinary system*. Frequency of micturition. Hesitancy. Poor stream. Dysuria. Colour of urine, e.g. haematuria. Thirst. Polyuria. Symptoms of uraemia – headache, drowsiness, fits, vomiting, peripheral oedema. Loin pain. Date of menarche or menopause. Menstruation. Dysmenorrhoea. Previous pregnancies and their complications. Breast symptoms – pain, lumps. Impotence. Dyspareunia.

4. *Past medical history*. Previous illnesses, operations or accidents. Diabetes. Rheumatic fever. Tuberculosis. Asthma. Hypertension. Sexually transmitted disease.
5. *Family history*. Cause of death of close relatives, e.g. parents, brothers and sisters. Enquire particularly about cardiovascular disease and malignancy. Check for familial illnesses, e.g. adult polycystic kidney disease.
6. *Social history*. Occupation – check fully the details of the occupation and make sure you understand exactly what the patient does. Housing. Travel abroad. Leisure activities. Marital status. Sexual habits. Smoking. Drinking. Eating habits.
7. *Drug history*. Check the patient's present medication. Make particular enquiries about steroids, anticoagulants and contraceptive pill. Drug abuse. Ask about allergies especially to antibiotics. Ask specifically 'does any drug bring you out in a rash?'

OBTAINING INFORMED CONSENT

Informed consent is required for all invasive procedures. At the time of writing, the trend is for consent to be obtained by the person who is actually going to carry out the procedure and certainly by somebody who is aware of the full details of the procedure. It is probably best that consent for major procedures is obtained either by the Consultant or with the Consultant present. It is a good practice that consent should be obtained for any procedure that can have a complication.

To give informed consent the patient must understand:

- the procedure
- the reasons for carrying it out
- any alternative treatments
- benefits of the procedure
- adverse effects or complications
- the outcome without any treatment.

Risks of operation may be general or specific to the operation. The general risks include the risks of anaesthesia and the risks of any operation, e.g. haemorrhage, wound infection, deep vein thrombosis. Examples of specific complications are recurrence after inguinal hernia repair, recurrent laryngeal nerve palsy after thyroid surgery, facial nerve palsy after superficial parotidectomy.

It is generally accepted that complications should be explained to the patient when they arise at a rate of 1% or greater. However, any devastating complication which may occur and has an incidence of less than 1% should be explained to the patient, e.g. paraplegia after aortic cross clamping.

BREAKING BAD NEWS

Breaking bad news to patients and their relatives is almost a daily occurrence. Most medical schools provide tutorials on breaking bad news as part of the course and much experience may be involved in role-play in such tutorials. However there is no substitute for the real thing and it is appropriate for a medical student to sit in when bad news is actually being broken to relatives or patients. A doctor who is explaining the bad news should always check with the patient or the relatives that it is appropriate for a medical student to be present at the time. It is understandable that some patient's relatives may find this obtrusive.

When we think of the nature of breaking bad news, we usually think in terms of explaining to someone that they have an inoperable condition. However, for some patients' relatives it is merely bad news that the patient actually requires surgery or even that as a result of curative surgery the patient needs a permanent colostomy. Usually, however, breaking bad news involves explaining inoperable and incurable cancer and the need to face death. A problem then arises about how much the patient needs to know, and occasionally, in some cases, whether the patient actually needs to know at all. The answer to the latter is that the patient should always be told. Unless the patient is fully aware of the facts, it is difficult to deal with subsequent management, particularly explaining palliative treatment, e.g. radiotherapy or the fact that the patient requires hospice care.

Occasionally relatives request that the patient is not told. This is not appropriate and this should be explained to the relatives, particularly the fact that if the patient finds out by other means (and the patient surely will, even through a careless word on a ward round), then trust is lost between patient and relative and patient and doctor. It is well recognized that most patients are told less than they would actually like to know. Occasionally even the medical profession will rationalize reasons for not wanting to tell the patient, e.g. the patient would not want to know. In fact, most patients are intelligent and shrewd and when you actually sit down to explain the bad news to them you will realize that they have already half suspected it and many will thank you for being honest with them. Always remember that patients have many affairs that they wish to put in order, and also explaining to them honestly about life expectancy will enable them to decide if further unpleasant palliative therapy is worthwhile.

It is always difficult to know how and what to tell the patient. It is probably best not to do this on a busy ward round but to take time to go back to the bed with the nurse who is looking after the patient, sit down and take time to explain. There is a balance to explaining bad news which is somewhere between giving a long explanation skirting round the problem without actually indicating how bad the problem is and the brusque honesty approach ('you have got incurable cancer and less then 3 months to live'). Do not leave the bedside immediately after giving bad news and worse still do not indicate that somebody else will come back shortly and re-explain what you have already said. It is best to wait a while to give patients a chance to ask any questions, and if they do not have any at the time, then to indicate that you will go back later when they have had a chance to let the bad news sink in and when they may have thought of some questions that they wish to ask. It is important to allow sufficient time to talk to patients and to talk to them sensitively and also indicate that you are prepared to talk to members of the family and explain things fully to them. Some patients would be grateful if members of the family are there when bad news is broken.

Accepting terminal illness often takes time and involves a number of well-defined stages, although not all these may occur in a particular patient. These include:

- shock and numbness
- denial
- anger
- grief
- acceptance.

It is important that every member of the team knows exactly what has been explained to the patient and also that the family doctor is aware. Over the days following the breaking of bad news, the patient and relatives may often have numerous questions and time must be taken to sit down and provide the answers to these.

DEATH AND THE CERTIFICATION OF DEATH

When you are qualified you will be required to diagnose death. The patient is pulseless, apnoeic, and has fixed dilated pupils.

Auscultation reveals no heart sounds or breath sounds. If the patient is on a ventilator, brain death may be diagnosed even though the heart is still beating. The preconditions and the criteria for testing for brain death are explained in Chapter 18. Do not forget that after death, organs and tissue may be donated for transplantation purposes. Any solid organ and tissues may be removed from a ventilated brain-dead patient but remember that kidneys may be removed within half an hour of death and other tissues such as cornea, bone, skin and heart valves may be removed within 24 hours after death.

Certification of death is important and should be carried out as soon as possible after death. This is not the same as certifying (or diagnosing) death, but is the official documentation of the patient's cause of death that must be delivered, usually by the next of kin, to the Registrar of Births and Deaths within 5 days of the death. In practice, death certification should normally be carried out on the day after death to allow the patient's relatives to make the funeral arrangements as soon as possible. Only a doctor who has seen the patient within 14 days prior to the death can legally fill in the certificate. In some cases, e.g. where the patient has died postoperatively, or after an emergency admission, or accident, the Coroner must be informed. If in any doubt, it is always best to ring the Coroner and discuss the case with him. If the Coroner decides to take the case, his department will deal with the certification of death.

BEREAVEMENT COUNSELLING

Explaining the death of loved ones to their relatives is never easy. It is best that the medical student attends a course in bereavement counselling and also, during attachments to both medical and surgical firms, accompanies the Houseman or Consultant when he or she is explaining death to relatives. The circumstances of death may cause different emotional reactions in relatives: some react with shock, others with anger and guilt, the latter being common emotions. Anger may be directed towards the deceased, other family members, or the medical profession involved in the patient's care. Support offered to the family both during the patient's illness and at the time of the patient's death not only helps them to cope better but may reduce the likelihood of future problems. Religious beliefs and cultural background may influence reactions and some individuals may resort to alcohol, drugs or denial as a way of coping with loss. In such cases, help of bereavement counsellors should be sought.

CAREERS IN SURGERY

During the undergraduate course, you may find yourself drawn to a particular speciality. It may be that this speciality is surgery or a branch of it. Particularly when you are nearing finals you may have some idea of what speciality you are going to choose and time passes extremely quickly and you will find that once you have started your house jobs, you have to start thinking about applying for senior house officer posts.

At the present time, training in surgery requires a minimum of 2 years of basic surgical training. This is usually on some form of rotation and involves 6 months of general surgery with emergency surgical take, 6 months of orthopaedic or trauma surgery with emergency take and either two 6-month or three 4-month periods in other surgical specialities, e.g. urology, neurosurgery, paediatric surgery, intensive care, accident and emergency. Candidates have to undertake a basic surgical skills course at this time, which is compulsory, and it is also strongly recommended that they register on an advanced trauma life support (ATLS) course during the period of basic surgical training. During this period, examinations have to be taken leading to the award of the Diploma of MRCS (Membership of the Royal College of Surgeons). This examination involves written papers consisting of multiple choice questions, clinical examination, and a viva voce examination consisting of three components, i.e. applied anatomy and operative surgery, applied physiology and critical care, and surgical pathology and the principles of surgery.

Because little basic science is taught in the undergraduate course nowadays and considerable knowledge of such science is required for the MRCS examination, it is appropriate that a candidate either obtains a rotation in which a period is spent in an anatomy department, or, prior to applying for a basic surgical training rotation, that the candidate spends a period of time as a demonstrator in an anatomy department. Such free-standing demonstrator posts are widely available.

After passing the MRCS examination it will be necessary to obtain a higher surgical training post at Specialist Registrar level. There is intense competition for these posts. The period of training in these posts depends upon the speciality, the time of training in general surgery being 6 years. Again during the tenure of an HST post, you will be required to take an examination to obtain the Diploma of FRCS. This is usually taken towards the end of higher surgical training and this diploma has to be obtained before a Certificate of Completion of Specialist Training (CCST) is awarded at the end of the period of higher surgical training. Having passed the FRCS examination and being within 3 months of the award of the CCST, a candidate may then apply for a Consultant appointment.

The Intercollegiate Speciality Examination leading to the award of the FRCS in General Surgery involves a clinical examination in the generality of surgery and also in the candidate's chosen speciality, e.g. colorectal surgery, endocrine surgery, breast surgery. It also involves a viva voce examination in the generality of surgery and the candidate's chosen speciality, and in addition there is an academic viva at which candidates present some of their own work and are also required to read two papers which they have to critically analyse in the presence of a pair of examiners.

SPECIFIC

The remainder of this chapter will describe various techniques which are part of the 'stock in' trade of the surgeon, and therefore of the student training in surgery.

SURGICAL INCISIONS

When choosing an incision the following points should be considered:

- *Access*: the incision must be appropriately placed, large enough and capable of extension.
- *Orientation*: if possible in the lines of skin tension (Langer's lines) or skin creases. This leads to minimal distortion and better healing.
- *Healing potential of tissues.*
- *Anatomy of underlying structures*, e.g. the avoidance of nerves.
- *Good cosmetic result.*
- *Abdominal incision*: the common abdominal incisions are shown in Figure 1.1 and the indications for such incisions are indicated on the diagram.

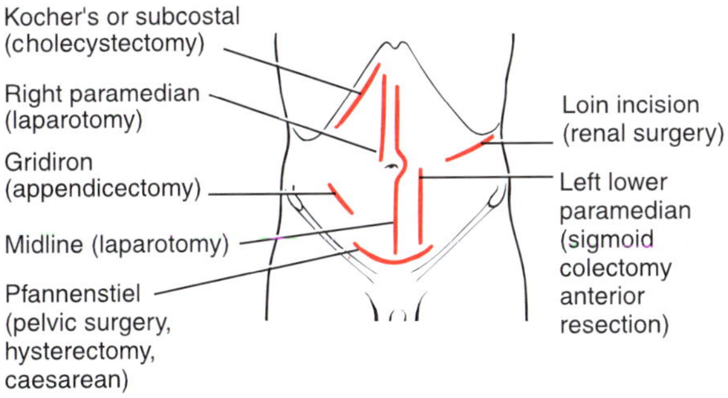

Fig. 1.1 Abdominal incisions.

SUTURES

Students are usually introduced to suturing during their A&E attachment. There is a wide range of suture materials. They may be broadly divided into absorbable and non-absorbable, natural and synthetic, braided and monofilament.

Absorbable

These are plain catgut (natural monofilament); chromic catgut (natural monofilament); polyglycolic acid (synthetic braided – Dexon); polyglactin (synthetic braided – Vicryl); polydioxanone (PDS – synthetic monofilament). The strength of absorbable sutures declines according to the material, catgut being the quickest to lose strength.

Non-absorbable

These include silk (natural braided); linen (natural braided); wire (stainless steel, usually monofilament); nylon (synthetic monofilament – Ethilon); polypropylene (synthetic monofilament – Prolene); expanded polytetrafluoroethylene (ePTFE – expanded monofilament). Non-absorbable sutures retain strength indefinitely and are used where strength is needed until repair is completed naturally, e.g. abdominal incisions and hernia repair. Non-absorbable sutures are often used for skin closure, synthetic monofilament used in subcuticular fashion giving the best cosmetic result.

Natural sutures

These are catgut, silk, linen, but their use is declining. Catgut is cheap but of variable strength. Silk handles well but as with linen it excites a strong inflammatory reaction.

Synthetic sutures

Types include Dexon, Vicryl, PDS, nylon, polypropylene and ePTFE. They are more expensive than natural sutures, but cause little tissue reaction. The degree of strength and absorbability can be controlled in manufacture.

Monofilament

These include catgut, polydioxanone, wire, polypropylene, nylon. They are smooth and pass easily through tissues and cause less tissue reaction. The disadvantage is that they are stiff, slippery, and difficult to knot.

Braided (polyfilament)

These include polyglycolic acid, polyglactin, silk, nylon, linen. They handle well, but interstices harbour bacteria.

Wire

This is useful for closing the sternum in cardiac procedures and for orthopaedic procedures. It is strong, inert, but subject to breakage and handles poorly.

GAUGE

Gauge is the calibre of the suture and is expressed in numbers. Originally, the finest gauge was '1' and the heaviest '4' but with the development of finer sutures a scale of '0s' was developed, the more 0s the finer the suture, e.g. '0', '00' (2/0), '000' (3/0). The finest suture is 10/0 used in eye surgery. The gauge used depends on the strength required, number of sutures, type of suture material being used and cosmetic requirements.

NEEDLES

Needles are cutting or round-bodied. They come in a variety of shapes and lengths and may be straight or curved. Cutting needles are usually triangular in cross-section, and are useful for skin, tendon, and breast tissue. Round-bodied are oval or round in cross-section. Round-bodied needles are useful for GI tract and vascular anastomoses.

METHODS OF SUTURING

Sutures may be interrupted, continuous, vertical mattress, horizontal mattress or subcuticular. The choice depends on the site and nature of the operation and surgeon's preference. Interrupted sutures may be used if there is a risk of infection where some individual sutures may be removed to allow drainage. Subcuticular sutures may be used to give good cosmetic results, especially when using synthetic monofilament. Synthetic absorbable subcuticular sutures (e.g. Vicryl) may be used in children to avoid the trauma of suture removal.

REMOVAL OF SUTURES

The timing is a balance between strength of healing and a good cosmetic result. Some areas are better vascularized, under less tension, and therefore heal quicker than others. The following is a rough guide for the time of removal for different areas: face and neck (3–4 days); scalp (5–7 days); limbs (5–7 days); hands and feet (10–14 days); abdomen (8–10 days).

ALTERNATIVES TO SUTURES

Alternatives include clips and staples. Michel clips appose the skin edges but do not penetrate the skin, and cosmetic results are good. Preloaded disposable staples have largely replaced Michel clips. Cosmetic results are excellent. Stapling devices are also available for GI anastomoses. Simple wounds in children can be closed with adhesive strips (Steristrips). Scalp lacerations in children can be closed using hairs adjacent to the wound edges as 'sutures'. The hairs are knotted across the wound.

DRAINS

Drains are used prophylactically to drain anticipated collections, e.g. haematomas, bile leaks, urine leaks, or therapeutically to remove collections of pus, blood or other body fluids. Most drains consist of latex-based material or silicone. Red rubber tube drains are still used occasionally. Red rubber and latex drains form better tracks than silicone by exciting more tissue reaction. Drainage may be open or closed, suction or non-suction.

Open drainage

This is drainage by capillary action or gravity into dressings or stoma bags. Drainage may depend on position of patient. Sepsis is commoner with open drains.

Closed drainage

This is drainage into a bag or bottle attached to the drain. Usually it is a suction system although it may be passive, working on the syphon system. Sepsis is less common with closed systems.

Suction drains

These help collapse down potential spaces as well as draining blood and other fluids. They are usually closed systems and therefore the risk of sepsis is less. Sump drains are open drains used in connection with suction. Sump drains contain an air inlet lumen which prevents blockage with soft tissue. Sepsis is a risk with sump drains.

Non-suction drains

These are used mainly intraperitoneally to drain GI and biliary anastomoses. They are usually left for up to 5 days. They are usually rubber, PVC or silastic. If prolonged drainage is necessary and there is need for a tract to be established, rubber drains should be used as they stimulate fibrosis.

COMPLICATIONS OF DRAINS

- Sepsis: commoner with open drains.
- Failure: especially suction drains which draw fat or omentum into the side holes.
- Pressure or suction necrosis of the bowel leading to leakage of the intestinal contents with peritonitis.
- Rarely, erosion into a vessel with haemorrhage.

STOMAS (-OSTOMIES)

Colostomy

A permanent colostomy usually opens onto the anterior abdominal wall in the LIF. It is flush with the skin and the contents of the bag are usually formed faeces. It is most commonly created following an operation for abdominoperineal resection of the rectum. A temporary colostomy in this position is usually consequent on a Hartmann's procedure. Colostomies may occasionally be seen in the upper abdomen, either to the right or left of the midline, when they are defunctioning colostomies fashioned in the transverse colon to protect a distal anastomosis, although defunctioning ileostomies are preferred nowadays.

Ileostomy

An ileostomy is usually in the RIF. It is *not* flush with the skin but overhangs as a 'spout' for about 2.5 cm. This is so that the liquid small bowel content, rich in pancreatic enzymes, does not come into contact with the skin of the abdominal wall, resulting in tryptic digestion of the skin. The contents of the bag are fluid and are of the consistency of porridge. An ileostomy usually results from total colectomy with excision of the rectum (panproctocolectomy) for ulcerative colitis. Defunctioning loop ileostomies are used to protect distal anastomoses.

Urostomy (ileal bladder)

A urostomy is usually in the RIF. It is a blind-ended loop of ileum which looks not dissimilar to an ileostomy, i.e. it is not flush with the skin edge but looks like a 'spout'. The ureters have been transplanted into the ileal loop. Urine drains from the ileal loop. It is usually created following total cystectomy for carcinoma of the bladder.

EXAMINATION OF A LUMP

History

1. When did the patient first notice the lump?
2. What brought the lump to the patient's notice, e.g. pain?
3. Is the lump symptomatic?
4. Has there been any change in size?
5. Does the lump ever disappear, e.g. a hernia may disappear on lying down or a sebaceous cyst may discharge and settle down only to fill up again at a later date?
6. Are there any other lumps on the body of similar nature, e.g. lipomas or neurofibromata may be multiple?
7. Does the patient know of any cause for the lump, e.g. trauma?

Examination

- *Site*: describe this in exact anatomical terms. It is best to measure it from a fixed bony point.
- *Shape*: e.g. is it spherical, does it have an irregular outline?
- *Size*: measure this accurately using a tape measure.
- *Surface*: is it smooth or irregular?
- *Edge*: is the edge of the lump clearly defined or indistinct?
- *Colour of overlying skin*: e.g. red and inflamed suggesting an inflammatory lesion.
- *Temperature*: is the skin overlying the lump hot or of normal temperature?
- *Tenderness*: is the lump tender?
- *Composition*: is the mass solid, fluid or gas? Check for consistence, fluctuation, fluid thrill, translucency, pulsation, compressibility and bruits.

Consistence A lump may vary from soft to bony hard. A simple scale of consistence is suggested: soft, e.g. subcutaneous lipoma; firm, e.g. Hodgkin's lymph node; hard, e.g. carcinoma of the breast; stoney hard, e.g. ivory osteoma of skull.

Fluctuation Demonstration of this sign indicates a fluid-filled cavity. Pressure on one side of a fluid-filled cavity causes the other surface to protrude because an increase in pressure within a cavity is transmitted equally and at right angles to all parts of its wall. The test should be carried out in two planes at right angles to each other.

Fluid thrill This detects the presence of free fluid in a cavity. A percussion wave can be conducted across the fluid. Tap one side of the lump and feel the transmitted vibration at the opposite extremity. This is a classical sign of ascites and to prevent a thrill being transmitted through the abdominal wall a second person should place the edge of a hand along the abdomen, midway between the percussing and palpating hands.

Translucency If a swelling transilluminates then it must contain clear fluid. Use a bright torch in a darkened room. Lumps which classically transilluminate brilliantly are hydroceles and cystic hygroma in children.

Resonance Solid and fluid-filled lumps are dull to percussion. Gas-filled swellings are resonant, e.g. distended obstructed bowel.

Pulsatility Rest your hand on every lump and make sure that it does not pulsate. If a pulse is present, distinguish between transmitted pulsation through a lump and an expansile pulsatile lump, i.e. an aneurysm. To do this, place a finger of either hand on opposite sides of the lump. If the fingers are pushed up and down in the same plane, it is a transmitted pulsation. If they are pushed upwards and apart, it is a true expansile pulsation, i.e. aneurysm.

Compressibility Try to empty a lump by gentle pressure and see if it refills spontaneously. This is the sign of compressibility, e.g. strawberry naevus, saphenovarix.

Bruit Listen over the lump. A systolic bruit may be heard over an aneurysm or a vascular goitre associated with thyrotoxicosis. A continuous machinery bruit may be heard over an arteriovenous fistula.

Reducibility This is a property of herniae. The lump may be gently compressed and reduced to the cavity in which it is normally contained. It will reappear by coughing or gravity (standing up).

Relation to surrounding structures Assess the mobility of the lump. Is it attached to the skin or is it attached to deep structures? Is it within the peritoneal cavity or the abdominal wall? Tensing the abdominal muscles by raising the head and shoulders will allow you to distinguish.

Regional lymph nodes Always remember to palpate the regional lymph nodes.

Surrounding tissues and extremities If the lump is on a limb, make sure that it is not interfering with the normal function of the limb, such as pressure on a nerve or interference with distal circulation, e.g. a popliteal artery aneurysm associated with distal ischaemia, or pressure on the common peroneal nerve.

General examination

Always remember to examine the whole of the patient, e.g. a lump in the breast may not only be associated with axillary lymphadenopathy but may be associated with a pleural effusion, and a malignant melanoma on the leg may be associated with hepatomegaly.

EXAMINATION OF AN ULCER

Definition

An ulcer is a break in the continuity of an epithelial surface. Many ulcers are occult in the GI tract and unfortunately many of these tend to be malignant. However, ulcers on the skin and in the oral cavity are easily noticed by the patient.

History

1. When did the patient first notice the ulcer?
2. What first made the patient notice the ulcer, e.g. was it painful or did it start as a different sort of lesion and then become ulcerated, e.g. malignant melanoma?
3. What are the symptoms of the ulcer?

4. Has the ulcer changed since it first appeared, e.g. has there been a chronic venous ulcer on the leg which has previously healed and then broken down again?
5. Has the patient ever had any other ulcers?
6. Is there any obvious cause for the ulcer, e.g. trauma?

Examination

Record accurately the site and size of the ulcer. Check for colour, tenderness, increased temperature, base, edge, depth, discharge, surrounding tissues. Check the state of the local lymph nodes and carry out a general examination.

Base Usually slough or granulation tissue. Some ulcers have a characteristic base, e.g. ischaemic ulcers often contain no granulation tissue but may contain black necrotic tissue, or tendons or bone may be seen in the base of the ulcer. Syphilitic ulcers have a classic slough that looks like a wash leather.

Edge Classically, five types are described. These are shown in Figure 1.2 together with their usual aetiologies.

Depth Record this accurately in millimetres.

Discharge This may be serous, sanguineous or purulent. It may be necessary to remove slough from the base of an ulcer to accurately assess it.

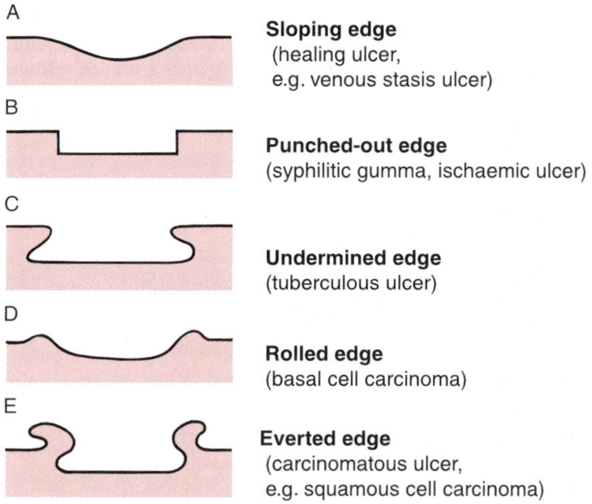

Fig. 1.2 Common types of ulcer edge.

Surrounding tissues Are the surrounding tissues pink and healthy? Is the innervation normal, e.g. neuropathic ulcer associated with diabetes? Are there black satellite nodules around the ulcer, e.g. malignant melanoma?

Examine the local lymph nodes

Carry out a general examination

CLASSIFICATION OF DISEASE

When initially starting your surgical training your knowledge will be limited. You will, therefore, find it difficult to reach a diagnosis. In order to do this you should go through a broad classification of the aetiology of disease as shown in the table (→ Table 1.1). This is sometimes known as the 'surgical sieve'. Ask yourself, is this lesion congenital (usually easy to decide) or is it acquired? If it is acquired then go through the 'sieve' and try and decide which classification it belongs to.. As you learn more pathology and more surgery you will still find this classification suitable when trying to reach a differential diagnosis. It is a good idea when you are first learning, with every disease, lump or ulcer you meet, to sit down and go through the 'surgical sieve' and decide which of these groups it belongs to.

Table 1.1
Classification of disease ('surgical sieve')

Congenital

Acquired

Traumatic

Inflammatory:
- physical stimuli
- chemical stimuli
- infection

Neoplastic:
- benign
- malignant

Degenerative

Vascular

Endocrine/metabolic

Autoimmune

Iatrogenic

Psychogenic

2

Investigative procedures

This chapter describes various investigative procedures used commonly in surgery. The procedures are described briefly together with their indications and possible complications.

CONVENTIONAL RADIOLOGY

Radiographs penetrate differentially through tissues of the body resulting in different exposure of the silver salts in the radiograph film. On a plain radiograph, gas and fat absorb few X-rays and consequently appear dark, while bone and calcified defects are poorly penetrated and appear white or radio-opaque.

A *plain* radiograph is one where no contrast medium is administered to the patient, e.g. routine CXR.

A *contrast* study involves administration of a contrast medium which outlines or delineates the structure under study, e.g. barium in GI studies or iodinated benzoic acid derivatives in arteriography.

PLAIN FILMS

Chest X-ray (CXR)

- Always check the name of the film and the right and left markers.
- Make sure the whole chest and diaphragm are clearly on the film. You may need to count the ribs to exclude a cervical rib.
- Check that the trachea is central.
- Check the mediastinal width.
- Check cardiothoracic ratio. Maximum width of heart divided by maximum 'bony' (rib-to-rib) diameter of chest should be less than 50% in normal adults.
- Check vascular pattern, e.g. reduced in recent pulmonary embolus; distension of upper lobe veins in pulmonary venous hypertension.
- Check lung fields, e.g. lobar collapse, pneumonic consolidation, bronchial carcinoma, pneumothorax.
- Check bony thoracic cage, e.g. fractures, secondary deposits, notching (coarctation of aorta).
- Check soft tissues, e.g. surgical emphysema, mastectomy.
- Check for free air under the diaphragm on erect chest X-ray.

Abdominal X-ray (AXR)

Check for the following:

- dilated hollow viscus with or without air/fluid levels, e.g. small and large bowel obstruction

- free intraperitoneal gas (check position in which film was taken, e.g. air under the diaphragm with perforated hollow viscus)
- abnormal gas patterns, e.g. air in biliary tree with cholecystoduodenal fistula and gallstone ileus, bladder with colovesical fistula
- calcified calculi – kidney, ureter, bladder, gallbladder; 10% of gallbladder stones are radio-opaque and 85% of renal stones are radio-opaque
- foreign bodies, e.g. swallowed keys etc.; trauma, e.g. bullet wounds; carelessness, e.g. swabs
- abnormal calcification, e.g. arteriosclerotic vessels, pancreatic calcification with carcinoma, uterine fibroids
- retroperitoneum, e.g. absence of psoas shadows with retroperitoneal haemorrhage, retroperitoneal gas with retroperitoneal perforation of a viscus
- bones, e.g. bony metastases, fractures, osteoarthritis (plain radiographs of the limbs and skulls are dealt with in the Chs 3, 17 and 18).

CONTRAST STUDIES

Gastrointestinal tract

Barium meal This investigation is used less commonly now in view of the increased use of endoscopy. Barium suspension is given orally together with sodium bicarbonate tablets to give a barium/air double-contrast study. The progress of barium is checked by screening, image intensification being used to show a moving image on a TV monitor. Areas of interest are noted and radiographs taken. The patient should not have any solid food overnight but sips of water are allowed prior to the investigation. A study is useful for diagnosis of pharyngeal lesions, e.g. pharyngeal pouch; oesophageal lesions, e.g. carcinoma, reflux, achalasia; stomach, e.g. ulcers and carcinoma; duodenum, e.g. duodenal ulcer and pyloric stenosis.

Barium enema Barium suspension is administered rectally. Rectal and lower sigmoid lesions should have first been excluded by sigmoidoscopy. Air is usually insufflated to give a double-contrast picture. Buscopan, an anticholinergic agent may be given intravenously to relax the bowel during the investigation.

Strict bowel preparation is required prior to barium enema. A laxative should be administered the evening prior to the enema and the occasional rectal washout is required if there is evidence of residual faecal loading. Barium enema should not be performed within 7 days of a rectal biopsy because of the risk of perforation. The study is useful for diagnosis of bowel carcinomas, polyps, diverticular disease and inflammatory bowel disease. Fine mucosal abnormalities may be missed. If a barium enema is equivocal, colonoscopy should be carried out.

Barium follow-through or small bowel enema Barium may be swallowed and followed through the small bowel into the colon. Alternatively, a duodenal tube may be positioned under radiographic control and barium injected into the duodenum and followed through the small bowel (a small bowel enema). This is useful for the diagnosis of Crohn's disease and small bowel tumours.

Barium should be avoided in the following situations:

- If there is a significant risk of peritoneal leakage, e.g. assessing the integrity of an anastomosis. Barium causes an intense peritoneal irritation and adhesion formation, and water soluble contrast media should be used in preference when checking an anastomosis, e.g. Gastrograffin.
- In bowel obstruction as the barium may rest at the site of a partial obstruction, solidify and cause a partial obstruction to become complete.

Biliary tree

Cholecystogram Iodinated contrast medium administered orally is excreted in the bile and concentrated in the gallbladder. Radiolucent stones show filling defects in the opacified bile. If the gallbladder is obstructed it will not opacify, i.e. a non-functioning gallbladder. An oral cholecystogram is of no value in the presence of jaundice. Oral cholecystography is rarely used at present, gallstones being diagnosed by ultrasound.

Endoscopic retrograde cholangiopancreatography (ERCP) Contrast medium is injected retrogradely through the ampulla of Vater via a side-viewing duodenoscope. The technique is described more fully in the section on endoscopy (→ p. 30).

Percutaneous transhepatic cholangiography (PTC) This is used for diagnosis of obstructive jaundice. A long fine needle (22G Chiba) is passed percutaneously into the liver until a duct is pierced, witnessed by the aspiration of bile. Contrast is then injected to outline the biliary tree. Jaundiced patients may have clotting defects, e.g. abnormal prothrombin time (PT), and therefore a clotting screen should be carried out prior to this investigation. Vitamin K or fresh frozen plasma (FFP) should be administered intravenously if the PT is abnormal. Complications include haemorrhage, bile peritonitis, cholangitis and septicaemia.

Operative cholangiogram At operation for cholecystectomy the ducts should be checked for stones. Contrast is injected via a cannula inserted into the common bile duct via the stump of the cystic duct and radiographs are carried out or the image intensifier used. The diameter of the ducts, presence of filling defects and failure of contrast to pass into the duodenum are significant.

T-tube cholangiogram If the common bile duct has been explored to exclude or remove stones, a latex T-tube is usually inserted. The horizontal bar of the T is in the duct and the vertical bar is brought out through the skin. Contrast is injected down the T-tube 8–10 days postoperatively to check for any residual stones, biliary leakage or stenosis prior to removal of the tube. There should be free flow of contrast medium into the duodenum and no filling defects.

Urinary tract

Intravenous urography (IVU) Intravenous contrast is administered which is excreted by the kidneys and eventually delineates the renal pelvis, ureters and bladder. A plain film is taken first so that any opacities seen can be compared with the films after contrast is given. It is useful for the diagnosis of obstruction, tumours, infection, congenital abnormalities and trauma. The only contra-indication is allergy to the contrast medium. Caution must be exercised in diabetes mellitus, renal failure, multiple myeloma and cardiac failure.

Cystography The patient is catheterized and the bladder filled with contrast medium. Bladder leaks, tumours, vesicoureteral reflux, and diverticulae can be diagnosed. A postmicturition film will diagnose residual urine. This technique has largely been superseded by ultrasonography.

Urethrography A gel-like contrast medium is injected per urethram. Ruptures of the urethra, strictures or tumours may be seen.

Retrograde pyelography This is carried out via cystoscopy by passing a ureteric catheter into each ureteric orifice. Clear views of the ureter and pelvicalyceal system are obtained. This test is used in patients with impaired renal function with poor concentration of contrast or if incomplete filling of the collecting structures is seen on IVU. The ureteric catheter may be left in situ to allow drainage of an obstructed system and for renal function tests to normalize prior to operative procedures.

Antegrade pyelography The pelvicalyceal system of the kidney is punctured with a fine 22G needle. Contrast is injected and allows accurate assessment of the ureter and pelvicalyceal system, as well as assessing drainage.

Vascular system

Arteriography Contrast medium is injected directly into the lumen of an artery. The catheter is usually introduced via the Seldinger wire technique into a suitable and easily accessible artery. The femoral artery at the groin is the usual portal of entry, although the brachial and axillary may be used. A careful history of allergies to contrast media needs to be ascertained. A clotting screen should be carried out prior to vascular radiology. With a catheter in situ, water soluble contrast medium is injected directly into the artery and images recorded in rapid sequences. Stenosis, thrombosis, embolism or aneurysm can be demonstrated. Complications include haemorrhage at the puncture site, dislodgement of atheromatous plaques, embolism, thrombosis.

Digital subtraction angiography (DSA) may be used. Vascular images may be obtained with lower concentrations of contrast medium. The digital images are processed by subtracting unnecessary background, e.g. bones, and enhancing contrast between the tissues. Where high resolution is not needed, the contrast can be given intravenously into a fast-flowing vein, e.g. via a central line or into the femoral vein, and the arteries imaged when the contrast reaches them. These studies are known as intravenous digital subtraction angiography (IVDSA) or digital intravenous angiography (DIVA).

Venography Contrast is injected into a superficial vein, i.e. a vein on the dorsum of the foot in the lower limb, and a tourniquet is placed around the ankle to direct the contrast into the deep veins. Lower limb venography is used to confirm or exclude DVT or to investigate deep venous insufficiency, i.e. it would demonstrate the site of incompetent perforating veins. This technique has been largely superseded by Doppler ultrasound.

ULTRASONOGRAPHY

Ultrasound works on the principle that the ultrasound emitted as a pulse from a transducer travels at constant velocity into tissue and is reflected by varying amounts from different tissue interfaces and travels back to the receiver at the same speed. The transducer is a piezoelectric crystal which both transmits and receives the ultrasound. The time required for the pulse to travel to the interface and back can be used to determine the depth of that interface. An image of the slice of the body is obtained by directing a narrow beam of high energy sound waves into the body and recording the manner in which the sound is reflected by different structures. Sound is transmitted well through any fluid but poorly or not at all through air or bone. Returning echoes are electronically converted into a video image on a monitor, the resulting picture being a wedge-shaped slice of the area of interest.

Advantages

These are:

- it does not employ ionizing radiation and therefore produces no biological injury in the tissues
- any plane can be employed to examine the region of interest
- it is less expensive than CT or MRI
- it can be used at the bedside if the patient is too ill to be moved.

Dimensions of organs or lesions can be measured and the volume of the bladder and the left ventricle can also be assessed. Stones cause marked changes in acoustic impedance with almost complete reflection of ultrasound, showing echogenic foci with fan-shaped acoustic shadowing.

Very little preparation is necessary. For pelvic ultrasound the bladder should be full, providing a fluid-filled non-reflective medium for the ultrasound to reach the pelvic organs. The patient should be starved for biliary ultrasound to allow the gallbladder to fill with bile and to minimize gas shadows.

Ultrasound is non-invasive, painless, safe and cheap in comparison with CT and MRI although it does not produce as sharp an image.

Ultrasound may be used for the following:

- assessment of abdominal masses
- distinguishing solid from cystic lesions, e.g. renal carcinoma from a renal cyst
- assessment of liver secondaries
- detecting stones in the gallbladder or urinary bladder
- measuring the size of lesions, e.g. the diameter of an abdominal aortic aneurysm or the width of a dilated bile duct
- guided biopsy, e.g. biopsy of liver secondary or other mass
- guided drainage, e.g. of localized collections of fluid or subphrenic or pelvis abscesses.

Disadvantages

Although limitations are few, lesions of the lower end of the common bile duct and head of the pancreas may be obscured by bowel gas. Bone completely reflects ultrasound and the method is therefore useless for studying organs encased by bone, e.g. brain and spinal cord.

DOPPLER ULTRASOUND

Doppler ultrasound is used in vascular monitoring to study blood flow. A beam of ultrasound is directed at a vessel using a special probe. Ultrasound is reflected from the red cells, which cause a frequency shift related to their velocity. The shift can be heard as a noise or recorded as a waveform or sonogram. The faster the flow of red cells past the probe the higher the sound pitch. The Doppler probe is coupled to the skin with acoustic gel and angled towards the direction of arterial flow. Stenoses and occlusions cause diminished signals distal to a proximal obstruction.

Uses of Doppler ultrasound

Measurement of systolic pressure in peripheral arteries A sphygmomanometer cuff is applied to occlude the artery. The probe is placed over the artery (dorsalis pedis, posterior tibial in the case of the lower limb), the tourniquet released and the pressure recorded when a signal is picked up. This pressure is compared with a normal brachial pressure, i.e. the ankle/brachial pressure index. The normal value is 1.0–1.2.

Other methods These include analysis of waveforms to assess stenoses and occlusions.

Duplex scanning

This combines real-time B-mode imaging with a pulsed Doppler spectral analysis of flow velocity pattern. Blood vessels are identified by their characteristic B-mode images with prominent wall echoes and dark sonar-lucent lumina. Calcified plaques shows bright echoes with acoustic shadowing behind. The pulsed Doppler beam is placed in the centre of the identified vessel and the spectral analysis allows classification of the degree of stenosis. Duplex scanning may be applied to analyse carotid disease, lower extremity arterial disease, intestinal arteries, renal arteries, and venous thromboses. Colour coding of flow direction may give further information.

COMPUTERIZED TOMOGRAPHY (CT)

CT produces cross-sectional images of the body, taking a series of transverse slices through the body. Sensitive X-ray detectors measure the X-ray attenuation through the patient in a large number of different directions, and a fast digital computer then uses the measurements to compute an image. These images are displayed on a screen and subsequently recorded on film. CT scanning may be used in conjunction with contrast medium enhancement. This may be given i.v. to show, for example, hepatic tumours, renal parenchyma and collecting system, aorta and IVC. It may enhance brain lesions when the blood–brain barrier is breached. Contrast may also be given by mouth or enema to outline the GI tract.

A new generation of spiral CT scanners are in use. The patient passes quickly through the scanner and a volume of data is obtained and analysed. Scanning is performed in a single breathold decreasing motion artefact and allowing accurate timing of intravascular contrast enhancement. Images are superior to conventional CT. Specific applications include CT angiography and imaging of pulmonary emboli.

Advantages

CT has many uses but is the investigation of choice in head injuries. It is also useful for studying the retroperitoneum, pancreas, mediastinum, and lungs. It can be used for staging tumours, e.g. lymphomas, and can be used for guided biopsy.

MAGNETIC RESONANCE IMAGING (MRI)

MRI is also known as nuclear magnetic resonance (NMR). MRI is based on the fact that certain atomic nuclei placed in a magnetic field and acted on by a suitable radiofrequency pulse undergo changes in their energy states which result in the emission of measurable radio signals. The signals are then manipulated in a computer to provide sectional radiographic images. No ionizing radiation is involved. The procedure is non-invasive and can be carried out as an outpatient procedure. It is relatively time consuming, with extensive studies taking in excess of 1 hour. MRI gives high soft tissue contrast and the body can be imaged in coronal, sagittal or transverse planes.

Advantages

The technique is particularly useful for studies of the CNS (lipids have a high hydrogen content), soft tissues of the pelvis, soft tissue tumours, and orthopaedic problems. Magnetic resonance angiography is also being increasingly used to assess the heart, renal arteries, and peripheral vessels. Magnetic resonance cholangiopancreatography (MRC) can also be used to image the biliary tract.

Disadvantages

These include high cost, limited availability, low patient throughput, poor detail of bone and calcified tissues, and image artefacts from respiratory and cardiac movement and bowel peristalsis. The patient is in the 'tube' for long periods and it is difficult to monitor the ill patient. Contraindications include patients with cardiac pacemakers, and cranial surgery with metal clips.

MAMMOGRAPHY

A mammogram is a soft tissue radiograph of the breast. The tissues constituting the breast have a very low inherent contrast. Soft tissue mammography depends on the fact that tumour tissue is denser than breast tissue, particularly in the older patient (age 40+) where glandular tissue has been replaced by fat. The study is uncomfortable and somewhat undignified for the patient, since compression of the breast is essential in order to 'spread' the breast over the film cassette, immobilize the breast and reduce the radiation dose. A radiolucent, translucent compression plate is used. Views are usually superoinferior and mediolateral. For screening programmes or follow-up usually only one oblique film is taken. Careful viewing of the film under high intensity light with magnification is essential. An infiltrating radio-opaque mass is suggestive of malignancy but fine-stippled calcification (like salt grains scattered on the film) strongly suggests the diagnosis. Mammography is used for the following:

- to assess palpable lumps
- to exclude lumps in other symptomatic patients, e.g. painful breasts
- for screening.

If a non-palpable lump is picked up on mammography, pre-operative localization with wires is undertaken via mammography. The wire is left in the breast and acts as a guide to the surgeon to the location of the radiological abnormality. When the specimen of breast tissue has been removed it is submitted to radiography to confirm that the abnormal area has in fact been excised.

RADIOISOTOPE SCANNING

A suitable tracer agent is given intravenously or orally. The tracer agent is a substance which is taken up by the target tissue. This substance is combined with a radioactive label, the most commonly used being technetium-99m (^{99m}Tc). A gamma camera is placed over the area of interest and simultaneously collects and counts the level of radioactivity. Dynamic imaging involves measuring the changing level of radioactivity over a period of time and storing this in a computer for later analysis. Renal blood flow measurement is an example of dynamic imaging. The following are applications of radioisotope scanning which are used in clinical practice.

Bone scans

Phosphates labelled with technetium are tracer agents. The tracer is taken up in areas of increased bone deposition and resorption.

Uptake occurs in sites of infection, secondary tumour and acute arthritis. Indications for bone scanning include suspected bony secondaries, suspected osteomyelitis, abnormal biochemical profiles suggesting bone disease, e.g. raised calcium or alkaline phosphatase.

Renal scans

Two isotopes are commonly used, i.e. diethylenetriaminepentacetic acid (DTPA) and dimercaptosuccinic acid (DMSA). DTPA is excreted like IVU contrast medium while DMSA remains in cortical tissue. They are useful in assessing asymmetrical renal function. Dynamic computer analysis allows assessment of renal blood flow as well as excretory activity. Mercaptoacetyltriglycine (Mag3) is now largely replacing DTPA. Practical applications include investigation of renal artery stenosis, and also differentiating ATN, renal ischaemia and obstruction in transplanted kidneys.

Lung scanning

This is important in the diagnosis of PE. Emboli obliterate areas of pulmonary arterial circulation but ventilation remains intact. A ventilation/perfusion scan (V/Q scan) is usually carried out. The perfusion scan involves the injection of radioactive particles small enough to temporarily block a small number of pulmonary capillaries. Technetium-labelled albumen microspheres are usually used. A ventilation scan using an inert radioactive gas, e.g. xenon, is performed simultaneously. The scans are compared. Areas that are ventilated and not perfused suggest embolism. Areas that are perfused but not ventilated suggest consolidation or collapse.

Scanning for infection

Ultrasonography or CT scanning will locate a collection of pus but in equivocal cases white cell scanning may help. The patient is bled and the white cells separated. These are then labelled with indium-111 (^{111}In) and reinjected. The body is then scanned and areas of interest noted. The test is useful in patients with pyrexia of unknown origin or septicaemia where other methods have failed to locate an area of sepsis.

Screening for GI bleeding

The patient's own red cells are labelled with technetium and reinjected. The abdomen is scanned at intervals over the next 24 hours. The investigation reveals only the general area of bleeding, e.g. stomach, right or left colon, rather than the exact site.

ENDOSCOPY

Endoscopy implies examination of part of the body through an instrument. This may be through a natural orifice, e.g. oesophagoscopy or sigmoidoscopy, or through a surgically created hole, e.g. laparoscopy or arthroscopy. Endoscopy may be carried out with a rigid instrument, e.g. oesophagoscopy or sigmoidoscopy, the latter two being the most commonly used rigid endoscopy instruments. More recently, fibreoptic instruments have become more sophisticated and more widely used, e.g. gastroscopy, colonoscopy.

USE OF ENDOSCOPES

Rigid endoscopes

Sigmoidoscope This is probably the most commonly used rigid endoscope. It is either 25 or 30 cm long. Examination is usually carried out in the left lateral position. The position of a lesion is usually indicated by measuring its distance in centimetres from the anal verge. Biopsies may be taken with long forceps inserted through the scope.

Oesophagoscopy This has largely been superseded by the flexible instrument. The rigid one, however, remains useful for removing large foreign bodies from the oesophagus.

Cystoscopy The rigid instrument has been widely used for many years but has now been largely superseded by the flexible scope. The rigid instrument remains useful for retrograde ureteric catheterization. Transurethral resection of the prostate has been carried out for many years via the rigid cystoscope.

Laparoscopy This technique was widely used by gynaecologists but is now being more widely used by the general surgeon, particularly for minimally invasive surgery. A cannula is introduced into the peritoneal cavity and the peritoneal cavity distended with carbon dioxide gas. It is useful not only for diagnosis and biopsy but invasive procedures are now being carried out through it, e.g. cholecystectomy, appendicectomy.

Flexible endoscopes

Gastroscope (oesophago-gastro-duodenoscope) This is used with intravenous sedation and a pharyngeal local anaesthetic spray. A clear view can be obtained of the oesophagus, stomach, duodenum, and with a side viewing scope the ampulla of Vater may be clearly seen. It is used for the identification and biopsy of lesions; tracing sources of GI haemorrhage; injection of oesophageal varices; lasering of bleeding lesions; dilatation of oesophageal strictures; cannulation of the ampulla of Vater for ERCP. With the technique of ERCP a diathermy wire can be used down the gastroscope for dividing the sphincter of Oddi and allowing stones to pass out into the GI tract.

Colonoscopy It is possible to inspect the whole of the colon after adequate bowel preparation. Biopsies can be carried out. Polyps can be removed by a wire snare or diathermy. Routine follow-up of patients having had previous carcinomas resected or ulcerative colitis can be carried out avoiding the need for repeated barium enemas.

Bronchoscopy Narrow fibreoptic bronchoscopes can be passed under local anaesthetic. They are mainly used for diagnostic purposes but can also be used postoperatively for removing mucous plugs which have caused segmental collapse.

Other flexible scopes These include cystoscopes, sigmoidoscopes, choledochoscopes (for inspecting the common bile duct at open surgery to assess for stones, tumours, etc.), and arterioscopes which will show areas of stenosis, embolus and allow inspection of arterial anastomoses for patency.

ADVANTAGES AND DISADVANTAGES OF ENDOSCOPY

Advantages

- Usually well tolerated. No need for general anaesthetic and therefore can be used on the elderly and unfit patient.
- Any lesion can be directly visualized and biopsy taken under direct view.
- More accurate than radiology.
- Flexible endoscopy is safer than rigid endoscopy.

Disadvantages

- Perforation of a hollow viscus.
- Tissue samples are usually small due to the size of the biopsy channel.
- Sterility of the instrument is paramount to offset the risk of HIV or hepatitis B.

Complications

The main complications include perforation, haemorrhage at the site of biopsy or operative procedure and pulmonary aspiration. Cardiovascular complications may be related to the medication.

TISSUE DIAGNOSIS

Biopsy

This is removal of a piece of tissue from the living to provide a diagnosis. *Incisional biopsy* is the surgical removal of a piece of accessible tissue. *Excisional biopsy* is the complete removal of a discrete lesion without a wide margin and without it being considered curative of the disease.

Lesions may be biopsied as follows:

- under direct vision, e.g. skin lesion
- by forceps via an endoscope, e.g. sigmoidoscopic biopsy of a rectal lesion
- percutaneously using a trucut punch needle, e.g. breast lesions
- percutaneously by guided needle under ultrasound or CT control
- laparoscopically
- by open surgical excision, e.g. lymph node biopsy.

Cytology

Specimens obtained by scraping or fine-needle aspiration are spread on a slide and stained. The earliest example of this technique was cervical smears stained by the Papanicolaou technique.

Cytological diagnosis requires a skilled pathologist. The method must be both specific and sensitive. False positives and false negatives may occur. Cytological diagnosis is useful in the following situations in general surgery:

- aspiration of ascites or pleural effusions
- aspiration of solid masses, e.g. breast, thyroid, pancreas or lymph nodes.

INTERVENTIONAL RADIOLOGY

Interventional radiology has increased markedly over the past decade and has probably been most marked in the areas of vascular radiology, urological radiology and the treatment of obstructive jaundice. The areas listed below have seen advances in interventional radiology.

Tissue diagnosis

- Trucut needle biopsy under ultrasound or CT control, e.g. liver biopsy.
- Fine-needle aspiration cytology (FNAC). A 22 gauge needle can usually be safely passed through most organs to aspirate the suspicious lesion under ultrasound or CT control, e.g. lesions in the head of the pancreas.

Biliary tract

In obstructive jaundice caused by malignant compression, either intrinsic (cholangiocarcinoma) or extrinsic (nodes at porta hepatis), the site can be accurately located by PTC and treated by stenting. A guide wire is passed through the stenosis and the stenosis dilated, following which a stent is passed over the guide wire to lie across the stenosis. This procedure may also be carried out at ERCP and is likely to be associated with fewer complications by the latter method.

Urinary tract

The renal pelvis can be punctured by percutaneous insertion of a needle under ultrasound or CT control. The tract can be dilated to allow tubes to be inserted and this allows for removal of stones from the renal pelvis or the insertion of nephrostomy tubes to drain the kidney prior to definitive treatment of a distal obstruction. The procedure is known as percutaneous nephrostomy.

Vascular system

Percutaneous transluminal angioplasty (PTA) Arteriography is carried out by the Seldinger technique. A flexible guide wire is then passed across the stenosis. A catheter with a rigid plastic inflatable balloon is then placed along the guide wire to lie within the stenosis and its position is checked under the image intensifier. The balloon is inflated to dilate the stenosis. Measurement of pressures above and below the site of the dilatation is used to assess the success of the procedure. The complications include arterial rupture, embolism, thrombosis or dissection. It is also possible to insert percutaneously a stent across the dilated stenosis in an attempt to prevent restenosis. A vascular surgeon should always be available to deal with any complications that may arise.

Thrombolysis Acute-on-chronic ischaemia of a limb without gross neurological deficit may be treated with thrombolytic therapy. Systemic thrombolysis carries dangers of haemorrhage, e.g. GI or cerebral, and local thrombolysis is safer. Arteriography is carried out to confirm the diagnosis. The tip of a catheter is then placed within the clot and a thrombolytic agent, e.g. streptokinase, urokinase or tissue plasminogen activator, is infused directly into the clot. Radiographs are repeated at 8- to 12-hour intervals to check progress. At each radiograph the catheter is advanced further into the dissolving clot. When the clot is cleared any stenoses demonstrated radiologically may be submitted to angioplasty if suitable.

Embolization This is suitable for highly vascular tissues, e.g. arteriovenous malformations or to treat lesions not amenable to surgery, e.g. liver metastases or extensive renal carcinoma. The main arterial supply is identified via arteriography and a catheter placed within it. An occlusive material is then injected. Suitable agents include gelatin foam or minute steel coils.

Prevention of pulmonary emboli Recurrent pulmonary emboli in the presence of adequate anticoagulation is an indication for interrupting the IVC. It is possible to insert a filter in the cava percutaneously via the internal jugular vein or femoral vein. A commonly used filter is the Greenfield which is shaped like a shuttlecock and is held closed with a special introducing catheter. This catheter is inserted through a sheath in the femoral vein. It is positioned in the inferior vena cava below the renal veins and released. The feet of the filter hook into the vein wall to prevent it becoming dislodged.

3

Shock and trauma

SHOCK

Shock is the clinical condition that results from inadequate tissue perfusion. Five types of shock may be encountered in surgical practice: hypovolaemic, septic, cardiogenic, neurogenic and anaphylactic.

HYPOVOLAEMIC SHOCK

This is due to decreased circulating plasma volume.

Causes
These include:

- haemorrhage, e.g. trauma, haematemesis, ruptured aortic aneurysm
- dehydration, e.g. severe vomiting or diarrhoea, sequestration of fluid in bowel obstruction
- burns resulting in massive loss of serum.

Symptoms and signs Pallor, cool moist skin, hypotension, tachycardia. Patients are often apprehensive and restless. Oliguria or anuria may be present. With severe shock, coma, cardiac arrhythmias and cardiac arrest may occur.

Treatment Shock is an acute emergency and needs rapid treatment.

1. Ensure an adequate airway. Deliver 100% oxygen by mask. If comatose, intubate.
2. Keep the patient recumbent and elevate the foot of the bed.
3. Establish vascular access with large intravenous catheters. If the cause of shock is haemorrhage, take blood for cross-matching. Also take blood for haemoglobin, haematocrit, U&Es. Restore circulating volume with crystalloid initially and with plasma expanders or blood as indicated.
4. Insert a central venous line to monitor CVP and to assess the response to fluid administration.
5. Insert a urinary catheter to monitor urinary output.
6. Establish basic observations of temperature, pulse, BP, respiratory rate and level of consciousness and urinary output.
7. The underlying cause of the shock should be ascertained and definitive treatment planned. Failure of resuscitation may be due to persistent massive haemorrhage. Surgical intervention is often necessary.

SEPTIC SHOCK

Septic shock is usually due to Gram-negative septicaemia. Circulating bacterial endotoxins give rise to widespread peripheral vasodilatation and increased capillary permeability with fluid leakage into the tissues. Peripheral arteriovenous shunting may occur and there may be a direct toxic effect on the heart.

Causes Surgery on the urinary, biliary or lower GI tract. Pulmonary infections, abscesses, invasive catheters. Diabetics, patients on corticosteroid therapy and immunosuppressive drugs are more susceptible.

Symptoms and signs There may be an obvious source of infection, together with a predisposing condition. The patient may be confused and restless; initially the skin is hot and flushed and the pulse characteristically 'bounding'. Vasoconstriction may develop later.

Treatment This is urgent and involves resuscitation, identification of the source of sepsis, appropriate antibiotic therapy and any necessary surgery to eradicate the focus of infection.

1. Ensure adequate airway and ventilation.
2. Restore circulating volume with plasma expanders while monitoring the venous pressure and urine output.
3. Obtain cultures of blood, sputum, urine and any drainage fluid.
4. Commence intravenous antibiotic. A combination of benzylpenicillin, metronidazole and gentamicin is an effective regime but the antibiotic therapy should be altered according to the appropriate culture and sensitivity results when available.
5. Carry out appropriate surgical intervention, e.g. drainage of abscess, peritoneal lavage.
6. Further supportive measures may be required, e.g. inotropic agents, ventilation.

Complications DIC and ARDS may occur. The mortality rate of septic shock is high especially in the elderly and very young.

CARDIOGENIC SHOCK

Cardiogenic shock may occur postoperatively especially in elderly patients and those with a previous history of cardiovascular disease. It may also occur in cardiac tamponade and tension pneumothorax.

Symptoms and signs May present as chest pain or collapse but occasionally clinical findings are absent or minimal. Patients may be grossly dyspnoeic with symptoms and signs of pulmonary oedema. The patient may have a tachycardia or a bradycardia and be hypotensive with pale, cold, sweaty skin.

Investigations • ECG • Cardiac enzymes • CXR.

Treatment

1. pain relief and refer to CCU
2. bed rest and oxygen administration
3. ECG monitoring
4. insertion of CVP line; avoid fluid overload
5. thrombolytic therapy is contraindicated in the postoperative period.

NEUROGENIC SHOCK

Neurogenic shock occurs because of a failure of arterial resistance usually from nervous stimuli, e.g. sudden pain or fright. The usual manifestation is a vasovagal attack where there is sudden autonomically mediated bradycardia and dilatation of the splanchnic vessels which give rise to transient hypotension and loss of consciousness. Other causes include spinal anaesthesia and spinal cord injury.

Symptoms and signs Pallor, cold sweaty skin, weakness, nausea and light-headedness. There is transient hypotension and bradycardia and the patient may faint.

Treatment Neurogenic shock is self-limiting. The patient should be recumbent in the head down position. If the patient is sitting down the head should be bent forward between the knees.

ANAPHYLACTIC SHOCK

Anaphylactic shock is a hypersensitivity reaction occurring in response to previous sensitization to an antigen. In surgical practice this usually occurs following administration of antibiotics, especially intravenously, or is due to radiological contrast media. Bee or wasp stings or occasionally food may be responsible.

Symptoms and signs Generalized urticaria, wheezing, laryngeal oedema, hypotension, loss of consciousness.

Treatment Anaphylaxis is a life-threatening condition requiring urgent treatment.

1. Ensure adequate airway and maintain oxygenation.
2. Drug therapy – administer 1 ml of 1 : 1000 adrenaline subcutaneously immediately. Other drug therapy which may be necessary includes intravenous antihistamines, intravenous steroids and aminophylline.

The importance of an adequate drug and sensitivity history cannot be overemphasized. Always make sure before giving parenteral injections that resuscitation equipment and drugs are available.

TRAUMA

Trauma is the main cause of death in people under the age of 35 years. It constitutes up to 20% of surgical admissions.

Mortality can be greatly reduced by appropriate handling of the injured in the following three settings:

1. Emergency medical teams which are capable of going to the scene of an accident and providing the necessary first aid.
2. A transportation system capable of rapid transport to a specified trauma centre.
3. A trauma centre with trained personnel who are capable of rapidly assessing the injuries with facilities capable of handling a large number of trauma cases with trained teams.

There must be a clear plan of management priorities for the patient with multiple injuries:

1. Rapid initial assessment of the degree of injuries.
2. Ensure a clear airway.

3. Ensure that the patient is breathing.
4. Maintain an adequate circulation.
5. Diagnosis of immediate life-threatening injuries followed by rapid treatment of such injuries.
6. Reassessment of the patient's status once the above have been dealt with.
7. Diagnosis of other significant injuries, e.g. fractures.
8. Definitive treatment, e.g. prophylactic antibiotics, tetanus prophylaxis and appropriate surgical management.

ABCDE of emergency management

A = Airway Ensure a clear airway. The mouth and upper airway should be inspected for foreign bodies and these removed. In the unconscious patient insert an airway to keep the tongue forward and maintain the oropharyngeal airway. Intubation may be necessary.

B = Breathing Check character and rate of ventilation. Check for cyanosis. Assess the thorax, e.g. flail chest, tension pneumothorax. Ventilation may be necessary, e.g. for serious head injuries or flail chest. Chest drains may be necessary to relieve tension pneumothorax or haemothorax.

C = Circulation Once the airway is clear and adequate ventilation has been established attention should turn to re-establishment of the circulation. Ensure an adequate circulation by controlling haemorrhage and administration of i.v. fluids. In the case of cardiac arrest, apply external cardiac massage. Occasionally, thoracotomy and direct massage of the heart may be necessary. Cardiac tamponade may be relieved by direct insertion of a needle into the pericardium.

D = Disability A rapid neurological evaluation should be performed. This establishes the patient's level of consciousness as well as pupillary size and reaction. The level of consciousness may be remembered by the mnemonic AVPU.

- **A** **A**lert
- **V** Response to **v**ocal stimuli
- **P** Responds only to **p**ainful stimuli
- **U** **U**nresponsive to all stimuli

E = Exposure/environmental control The patient should be completely undressed and fully exposed for examination. After the patient's clothing is removed and assessment completed, the patient should be covered with warm blankets or a warming device to prevent hypothermia. Intravenous fluids should be warm before infusion and the warm environment should be maintained.

ACCIDENT AND EMERGENCY (A&E) DEPARTMENT

The A&E Department should have a clear plan for the management of trauma patients:

1. Notification by ambulance or police of impending arrival of seriously injured patients.
2. Alert casualty surgical and anaesthetic teams.
3. Prepare resuscitation rooms, e.g. set up infusions, prepare drugs.
4. One member of the medical team to take overall responsibility for deciding priorities.
5. Major disaster plan, e.g. for major road traffic accidents, explosions, train crashes. Rehearsals for major disasters should be held on a regular basis so that the responsibility of individuals is clearly demarcated and understood.
6. Triage. This is a process of sorting patients on arrival into priority groups as far as management is concerned. The usual categories are immediate surgery, requires surgery but can wait, minor injury and dead.

ASSESSMENT OF THE TRAUMA PATIENT

This should follow ATLS (advanced trauma life support) guidelines. Initial assessment and management is based on a primary survey where patients are assessed and their treatment priorities established based on their injuries, their vital signs, and the injury mechanism. This is followed by a secondary survey which does not begin until the primary survey (ABCDE) is completed, resuscitative efforts are well established, and the patient is demonstrating stabilization of vital functions.

Primary survey

This process constitutes the ABCDE (see above) of trauma care and identifies life-threatening conditions by adhering to the following sequence:

A Airway maintenance with cervical spine protection
B Breathing and ventilation
C Circulation with control of haemorrhage
D Disability – neurological status
E Exposure/environmental control: completely undress the patient but prevent hypothermia.

Secondary survey

The secondary survey is a head-to-toe evaluation of the trauma patient, i.e. a complete history and physical examination including a reassessment of all vital signs. Each area of the body should be completely examined. A full neurological examination is carried out including a GCS (Glasgow Coma Score) determination (→ Table 3.1). At this time appropriate X-rays and blood tests are obtained.

History This is obtained from the patient (if possible), ambulance staff or other witnesses. Ascertain the time of the accident, the type of accident, the conscious level of the patient at the time of the accident and any change since, any blood loss, details of drugs administered at the scene of accident, previous medical history including drugs and allergies, details of food, alcohol and drug intake. A way of remembering this is to take an 'AMPLE' history:

- Allergies
- Medications

Table 3.1
Glasgow Coma Scale (GCS)

Responses	Score
Eye-opening response	
Spontaneuous	4
To voice	3
To pain	2
None	1
Best verbal response	
Orientated	5
Confused	4
Inappropriate speech	3
Incomprehensible speech	2
None	1
Best motor response	
Obeys commands	6
Localizes pain	5
Withdraws to pain	4
Flexion to pain	3
Extension to pain	2
None	1
Total	3–15

A score of 3 indicates a severe injury with a poor prognosis.
A score of 13–15 indicates minor injury with a good prognosis

- Previous illnesses
- Last meal
- Events surrounding injury.

Examination An initial rapid preliminary examination will have been made during the primary survey. A full examination is carried out during the secondary survey looking for head injuries, maxillofacial injuries, cervical spine injuries, chest injuries, abdominal and perineal injuries, musculoskeletal injuries, and neurological trauma.

Investigations The timing of the investigations depends on the clinical state of the patient • Routine blood tests including haemoglobin • U&Es • Glucose • Blood for grouping and cross-matching should be taken • ABGs may be required • Radiographs of the skull, cervical spine, chest and any other obvious sites of injury • CT/MRI scans • Contrast studies of the urinary tract or angiography may also be required. Diagnostic imaging should only be carried out once the patient's condition has been stabilized and life-threatening conditions dealt with.

HEAD INJURY (→ Ch. 18)

Primary brain damage occurring at the time of injury cannot be repaired. Management should be aimed at preventing secondary injury.

Management The management of specific head injury is dealt with in the section on neurosurgery (→ p. 434) but the basic principles are outlined here as far as trauma management is concerned.

Treat hypoxia, hypercapnia, hypovolaemic shock, and anaemia to prevent further neurological deterioration. Primary neurological management is identification and rapid treatment of localized lesions and intracranial haemorrhage, cerebral debridement and prevention of raised ICP.

Hypotension does not usually accompany head injury alone and must be assumed to be related to blood loss. The scalp should be examined for lacerations and boggy wounds. Observation should be made for bleeding and CSF leakage from the ear and nose. The cranial nerves should be checked and the limbs examined. Radiographs of the skull, cervical spine and chest are required as is a CT scan.

→

Immediate management depends on severity. The presence of abnormal pupillary reflexes, asymmetrical motor signs or deteriorating level of consciousness is an immediate indication for treatment.

Immediate measures:

1. intubate
2. ventilate with 100% oxygen
3. intravenous mannitol to produce a diuresis and reduce cerebral oedema
4. maintain normovolaemia
5. immediate transfer to theatre for burr holes and evacuation of haematoma.

Less urgent management is required where there are focal lesions without brainstem compression and with an unconscious patient without focal neurological observations.

THORACIC TRAUMA

Blunt and penetrating thoracic trauma are responsible for 25% of deaths due to trauma, but less than 20% of patients require thoracotomy for the treatment of their injuries.

Management Most patients with thoracic trauma can be managed as follows:

1. adequate resuscitation
2. respiratory support
3. chest drain.

Rapidly fatal complications of thoracic trauma needing immediate treatment are:

- cardiac tamponade
- tension pneumothorax
- haemorrhage from the heart and major vessels.

Other life-threatening complications include:

- airway obstruction
- open pneumothorax
- disruption of trachea or larynx
- flail chest
- air embolus.

Management of these are further covered in Chapter 9.

ABDOMINAL TRAUMA

Abdominal trauma may be *penetrating*, e.g. stab wound, bullet wound, or *blunt*, e.g. seatbelt injury in road traffic accident (RTA). *Injury to an abdominal viscus* should be suspected in any blunt injury to the thorax or abdomen or in penetrating injuries anywhere between the nipple and perineum.

Obtain information about the injury from the patient, relatives or ambulance personnel.

Signs Skin bruising, clothing imprints on skin suggest sufficient impact to cause major internal damage. Hypotension. Abdominal tenderness and distension. Fractures of left lower ribs suggest ruptured spleen. Pelvic fractures may be associated with bladder and urethral injuries. Haematuria suggests injury to the urinary tract.

Penetrating trauma

1. Look carefully for the wound. This may not always be obvious. Look for an exit site diametrically opposite.
2. The size of the skin wound is no guide to the extent of internal injury.
3. High-velocity bullet wounds injure widely and deeply. Damage in low-velocity bullet wounds is usually confined to the tissues along the track.
4. As a general principle all penetrating abdominal wounds should be explored under general anaesthetic.

Investigations • Plain radiographs. Look for free gas, pelvic fractures, rib fractures, obliteration of psoas shadows owing to retroperitoneal bleed • CXR. Look for rib fractures, pneumothorax, haemothorax • Peritoneal lavage. Run in 500 ml of normal saline via a rigid peritoneal dialysis catheter. Syphon out. *Heavy* blood staining indicates intra-abdominal injury. Bile staining, cloudiness or particulate matter suggests ruptured viscus • USS. Useful for liver, spleen or kidney injuries • CT. Injuries to liver, spleen or kidneys • IVU. If haematuria present • Urethrography. If suspected urethral injury.

Treatment

1. Treat shock as described earlier in the chapter.
2. Prophylactic antibiotics; and tetanus prophylaxis for penetrating injuries.
3. Explore all penetrating injuries.
4. Explore blunt trauma if there is evidence of intraperitoneal bleeding or ruptured viscus.

→

5. Laparotomy. Principles:
   - control bleeding
   - remove source of bleeding if necessary and feasible, e.g. ruptured spleen
   - check carefully for perforated viscus
   - peritoneal irrigation with saline especially if perforated viscus.

Injury to specific organs

Solid organs

Spleen Treatment is by splenectomy. If small capsular tear is present, suture.

Liver Small lacerations require suture only, major lacerations may be safely treated with tight packing with large gauze rolls. The packs should be removed under general anaesthetic 48 hours later. Complete disruption of a lobe may be best treated with hepatic lobectomy.

Pancreas This usually splits vertically across the vertebral column. Treatment is via a distal pancreatectomy. Crushing injuries may be treated with simple drainage and subsequent treatment is as for acute pancreatitis.

Hollow viscus

Stomach, duodenum, small bowel Simple suture for knife wounds and low-velocity bullet wounds. High-velocity bullet wounds and blunt trauma require resection either with end-to-end anastomosis or exteriorization of bowel.

Large bowel Antibiotic on induction of anaesthesia.

- Right colon: limited or full right hemicolectomy with primary anastomosis unless gross contamination.
- Left colon: small wounds may be exteriorized as a colostomy. Large wounds need bowel resection and ends of bowel brought out as colostomy and mucous fistula. Re-anastomosis is performed later. Rectal injuries may be sutured and protected by a defunctioning sigmoid colostomy. Thorough peritoneal lavage and drainage is required.

URINARY TRACT TRAUMA

Injuries to the urinary tract are divided into those of the upper and lower urinary tract. Most injuries are caused by blunt trauma.

Upper urinary tract

Injuries to the kidneys should be treated expectantly with blood transfusion and bed rest and antibiotics until haematuria subsides. Indications for surgery include shock, persistent haematuria and infection. Procedures include simple suture of a laceration, and partial or total nephrectomy. Ureteric injury is rare with external trauma. Most ureteric injuries are iatrogenic at surgery. Surgical repair is required.

Lower urinary tract

Intraperitoneal rupture of the bladder is repaired at laparotomy and a suprapubic catheter inserted. Extraperitoneal rupture may be treated by catheterization. Partial urethral injuries may be treated by catheterization. Complete injuries are treated by suprapubic catheterization and by immediate or delayed repair of the tear.

LIMB TRAUMA

This involves injury to: soft tissues; blood vessels (→ Ch. 15); nerves; bones (→ Ch. 17).

Soft tissue injuries

These range from minor cuts to extensive deep contaminated wounds and crushed muscle.

Abrasion Loss of superficial epithelium caused by friction. Treatment is by cleansing to remove any dirt or gravel, especially with wounds of the face. Application of sterile dressings.

Bruising Exclude underlying fracture. Icepacks are helpful. Rarely need to evacuate haematoma.

Laceration This is tear or cut in soft tissue. General principles of management include:

1. thorough search for associated nerve, vessel or tendon injury
2. careful check for tissue viability with debridement as necessary
3. cleansing and irrigation of the wound
4. delayed primary sutures used where the wound is contaminated or there has been excision of necrotic tissue; occasionally healing is allowed to occur by secondary intention
5. primary closure, i.e. immediate suture is undertaken where the wound is clean
6. antibiotics (benzylpenicillin) in contaminated wounds or where dead tissue has been excised; prophylaxis against gas

gangrene is required in contaminated wounds involving muscle
7. tetanus prophylaxis given especially in deep soil-contaminated wounds.

Foreign bodies Any open wound may contain a foreign body. Common materials include glass, wood splinters, road dirt or gravel, clothing or metal fragments. Radiograph in two planes with a marker may be required to accurately locate the foreign body. Metal and glass will usually be seen although a negative radiograph does not always exclude glass fragments. Foreign bodies should be removed if they protrude through the skin, cause pain or wound infection, or have material that may cause contamination, e.g. clothing particles. Foreign bodies may migrate and cause pressure on other structures, e.g. nerves, and then require removal.

Nerve injuries

Classification

Neurapraxia A condition of transient physiological block without degeneration. There is continuity of the axons and the myelin sheaths remain intact. Function returns spontaneously in about 6 weeks.

Axonotmesis Usually the result of compression or traction injuries which causes disruption of the axons with intact myelin sheaths. The distal axons shows degeneration but since the myelin sheaths are intact, return of function can be anticipated. The axons regenerate at the rate of about 1 mm a day. Return of function can be anticipated but may take many months.

Neurotmesis This is division of the nerve in whole or in part which occurs after incised or lacerated wounds or maybe a complication of a fracture. There is complete disruption of both the axon and the myelin sheath. Surgical repair is required. Residual neurological deficit is likely and neuroma may occur.

Management

- Peripheral nerve injuries are frequently associated with limb trauma.
- A thorough inspection and examination of the limb should be carried out to establish the presence of a nerve lesion before any treatment is undertaken. This is important for medicolegal reasons.
- Nerve injuries associated with closed trauma do not usually require exploration. Physiotherapy will be needed to prevent contractures and muscle wasting while nerve recovery occurs.
- Penetrating injuries should be explored and nerve repair undertaken. Immediate surgical repair should be undertaken

for digital nerves in clean wounds involving sharp lacerations. In contaminated wounds, repair may be delayed. It is wise to mark the nerve at the time of initial exploration with a suture to facilitate later identification. In extensive wounds with contusion and extensive tissue damage, e.g. gunshot wounds, nerve grafting may be necessary.

4

Preoperative and postoperative care

PREOPERATIVE PREPARATION

The purpose of preoperative evaluation is to identify the problems which may increase the operative risk and predispose to postoperative problems.

Assessment

1. *Full history*: present illness; past illnesses; bleeding tendencies; medication, allergies.
2. *Examination*: directed not only at the presenting complaint but also including a thorough examination of all systems, especially the cardiovascular and respiratory.
3. *Laboratory tests*: Hb, FBC for all but the most minor surgery.
4. *Radiographs*: CXR should be obtained in all patients with cancer, and cardiac, respiratory and renal disease. A routine preoperative CXR is unnecessary in young patients unless there are abnormalities on auscultation.
5. *ECG*: Obtain in all patients over the age of 40 and in those with a history of cardiac, respiratory or renal disease.

Principles of preoperative preparation

1. Correct any abnormalities that affect surgical risk.
2. Obtain informed consent. Explain all forms of possible treatment available for the condition. Explain the likely outcome without surgery. Explain the nature of the operation and the risks. Obtain the signature of the patient, parent or legal guardian. There is a special consent form for Jehovah's Witnesses.
3. Details of preparation:
   - nil by mouth for 4–6 hours preoperatively
   - i.v. fluids
   - nasogastric aspiration
   - bowel preparation
   - medication planning, e.g. steroids, insulin, antihypertensives.
4. Laboratory investigations, e.g. blood sugar in diabetes, K^+ in renal failure.
5. Cross-match of blood if major operation with expected blood loss.
6. Physiotherapy – breathing exercises.
7. DVT prophylaxis, e.g. graded compression stockings (TED), subcutaneous low molecular weight heparin, e.g. clexane.
8. Anaesthetic premedication.

POSTOPERATIVE CARE

Monitor the patient's progress at least daily postoperatively and more frequently if indicated. Record in the notes at least daily.

1. *Detailed operation note* including intraoperative drugs; postoperative instructions should accompany the patient to the ward.
2. *Monitoring of vital signs*. Monitor BP, pulse and respiratory rate every 15 minutes until the patient is stable and thereafter hourly for 24 hours. Monitor CVP after major surgery in the elderly and those with cardiac disease. Continuous ECG monitoring is advisable in those with cardiac disease or elderly patients undergoing major surgery.
3. *Early mobilization*. Patients requiring prolonged bed rest should be turned regularly from side to side to avoid pressure sores. Nurse on sheepskin or airbed. Protect sacrum and heels especially in diabetics.
4. *Diet*. Where an NG tube is used, sips of water may be administered when peristalsis returns as evidenced by bowel sounds. When fluids are tolerated remove the nasogastric tube and introduce full diet gradually. In operations not involving the GI tract, the patient may drink when fully awake after a GA.
5. *Intravenous fluids*. Administer according to requirements which are monitored by clinical examination, urine output and CVP.
6. *Intake/output chart*. Monitor closely to avoid dehydration or fluid overload.
7. *Urinary output*. If the patient is catheterized monitoring is easy. If the urine output falls below 30 ml/hour action is required. If the patient is not catheterized inform the surgeon if urine has not been passed within 8 hours postoperatively.
8. *Medication*:
    - analgesics – the dose, frequency, and route of administration should be clearly indicated
    - antibiotics as indicated
    - routine medication as indicated; if the patient is 'nil by mouth', essential medication should be given parenterally.
9. *Laboratory tests*. After major procedures, the Hb, FBC and U&Es should be checked 24 hours postoperatively and thereafter according to indications.
10. *Radiographs and ECG*. Carry out according to indications and not as routine. CXR may be necessary if pyrexia continues after 24 hours postoperatively, if there is sputum production or chest signs.

PROGRESS

The following points should be noted:

- general condition, e.g. well, ill, improving, deteriorating; pain
- vital signs, e.g. pyrexia, tachycardia
- mobility
- chest, e.g. clear, reduced air entry, consolidation
- abdomen, e.g. distended, bowel sounds, tender
- legs, e.g. DVT
- wound, e.g. discharge, infection
- intake/output
- diet
- results of any laboratory tests.

CONDITIONS AFFECTING SURGICAL RISK (→ Table 4.1)

GENERAL CONDITIONS IN SURGICAL PATIENTS

Age

Problems occur at extremes of life. There are limits to cardiac and renal reserves in the elderly. Avoid fluid overload. Smaller doses of narcotics, sedatives and analgesics are needed.

Obesity

This often results in poor wound healing and a higher incidence

Table 4.1
Conditions affecting surgical risk

General	Age Obesity Compromised host: • malnutrition • immunosuppression • vitamin deficiency Allergies Drugs
Medical problems in surgical patients	Cardiac Respiratory Renal Hepatic Haematological Endocrine

of respiratory problems. DVT and PE are more common. Pressure sores can develop. Delay elective surgery until the patient loses weight.

Compromised host

There is reduced response to trauma and infection, e.g. immunosuppressive drugs or uraemia. Malnutrition, e.g. vitamin deficiencies or liver disease, can also be a factor.

Allergies

Check for these preoperatively. Unsuspected reactions may occur. In severe cases anaphylactic shock may result. Sensitivity to surgical dressings (e.g. Elastoplast) may occur.

Drugs

Current drugs should be monitored carefully, e.g. insulin and steroids. Adjust anticoagulant therapy, e.g. conversion from warfarin to heparin over the perioperative period.

MEDICAL PROBLEMS IN SURGICAL PATIENTS

Cardiovascular

In elderly patients the following are common: angina, cardiac failure, arrhythmias, valvular heart disease, hypertension, cerebrovascular disease, peripheral vascular disease. It is necessary to obtain a cardiology opinion, optimize medical treatment and assess operative risk. The decision to operate rests with the surgeon and anaesthetist.

Angina Unstable angina and recent MI greatly increase the operative risk. Emergency surgery following recent MI has a mortality of 30%. Delay elective surgery for 6 months.

Cardiac failure Treat prior to surgery. Stabilize at least 1 month prior to surgery. Digoxin. Diuretic. Check K^+ prior to surgery. Mild CCF well controlled with digoxin and diuretics carries little risk. CCF with dyspnoea on exertion, orthopnoea and PND carries a significant risk.

Arrhythmias Uncontrolled AF may cause perioperative CCF. Digitalize adequately preoperatively. Some degrees of heart block require a prophylactic temporary transvenous pacemaker. Check digoxin levels in patients who have bradycardia. Arrhythmias developing during surgery may be due to hypoxia, hypercapnia or high or low K^+.

Valvular heart disease May result in MI, CCF, arrhythmias, embolism or bacterial endocarditis in the perioperative period. Newly discovered murmurs require a cardiology opinion.

Elective cases should be deferred until the murmur has been evaluated. Prophylactic antibiotics are important in the perioperative period and for patients with prosthetic valves. Check if patient is on anticoagulants.

Hypertension Mild hypertension without renal or cardiac complications does not significantly affect surgical risk. Control BP at or below 160/95. Defer and investigate elective cases with newly diagnosed hypertension. Check K^+ in patients on diuretics. Severe and poorly controlled hypertension should be adequately controlled prior to surgery.

Cerebrovascular disease High risk of intraoperative CVA. Previous history of TIAs or stroke. Carotid bruits. Aspirin may be protective. Avoid intraoperative hypotension.

Peripheral vascular disease Patients with peripheral ischaemia may develop arterial thrombosis if hypotensive. Take care to avoid pressure sores which may not heal and lead to the need for amputation.

Respiratory disease

This is a major cause of postoperative morbidity and mortality in the elderly. COPD, asthma, and bronchiectasis are precipitating causes. Smoking, obesity, old age, general debility and cardiac disease are contributory. Preoperative investigations include CXR, lung function tests (e.g. FEV_1, peak expiratory flow rate, spirometry), sputum culture, ABG.

Perioperative management of respiratory disease

- Stop smoking. Preferably 4 weeks prior to surgery.
- Preoperative chest physiotherapy and breathing exercises.
- Drugs, e.g. bronchodilators, nebulized salbutamol, antibiotics.
- Anaesthetic – local or spinal if possible.
- Analgesia. Avoid narcotic analgesics which may lead to respiratory depression. Consider epidural pain relief.
- Postoperative physiotherapy.
- Early mobilization.

Renal disease

This should be managed jointly with a nephrologist. Symptoms of renal failure do not usually become apparent until 80–90% of renal function has been lost and there is little renal reserve.

Mild impairment of renal function Mildly raised urea or creatinine. Refer to a nephrologist and delay elective surgery until a diagnosis has been reached and appropriate treatment instituted. Deterioration of renal function may occur after major surgery especially if dehydration is allowed to occur. Adequate preoperative rehydration. Monitor CVP. Caution with nephrotoxic drugs, e.g. gentamicin.

Grossly impaired renal function (non-dialysis dependent) Inadequate management may precipitate end-stage renal failure. Problems include fluid overload, dehydration, hyperkalaemia, metabolic acidosis. Chronic anaemia occurs but patients are well adapted to this. Uraemia is immunosuppressive and prophylactic antibiotics are required. Uraemia alters platelet function and bleeding may be a problem.

Dialysis-dependent renal failure

Haemodialysis Dialysis should take place 24 hours prior to surgery to allow the effects of heparin to wear off. Check U&Es, creatinine, and HCO_3 postdialysis. CXR to exclude pulmonary oedema. Check K^+ postoperatively as hyperkalaemia may occur following surgery under GA. If possible, delay postoperative dialysis for 24 hours in view of risk of bleeding with heparin.

Continuous ambulatory peritoneal dialysis (CAPD) Check U&Es prior to surgery. If abdominal surgery, CAPD may need to be discontinued and patient instituted on haemodialysis via a subclavian line until intra-abdominal healing has occurred.

Hepatic disease

There is a high incidence of morbidity and mortality with cirrhosis. Predisposing factors are anaemia, electrolyte disturbances, abnormal clotting, malnutrition, abnormal drug metabolism, ascites, portal hypertension. Defective synthesis of clotting factors in the liver and thrombocytopenia due to hypersplenism may result in excessive bleeding.

Care must be taken to assess a past history of jaundice. This may be due to hepatitis, obstructive jaundice, halothane jaundice or haemolytic disease.

Hepatitis Hepatitis A in the past carries little risk; hepatitis B and C may be carried permanently. Check HBsAg.

Obstructive jaundice There is usually a clear history. Surgery will usually have been necessary to deal with the problem.

Halothane jaundice It is due to the anaesthetic agent, halothane. Past history should be clearly recorded in the notes. A second exposure carries a greater risk.

Haemolytic disease It may cause jaundice.

Perioperative management of patients with liver disease

1. Full clinical examination.
2. Hb, FBC, U&Es, Cr, LFTs, PT, glucose.
3. Correct hypoglycaemia.
4. Correct coagulation defect, e.g. vitamin K parenterally, but in severe disease FFP may be required. Platelet transfusion.

5. Avoid saline infusions (risk of hypernatraemia).
6. Avoid hepatotoxic drugs.
7. Avoid drugs metabolized by liver, e.g. opiates.
8. Correct protein deficiency.
9. Antibiotics.

The main postoperative problems are bleeding, infection, and poor wound healing.

Haematological disease

Anaemia Mild anaemia, e.g. Hb greater than 10 g/dl, imposes little risk. Anaemia may be related to the condition for which surgery is being undertaken, e.g. GI cancer. Hb less than 10 g/dl should be treated by preoperative iron therapy or transfusion. Unsuspected anaemia noted prior to elective surgery should be investigated and the operation deferred.

Polycythaemia Hb greater than 18 g/dl. PCV (↑). Risks of arterial and venous thrombosis. Venesect prior to surgery. Myelosuppressive drugs may be required.

Bleeding disorders

Inherited Haemophilia is treated with cryoprecipitate preoperatively and until the danger of postoperative haemorrhage is over. Von Willebrand's disease is treated with FFP or cryoprecipitate.

Anticoagulant therapy Warfarin. The patient may have a history of thromboembolic disease, valvular heart disease or prosthetic heart valves. Anticoagulation may need to be continued during surgery, albeit at a reduced level. The safest procedure is to discontinue warfarin 3–4 days preoperatively and start heparin i.v. This can be more readily adjusted and is more easily reversed (with i.v. protamine sulphate) if bleeding occurs.

Disseminated intravascular coagulation (DIC) Coagulation and fibrinolysis occur simultaneously. Surgically important causes precipitating the condition include Gram-negative septicaemia, acute pancreatitis, malignancy, major surgery, e.g. ruptured aortic aneurysm. Clinical features include extensive bruising, oozing from drip and venepuncture sites, oozing from the wound, tracheostomy or bowel occurring in a severely ill patient. Diagnosis is confirmed by PT (prolonged); PTT (prolonged); thrombocytopenia; decreased fibrinogen level, raised FDPs. Treatment is by FFP, platelets and cryoprecipitate. Heparin i.v. may halt the coagulation element. Aggressive treatment of the underlying disease.

Endocrine disease

Diabetes This poses numerous risks, and affects many systems. Complications include:

- vasculopathy: heart – increased risk of MI; peripheral vascular disease (PVD) – risk of lower limb ischaemia with ulcers and gangrene; risk of stroke
- nephropathy – risk of CRF
- neuropathy – peripheral neuropathy with risk of pressure ulcers on heels and autonomic neuropathy with risk of cardiac arrest and gastric stasis with aspiration
- retinopathy leading to blindness – problems with management of blind patient in unfamiliar surroundings; anticoagulation, if needed, may make retinal haemorrhages worse
- increased incidence of infection.

The principles of management of diabetes in the perioperative period depend on whether patients are insulin dependent, on oral hypoglycaemics or controlled by diet.

Insulin-dependent

1. Admit 2 days preoperatively: CXR, ECG, FBC, U&Es, glucose, glycosylated Hb (HbA_1c).
2. Establish good diabetic control (glucose 4–10 mmol/l).
3. First on morning list. Check glucose.
4. Dextrose/insulin/K^+ infusion.
5. Check glucose intraoperatively and U&Es postoperatively.
6. Monitor glucose regularly in early postoperative period.
7. Continue infusion until full oral diet is established and then reinstitute normal insulin regime.

Oral hypoglycaemics

1. Review control.
2. Major surgery: convert to insulin/glucose/K^+ infusion as above.
3. Minor surgery: omit oral hypoglycaemic agent. Check blood sugar. If greater than 13 mmol/l give small dose of subcutaneous insulin.

Diabetics controlled by diet alone

1. Review control.
2. If preoperative control is adequate, no other measure required other than routine check of blood sugar pre- and postoperatively.

AMERICAN SOCIETY OF ANESTHESIOLOGISTS' CLASSIFICATION OF PHYSICAL STATUS (ASA GRADING)

When an operation is planned and there are problems concerning the patient's fitness for anaesthetic, then the anaesthetist should be involved as soon as possible. The American Society of Anesthesiologists has produced a grading system which attempts to quantify the risks of anaesthetizing patients with various clinical conditions. (→ Table 4.2).

Table 4.2
Grading system for quantifying anaesthetic risk

Class	Description
I	A healthy patient with no systemic disease process, e.g. a fit patient with an inguinal hernia
II	A patient with mild to moderate systemic disease process caused either by the condition to be treated surgically or by other pathological process which does not limit the patient's activity in any way, e.g. mild diabetic, treated hypertensive
III	A patient with a severe systemic disturbance from any cause, and which imposes a definite functional limitation on the patient, e.g. severely limiting organic heart disease, severe diabetes with vascular complications, severe chronic airways disease
IV	A patient with severe systemic disease which is a constant threat to life, e.g. severe unstable angina, advanced chronic liver failure
V	A moribund patient who is unlikely to survive 24 hours with or without surgery, e.g. ruptured aortic aneurysm in a patient with severe COPD

POSTOPERATIVE COMPLICATIONS

All operations carry a risk of complications. A classification is shown in Table 4.3. Complications may be divided into:

- general complications of any operation
- specific complications of individual operations.

The latter are discussed in relation to the specific operations and conditions in the various chapters.

Table 4.3
Postoperative complications

Haemorrhage	Early postoperative Secondary haemorrhage
Wound	Infection Bleeding Haematoma Seroma Suture sinus Breakdown: • burst abdomen • incisional hernia • anastomotic breakdown: peritonitis, abscess, fistula
Cardiovascular	Cardiac arrest MI Pulmonary oedema Arrhythmias DVT
Lung	Atelectasis Aspiration Pneumonia PE Pulmonary oedema Pneumothorax ARDS
Cerebral	Confusion: • sepsis • electrolyte/glucose • hypoxia • alcohol withdrawal Stroke
Urinary	Acute retention UTI Acute renal failure
Gastrointestinal	Paralytic ileus Mechanical obstruction Acute gastric dilatation Constipation
Other	Pressure sores

HAEMORRHAGE

Early postoperative

Inadequate haemostasis, unrecognized damage to blood vessels, defective vascular anastomosis, slipped ligature, massive blood transfusion without adequate clotting factors, use of intraoperative anticoagulants, e.g. in vascular surgery. Treatment depends on cause. Check clotting screen. Surgical re-exploration is usually required.

Secondary haemorrhage

Several days postoperatively. Related to infection which erodes vessel. Treatment of the infection and appropriate surgery to deal with the bleeding.

WOUND PROBLEMS

Infection

Incidence varies according to type of surgery and potential for contamination (→ also Ch. 5). Factors leading to increased risk of wound infection include: haematoma, poor nutritional state, diabetes mellitus, reduced immunity, nasal carriage of *Staphylococcus aureus*.

Symptoms and signs Painful red incision with discharge. General malaise. Examination reveals pyrexia, red, hot, tender wound. A purulent discharge may be apparent.

Treatment

1. If pus is present, it should be evacuated.
2. Culture and sensitivity of pus.
3. Appropriate antibiotic if cellulitis present or compromised patient, e.g. diabetic, steroids.
4. If cavity present, pack with antiseptic-soaked gauze to allow healing from base.

Wound breakdown

Factors which delay wound healing include old age, obesity, malnutrition, poor vascularity, sepsis, carcinoma, jaundice, uraemia, steroids, haematomas, raised intra-abdominal pressure.

Burst abdomen

This is a sudden bursting of the wound, revealing bowel. Usual cause is inadequate suturing of abdominal wall. Coughing, straining at stool, may be contributory. Cover the abdominal contents with sterile saline-soaked packs. Return the patient to theatre and repair with large bites of whole thickness of the abdominal wall using deep tension sutures.

Incisional hernia

The overall incidence is about 10%. In addition to factors which delay wound healing, causes include poor suture technique, raised intra-abdominal pressure (e.g. paralytic ileus), coughing, straining (e.g. constipation), prostatism. Rarely a broken suture is responsible. These herniae often have a wide neck and strangulation is rare.

Treatment If the patient is unfit, a surgical belt may be worn. If the patient is fit, surgical repair should be carried out.

Anastomotic breakdown

It is a major cause of postoperative morbidity and mortality after bowel surgery.

Causes

These include:

- poor surgical technique
- ischaemia at the anastomosis
- preoperative sepsis
- distal obstruction
- residual inflammatory disease, e.g. Crohn's or malignant disease
- general condition, e.g. uraemia, jaundice, malnutrition, steroids.

Anastomotic breakdown may result in generalized peritonitis, paracolic abscess, abscesses between loops of bowel or fistula formation. (For management of these conditions → Chs 5 and 14.)

Haematoma

This is a localized collection of blood beneath the wound. May be obvious tender mass with surrounding bruising. Treatment is by aspiration percutaneously or may require opening of the wound and clot evacuation.

Seroma

This is a localized collection of serous fluid. Often where skin flaps have been raised, e.g. chest wall in mastectomy, or where lymphatics have been divided, e.g. groin or axilla. Examination reveals a non-tender fluctuant mass. Small areas may be left and may absorb spontaneously or they may be needled percutaneously. Large ones may need formal drainage.

Stitch sinus

Sutures may act as nidus of infection especially at the knot. Less common since absorbable sutures and monofilament nylons replaced silk. Often the suture will extrude through the sinus spontaneously and the sinus will then heal. Occasionally, exploration and removal of the suture is required.

CARDIOVASCULAR PROBLEMS

Cardiac arrest following surgery is usually due to an underlying cardiac condition aggravated by a precipitating cause, e.g. hypoxia, shock, MI, anaesthetic overdose, hyperkalaemia, hypokalaemia or drug reactions. Cardiac arrest may follow respiratory arrest, e.g. following an obstructed airway (laryngeal oedema or tongue blocking airway) or inhalation of vomit. DVT may follow prolonged bed rest.

LUNG PROBLEMS

Lung complications are a common postoperative problem. They include atelectasis, aspiration, pneumonia, PE, pulmonary oedema, pneumothorax, and ARDS.

Atelectasis

Mucus is retained in the bronchial tree, blocking the smaller bronchi resulting in absorption of alveolar air with collapse of an area of lung. Infection may then occur. Minor degrees are common. Smoking, COPD, are predisposing factors. Anaesthesia may increase bronchial secretions and depress ciliary action. Post-operative abdominal pain inhibits coughing and allows secretions to accumulate.

Symptoms and signs Minor atelectasis may be accompanied by mild pyrexia alone; greater degrees are accompanied by dyspnoea, tachypnoea, rapid pulse and elevated temperature. Major degrees may be accompanied by cyanosis and respiratory collapse. The signs include widespread rales, reduced air entry and dullness to percussion.

Diagnosis Clinical: • CXR • ABG • Sputum culture.

Treatment Minor degrees require only chest physiotherapy. Adequate pain relief facilitates mobility and physiotherapy. Nebulized bronchodilators. More severe degrees may require bronchoscopy to remove mucus plugs. The most severe case may require intubation and ventilation.

Aspiration

Aspiration pneumonitis following inhalation of acidic gastric contents is known as Mendelson's syndrome. Aspiration may occur during induction, or at the termination, of anaesthesia. It may also occur in patients with bowel obstruction or paralytic ileus who vomit in the early postoperative period. Prevention includes preoperative 'nil by mouth' in elective cases, nasogastric suction in the emergency case and cricoid compression in 'crash' induction. If aspiration occurs, suction, intubation and saline lavage should be carried out. Steroids may help. Antibiotics will prevent super-added infection. Oxygen by mask.

Pneumonia

Predisposing factors include smoking, atelectasis, COPD, aspiration, debilitated patients.

Symptoms and signs Cough, respiratory distress, sputum. Signs include fever, tachypnoea, tachycardia, cyanosis, consolidation and rales.

Diagnosis • Sputum culture • CXR • ABG.

Treatment Chest physiotherapy. Antibiotics, e.g. amoxycillin or septrin until results of culture are known. Oxygen by mask.

Pulmonary oedema

Usually elderly patient with compromised cardiac function or young patient with history of cardiac or renal disease.

Symptoms and signs Tachypnoea, tachycardia, orthopnoea, raised JVP, pink frothy sputum, widespread crepitations.

Diagnosis • CXR • Raised JVP • Elevated CVP.

Treatment Stop i.v. fluids. Sit patient upright. Oxygen by face mask. i.v. frusemide. Small doses of opiates.

Pulmonary embolus (PE)

Complication of silent or overt DVT. Passage of a clot from pelvic or leg veins into the pulmonary artery. Major PE with overt DVT is usually obvious clinically. In some cases, diagnosis relies on a high index of clinical suspicion.

Symptoms and signs Usually 4–10 days postoperatively. Sudden dyspnoea and collapse. Hypotension. Pleuritic chest pain. Haemoptysis. Pleural rub.

Diagnosis • CXR: wedge-shaped collapse • ECG: right heart strain • S1, Q3, T3 pattern • ABG: hypoxia • V/Q scan: mismatch of ventilation/perfusion areas, i.e. ventilation normal but perfusion deficient • Pulmonary angiography is most accurate – used prior to surgery or thrombolysis.

Treatment

Patients without shock They may be treated by i.v. heparin sufficient to maintain the APTT at 2.5 times normal. Start warfarin after 5 days of heparin and continue for 6–9 months. With recurrent pulmonary emboli it should be continued for life.

Profound shock Inotropic support. Urgent pulmonary angiography. Thrombolytic therapy or pulmonary embolectomy.

Recurrent pulmonary embolus This should be treated by insertion of a filter, e.g. Greenfield filter percutaneously via the venous route into the IVC.

Pneumothorax

Rare complication of surgery. Rupture of subpleural bulla or complication of insertion of central line perioperatively.

Symptoms and signs Respiratory distress. Reduced breath sounds and hyperresonance to percussion of affected side.

Treatment Small: treat expectantly. Large: chest drain.

Adult respiratory distress syndrome (ARDS; shock lung)

This is acute respiratory failure with tachypnoea, hypoxia, decreased lung compliance, and diffuse pulmonary infiltrates on CXR. The exact aetiology is unknown but there is interference

Table 4.4
Causes of ARDS

Infection	Septicaemia
Inhalation	Smoke, vomit, water, high O_2 concentrations, chlorine, ammonia
Embolism	Fat, amniotic fluid, air
Cerebral	Head injury, cerebral haemorrhage
Drugs	Opiates, barbiturates
Others	Pancreatitis, DIC, blood transfusion, cardiopulmonary bypass, major trauma with shock

with the pulmonary epithelial/endothelial cell interface with increased interstitial oedema, vascular congestion and ultimately fibrosis. (For causes → Table 4.4.)

Symptoms and signs Present a few days after diagnosis of a serious underlying condition. Breathlessness, deterioration in clinical condition.

Investigations • CXR shows whiteout with sparing of costophrenic angles • ABG: hypoxia resistant to oxygen administration • May be difficult to distinguish from pulmonary oedema in early stages but latter usually shows cardiomegaly on CXR and response to diuretics.

Treatment
1. Treat the underlying disease, e.g. septicaemia.
2. Treat the pulmonary problem:
   - Mechanical ventilation to maintain $Pa\text{O}_2$. PEEP may be necessary.
   - Monitor fluid balance. CVP to monitor right atrial pressure. Left atrial pressure is monitored as pulmonary wedge pressure with a Swann–Ganz catheter.
   - Careful monitoring for development of secondary lung infection. Administration of appropriate antibiotics.
   - Renal failure is a common complication. Early administration of dopamine in renal doses may be appropriate.

The mortality rate for ARDS is between 70 and 90%.

CEREBRAL PROBLEMS

Confusion

Confusion postoperatively is not uncommon especially at night in the elderly. However, there may be an underlying cause, e.g. sepsis, hypoxia, alcohol withdrawal, electrolyte or glucose imbalance, cerebral bleed, postoperative pancreatitis, opiate analgesia.

Investigations • Hb • FBC • U&Es • Glucose • Amylase • ABGs • Blood culture • Urine analysis • Sputum culture • CXR • Brain scan.

Treatment
- Correct electrolyte or glucose disturbance.
- Correct hypoxia. 35% oxygen by mask or nasal cannula.
- Investigate and treat any sepsis.
- Tranquillizers may be required, e.g. chlorpromazine or haloperidol.
- For acute alcohol withdrawal, i.v. chlormethiazole and parenteral vitamin B may be used, although 60 ml of medicinal brandy may be more appropriate.

Stroke

May occur in the elderly postoperatively. Avoid intraoperative hypotension in patients with TIAs or carotid bruits.

URINARY TRACT PROBLEMS

Acute retention

Common postoperatively especially in elderly males.

Symptoms and signs Usually suprapubic discomfort although this may not be apparent because the patient has been given analgesia postoperatively. Usually nurse reports that patient has not passed urine for several hours postoperatively. Examination reveals a palpable bladder dull to percussion. If the patient has no desire to micturate and the bladder is not palpable, oliguria must be considered and corrected.

Treatment Conservative. Ensure adequate analgesics. Stand patient up. If no benefit, and the patient is fit enough, take to bathroom and leave tap running to encourage micturition. If conservative measures fail, pass a urinary catheter.

Urinary tract infection (UTI)

This is common, especially in females. Catheterization may predispose.

Symptoms and signs Dysuria/frequency/dribbling/smelly urine. May be found in investigation of undiagnosed pyrexia postoperatively.

Investigations • MSSU.

Treatment Appropriate antibiotic.

Acute renal failure (ARF)

Oliguria is passage of less than 30 ml of urine per hour. Anuria is failure to pass any urine.

Causes

Prerenal Reduced cardiac output, shock, e.g. hypovolaemic, cardiogenic, septic.

Renal Pre-existing renal disease, e.g. diabetes, glomerulonephritis. Nephrotoxic drugs, e.g. gentamicin. Myoglobinuria in crush syndrome. Haemoglobinuria with haemolysis.

Postrenal Obstruction, e.g. damage to ureters, benign prostatic hypertrophy.

Treatment of anuria/oliguria

1. Check that the catheter is patent. If patient not catheterized, then pass catheter.
2. Check BP to exclude hypotension.
3. Fluid challenge, e.g. 1 litre normal saline over 1 hour. Give sufficient fluid to restore CVP. If elderly patient, a fluid challenge is best done with CVP monitoring.
4. If no improvement in urine output, give bolus dose of loop diuretic, e.g. 120 mg of frusemide i.v.
5. If no improvement, give renal dose of dopamine.
6. If no response, check K^+ and HCO_3^-. ECG (signs of hyperkalaemia).
7. Contact renal physician and manage jointly. In the presence of hyperkalaemia and metabolic acidosis, dialysis will be required until a diuresis ensues. Fluid overload may be treated with CVVH.

GASTROINTESTINAL PROBLEMS

Paralytic ileus

This is the cessation of GI motility. Aetiological factors include fractures of the spine and pelvis, retroperitoneal haemorrhage, peritonitis, hypokalaemia, drugs, e.g. ganglion blockers and anticholinergic agents, abdominal surgery, immobilization. Atony of the bowel may be expected for 24–48 hours postoperatively.

Table 4.5
Factors distinguishing paralytic ileus and mechanical obstruction

	Ileus	Obstruction
Time	Usually settles in 3–4 days	May persist longer
Bowel sounds	Absent	High-pitched and 'tinkling'
Pain	Painless	Colicky abdominal pain
AXR	General gaseous dilatation of small and large bowel	Localized small-bowel distension with absent gas in colon and rectum

Paralytic ileus continuing after 48 hours may have an underlying cause.

Symptoms and signs Abdominal distension, vomiting, constipation. Tense tympanitic abdomen. Absent bowel sounds. (For distinguishing features between obstruction and ileus → Table 4.5).

Investigations • AXR: gaseous distension with fluid levels throughout the large and small bowel.

Treatment

1. Pass NG tube and aspirate hourly.
2. Ensure adequate hydration.
3. Correct any potassium imbalance.
4. Paralytic ileus rarely lasts for more than 4 days.
5. If symptoms persist, look for continuing cause and exclude mechanical obstruction.

Mechanical obstruction

Early (within 2 weeks of surgery) May be due to *fibrinous* adhesions. Obstruction may settle with i.v. fluids and nasogastric suction or it may progress and require laparotomy.

Late (after 2 weeks) May be due to obstruction by adhesions which are fibrous bands arising as part of peritoneal healing. Symptoms may settle with i.v. fluids and nasogastric suction. If they do not or signs of strangulation appear, laparotomy will be necessary.

Gastric dilatation

Acute gastric dilatation may occur in the early postoperative period and may be associated with shock. Vomiting with aspiration may occur.

Treatment This is with NG suction which may aspirate several litres of brownish/black fluid with altered blood. Fluid and electrolyte losses must be replaced.

Constipation

Uncomfortable for patient. Precipitating factors include starvation, dehydration, inactivity, opiates.

Treatment

1. Check daily if patient has had bowels open. Do not delay treatment.
2. Lactulose should be given as soon as the patient is eating.
3. Glycerine suppositories. PR to exclude faecal impaction.

→

4. Enemas may be required. With faecal impaction, oil enemas may be necessary.
5. Attention to diet. High-fibre diet or bulking agent.

POSTOPERATIVE PAIN RELIEF

Pain must be expected from most surgical procedures but it usually subsides gradually over the first few days. Patients respond differently to pain. However, excess pain in the post-operative period may be a symptom of a developing complication.

METHODS OF POSTOPERATIVE PAIN CONTROL

1. Full explanation of the operation and postoperative course and an attempt to relieve preoperative anxiety may reduce the severity of postoperative pain.
2. Oral analgesics. These are suitable for mild to moderate pain, e.g. groin hernia repair or varicose vein surgery. Paracetamol or codeine tablets are suitable agents. For moderate pain, NSAIDs, paracetamol and dextropropoxyphene (coproxamol) are suitable. For severe pain, sublingual buprenorphine or slow-release morphine tablets may be given.

Parenteral analgesia

Intermittent intramuscular opiates Most commonly used. Usually given p.r.n., 4-hourly. Many patients still complain of pain.

Continuous subcutaneous infusion of opiates Given via a subcutaneous butterfly needle. Avoids painful i.m. injections. Venous access not required. Respiratory rate should be monitored and the rate of infusion reduced if it falls below 8 breaths per minute.

Continuous i.v. infusion of opiates Reliable venous access and expensive equipment required. Respirations must be monitored as above.

PCA pump This device allows the patient to self-administer a preset dose of an analgesic drug by pressing a button connected to a pump. This in turn is connected to an i.v. cannula. There is a preset interval before the infusion equipment will deliver another dose, i.e. the 'lock-out' time. This is a very effective method of pain control but is expensive.

Spinal opioids

Insert indwelling intrathecal or epidural catheters at the time of surgery. Surgery may then be performed with local anaesthetic and opioids given by the spinal or epidural route. When the local anaesthetic has worn off, the longer-acting opioid continues to provide analgesia. This may be topped up.

Intercostal nerve blocks

These are useful for upper abdominal surgery.

Direct infiltration

Bupivacaine, a long-acting local anaesthetic, can be injected directly into the wound, e.g. for repair of an inguinal hernia. It may be also injected around the nerve supplying the area of the wound, e.g. the ilioinguinal nerve in hernia repair.

BLOOD TRANSFUSION

Blood transfusion is not without risk. The decision to transfuse blood must have clear indications and, if possible, alternative therapies, e.g. plasma substitutes for hypovolaemia, or iron therapy for anaemia should be used. Screening programmes for HIV, hepatitis B and C have made transfusion safer.

BLOOD, BLOOD PRODUCTS, BLOOD SUBSTITUTES

- *Whole blood*. It is used for major haemorrhage, e.g. trauma, surgery, bleeding ulcers.
- *Packed cells*. These are used to correct anaemia where there is a risk of overload.
- *Human albumin (4.5%)*. It is used to replace plasma, e.g. burns.
- *FFP*. It is separated from blood and snap-frozen to preserve clotting factors. Given in liver disease, to reverse anticoagulants, and in DIC.
- *Platelet concentrates*. These are given for thrombocytopenia and to cover massive blood transfusions.
- *Cryoprecipitate*. This is used in haemophilia.
- *Fibrinogen*. It is used in DIC.
- *Plasma substitutes*. These include gelatin solutions (gelofusin, Haemaccel). They are used to restore circulating volume until blood becomes available.

CLINICAL ASPECTS OF BLOOD TRANSFUSION

1. The patient's ABO and Rh groups are established.
2. Each unit of group compatible blood is then cross-matched against the recipient's serum.

3. Minor incompatibilities may occur and require further cross-matching.
4. If blood is required urgently, O negative (universal donor) may be given in an emergency with comparative safety.
5. 'Group and save'. In some operations transfusion is unlikely but occasionally possible. Blood is taken preoperatively and grouping assessed. The serum is retained in the laboratory and blood is cross-matched as required.
6. For some operations, blood should be immediately available. Blood is grouped, cross-matched and available on the day of surgery.
7. Mistakes with mismatched transfusions often have serious and occasionally fatal consequences. To avoid mistakes, blood specimens sent to the laboratory must be carefully labelled with the name, date of birth and hospital unit number of the patient.
8. Each unit of blood subsequently transfused must be carefully matched to make sure that the label of the bag of blood corresponds with the name, blood group and hospital number of the patient.

COMPLICATIONS OF BLOOD TRANSFUSION

Incompatibility

This is usually due to human error. Always administer blood slowly (unless life-saving emergency), and monitor pulse, BP, temperature and urine output.

Symptoms and signs Pyrexia, dyspnoea, rigors, loin pain, hypotension, oliguria with haemoglobinuria, jaundice.

Investigations • Check identity of patient • Check blood group and the donor blood group • Take blood for haemolytic screen and FBC.

Treatment Stop transfusion immediately. Return bag of blood and specimen of patient's blood to BTS. Give mannitol i.v. to induce diuresis. ARF may occur and should be treated appropriately.

Febrile reactions

Common, due to pyrogens. Mild fever is not a contraindication to continuing transfusion. High fever and rigors demand cessation of transfusion and a check of compatibility.

Allergic reactions

These include itching, skin rashes, urticaria. Discontinue transfusion and administer antihistamine.

Infection

This is unlikely with the present testing in the UK. Hepatitis B and C, HIV, syphilis, CMV may be a problem where testing is not carried out.

Massive transfusions

These may be complicated by fluid overload, hypothermia, arrhythmias, hyperkalaemia, citrate intoxication, ARDS and haemorrhage (unless FFP and platelets administered simultaneously).

FLUID AND ELECTROLYTE BALANCE

The basic principle of fluid and electrolyte balance is that which is lost must be replaced.

WATER

Water losses amount to an average of 2500 ml/day. This occurs via the skin (sensible and insensible sweating); lungs as water vapour in expired air; kidney as urine; GI tract as faeces.

Insensible losses are higher than normal postoperatively, especially in the febrile patient. Increased environmental temperature causes increased sweating. In the absence of any other problem, e.g. vomiting or diarrhoea, 3 litres of fluid replacement will be adequate replacement for normal water loss, i.e. an average of 40 ml/kg/day.

ELECTROLYTES

The main ones to consider are Na^+ or K^+. The loss of Na^+ averages approximately 100 mmol/day mainly in the urine but about 40 mmol/l is lost in sweat. The loss of K^+ averages approximately 80 mmol/day mainly in urine but a small amount is lost in the faeces. Approximately these amounts of electrolytes should be added to the water requirement. There is a tendency to overestimate the Na^+ replacement and underestimate the K^+ replacement in most fluid replacement regimens but if the patient has normal renal function the body will deal with this. U&Es should be checked at least daily while patients are on i.v. fluids and adjustments made in electrolyte replacement should be based on these results.

Examples of daily fluid and electrolyte regimens are shown below. Each 500 ml bag of fluid is given over 4 hours.

- 500 ml normal saline plus 20 mmol KCl
- 500 ml 5% dextrose

- 500 ml 5% dextrose plus 20 mmol KCl
- 500 ml normal saline
- 500 ml 5% dextrose plus 20 mmol KCl
- 500 ml 5% dextrose

This gives 3 litres of fluid plus 150 mmol Na^+ plus 60 mmol K^+.

- 500 ml 5% dextrose/1/5 normal saline plus 20 mmol KCl
- 500 ml 5% dextrose/1/5 normal saline
- 500 ml 5% dextrose/1/5 normal saline plus 20 mmol KCl
- 500 ml 5% dextrose/1/5 normal saline
- 500 ml 5% dextrose/1/5 normal saline plus 20 mmol KCl
- 500 ml 5% dextrose/1/5 normal saline

This gives 3 litres of fluid plus 90 mmol Na^+ plus 60 mmol K^+. This regimen is probably safer in patients with cardiac impairment. It is also probably best given in the first 24 hours postoperatively when the adrenal response to surgery causes Na^+ retention.

Fluid and electrolyte depletion

Surgical patients may suffer large losses of fluid and electrolytes as part of the disease process, operation, or postoperative complications. In addition to obvious losses, e.g. vomiting and diarrhoea, fluid may be lost into 'new' spaces resulting from the disease process, e.g. the intestine during paralytic ileus, the peritoneum in peritonitis, the retroperitoneum in acute pancreatitis or intracellular shifts in shock. These losses are called 'third space' losses. These losses must be promptly replaced as the problems they cause are just as important as external losses. These fluids are eventually reabsorbed and care must be taken that circulatory overload does not occur.

Management of Na^+ and K^+ imbalance

Hyponatraemia (i.e. low Na^+) In a surgical patient this is usually due to water overload and results from administration of inappropriate amounts of 5% dextrose. If the hyponatraemia associated with fluid overload is mild, it is best treated by restricted fluid intake, avoiding the administration of saline, and giving frusemide i.v. to force a diuresis. Electrolytes should be checked twice daily. Hyponatraemia is associated with symptoms, e.g. confusion, convulsions, coma, if the Na^+ falls below 120 mmol/l. In hyponatraemia with hypovolaemia, saline should be given.

Hypernatraemia (i.e. high Na^+) This is uncommon in the surgical patient. It may occur during dehydration and in the postoperative period if too much saline is given at a time when aldosterone secretion is high and sodium is being conserved. Rarely it may be caused by Conn's syndrome (→ Ch. 11). If the cause is dehydration (i.e. clinically dry with low CVP and oliguria), the patient will need water replacement, whereas in the postoperative period with normovolaemia, sodium restriction is required.

Hypokalaemia (i.e. low K^+) Preoperatively this may be due to diuretic therapy, diarrhoea, fistula or excessive mucus loss from a villous adenoma of the rectum. Postoperatively it is usually due to inadequate K^+ replacement. It may occur with pyloric stenosis (with an associated metabolic alkalosis). Symptoms include muscle weakness, cardiac arrhythmias (T wave flattening on ECG) and paralytic ileus. Treatment is by K^+ replacement but this should not exceed 15 mmol/hour as cardiac arrhythmias may arise with high infusion rates.

Hyperkalaemia (i.e. high K^+) Preoperatively this may be due to CRF, crush injuries or absorption from massive haematomas. Massive transfusions of stored blood may also cause hyperkalaemia. Postoperatively it is usually due to excessive administration and is usually asymptomatic. A K^+ above 7 mmol/l is an emergency. Intravenous insulin and glucose should be given and the K^+ checked. ECG changes include elevated T waves. If ECG changes are marked, calcium gluconate should be given i.v. Other methods of reducing the serum K^+ include calcium resonium orally or rectally, and if renal function is compromised, dialysis.

Acid–base balance

Abnormalities of acid–base balance usually occur in seriously ill patients and include:

Metabolic acidosis Severe tissue hypoxia, e.g. septicaemia, hypovolaemia or cardiogenic shock; renal failure; diabetic ketoacidosis; and after aortic surgery when the clamp is removed. The patient compensates by rapid deep respiration to 'blow off' CO_2. Excretes acid urine. ABGs show pH (↓), HCO_3 (↓), $P\text{CO}_2$ (↓). Management involves treatment of the underlying condition. Bicarbonate infusion may be necessary in severe cases.

Metabolic alkalosis This occurs with prolonged vomiting or nasogastric aspiration. Pyloric stenosis. In order to compensate, the kidney conserves hydrogen ions at the expense of K^+ excretion. ABGs show pH (↑), $P\text{CO}_2$ (↑). Low K^+. Treatment is by rehydration with normal saline with potassium supplements and treatment of the underlying condition.

Respiratory acidosis This results from CO_2 retention. After surgery this is usually due to severe chest complications, e.g. atelectasis from sputum retention or respiratory depression due to narcotics. Respiratory acidosis is compensated for by H^+ being excreted by the renal tubules and HCO_3^- being reabsorbed. ABGs show pH (↓), $P\text{CO}_2$ (↑). Treatment is of the underlying cause.

Respiratory alkalosis Hyperventilation due to anxiety. Excessive mechanical ventilation. Compensation occurs by renal excretion of HCO_3^-. ABGs show pH (↑), $P\text{CO}_2$ (↓). Treatment is of the underlying condition.

NUTRITIONAL SUPPORT

Poor nutrition results in increased postoperative morbidity and mortality. Poor wound healing occurs and there is a reduced resistance to infection. General examination of the patient will show evidence of weight loss, e.g. general appearance, loose skin folds. The patient will often be aware of how much weight has been lost and over what time period.

CAUSES OF MALNUTRITION

- Increased catabolism, e.g. sepsis, major surgery with complications.
- Increased losses, e.g. chronic liver disease with loss of albumin, protein-losing enteropathy.
- Decreased intake, e.g. dysphagia, vomiting, general debility.
- Decreased absorption, e.g. intestinal fistulae, short bowel syndrome.
- Other causes, e.g. major trauma, chemotherapy, radiotherapy.

INDICATIONS FOR NUTRITIONAL SUPPORT

Most patients requiring surgery are well nourished and will stand a few days starvation. They will recover from surgery sufficiently to resume eating before they become malnourished. Some patients will be clearly malnourished prior to surgery while others may develop complications which delay resumption of normal diet and require parenteral nutrition. Others may have conditions, e.g. short-bowel syndrome, which require long-term or permanent nutritional support.

Other indications for nutritional support include:

- preoperatively in malnourished patients
- postoperatively in malnourished patients and those who develop malnutrition because of complications
- patients with sepsis or major postoperative complications
- patients with fistulae
- patients with chronic liver disease
- patients undergoing chemotherapy or radiotherapy for certain tumours
- patients with short-bowel syndrome or malabsorption syndrome.

EVALUATION OF NUTRITIONAL STATUS

1. History: duration of illness, weight loss, change in appetite, dietary habits.
2. Physical examination: general appearance, loose skin folds, loss of skin contours over bony prominences, muscle wasting, peripheral oedema.
3. Weight: in relation to height.
4. Anthropometric measurements: e.g. triceps skin fold thickness.
5. Laboratory tests: e.g. Hb, serum albumin, serum iron.

ADMINISTRATION OF NUTRITIONAL SUPPORT

Oral nutrition

This is the most efficient, least expensive, most pleasant and safest route for the patient. If the GI tract is available and the patient able to take oral nutrition, then this method is the most appropriate. Liquidized food, Clinifeed or supplements may be given this way.

Enteral nutrition

This is used for patients with a functioning small bowel unable to take nutrients by mouth, e.g. those who are seriously ill, unable to swallow or have a mouth lesion, e.g. herpes.

Fine-bore NG tubes Liquidized food, Clinifeed or supplements are given via a tube passed via the nose into the stomach.

Surgically created gastrostomy or jejunostomy These are appropriate for long-term enteric feeding.

In both the above methods the feed is dripped slowly into the GI tract. Bolus feeding should be avoided as it gives marked diarrhoea and if given via a nasogastric tube in large volumes, may result in regurgitation and aspiration pneumonia.

Parenteral nutrition

This is used where GI function is inadequate and nutrition is administered via the venous system.

Peripheral line Short-term feeding (up to 5 days) may be given via drip in a peripheral vein. Solutions used with this method must be of a special type which causes little thrombophlebitis. This method may be used preoperatively for patients with malnutrition of moderate degree for which oral nutrition is unsatisfactory, e.g. malignant strictures of the oesophagus.

Central line This is the most appropriate route and is used for total parenteral nutrition (TPN). For short-term use, a percutaneous internal jugular line may be used. For longer-term and permanent nutrition, a tunnelled subcutaneous line (Hickman or Broviac) should be used. Hypertonic solutions are infused via the catheter into a large-bore vein with good flow to prevent thrombophlebitis.

TOTAL PARENTERAL NUTRITION (TPN)

This is usually provided in 3-litre bags either prepared in the hospital pharmacy or bought commercially. This provides all the nutrients required for a 24-hour period. Controlled rates of administration are essential and this is achieved either by a special counting device attached to the drip line or via an infusion pump. Any additional fluid and electrolyte to restore losses, or administration of drugs, should be via a separate peripheral line.

Components of TPN

- Calories: these are supplied as a combination of carbohydrate and fat. Most patients require approximately 2000 kcal/day or more if they have sepsis or burns.
- Protein: this is supplied as amino acids. Nitrogen requirements are about 15 g/day but may be as high as 30 g/day in hypercatabolic states.
- Water.
- Vitamins.
- Electrolytes, e.g. Na^+, K^+, calcium, phosphate, magnesium.
- Trace elements, e.g. zinc, copper, manganese.

Monitoring TPN

Blood sugar, U&Es should be checked daily. Until fluid and nitrogen balance is obtained the blood sugar should be monitored 6-hourly by BM stix. LFTs, calcium, phosphate, and FBC should be checked twice weekly. If the patient becomes pyrexial, blood cultures should be obtained. The site of catheter insertion should be dressed twice weekly under aseptic conditions. If the patient develops a pyrexia and no other cause is found, it may be necessary to remove the catheter and send the tip for culture. The catheter should be used for feeding only. Any other substances, e.g. additional electrolytes or drugs, should be given via a separate peripheral line.

Complications of TPN

Catheter related Pneumothorax or arterial puncture may occur during insertion. If the catheter is not correctly positioned in a large vein but is in a chamber of the heart, arrhythmias may occur. Rarely the catheter may erode through a vessel wall and give rise to haemopericardium. Air embolus may occur when manipulating the line and this should be avoided by keeping the patient supine. Thrombosis of a central vein may occur. Prophylactic heparin 1000 units/l of the infusion is useful prophylaxis.

Metabolic Too much or too little of components of i.v. feeding may be given. Careful monitoring for the following is required:

- fluid overload
- hyperglycaemia
- hypoglycaemia may occur if infusion of hypertonic glucose is suddenly stopped
- electrolyte abnormalities
- hepatic cholestasis.

Home TPN

Long-term TPN in ambulatory patients is practicable providing it is properly monitored. Patients with short-bowel syndrome are the most appropriate. The patient or a partner is taught the technique and back-up is provided by a specially trained team who are able to provide regular biochemical monitoring. A Broviac or Hickman tunnelled central line is used. The feeding solution may be administered overnight and the catheter disconnected to allow activity during the day. Alternatively it may need to be administered throughout 24 hours, depending on the patient's requirements.

5

Infection and surgery

PRINCIPLES OF WOUND MANAGEMENT

Healing by first intention

When appropriate, the wound edges are approximated as soon after the injury as possible, e.g. clean traumatic wounds or surgical incisions. This is known as primary closure and the wound heals by first intention.

Healing by second intention

The wound edges are not apposed and the wound is left to heal by second intention. Granulation tissue grows up from the base of the wound and the skin grows over in a centripetal manner. This type of healing is appropriate for large, grossly contaminated wounds.

Delayed primary closure

The wound is left open and observed for several days. If the wound then appears healthy it may be closed as for a primary closure. This type of closure is suitable for wounds that have low-grade infection or for surgical incisions where infection may be expected, e.g. abdominal incisions following operations for gross faecal peritonitis.

Skin grafts (→ Ch. 19)

These may be used to cover large, open wounds where primary closure is impossible. Grafts are placed on healthy granulation tissue.

Factors affecting wound healing

Age Younger patients heal better than older patients.

Nutritional state Malnutrition impedes wound healing. Patients who are poorly nourished should be given appropriate feeding, e.g. TPN prior to surgery.

Drugs Steroids delay wound healing.

Tissue oxygenation and vascularity Hypoxaemia and ischaemia delay wound healing. Highly vascular areas, e.g. face, heal better than poorly vascularized areas, e.g. shin.

Radiotherapy Causes endarteritis obliterans of small vessels resulting in local ischaemia and poor healing.

Local sepsis This is probably the commonest cause of delayed healing.

Classification

Surgical wounds may be classified by their potential for infection.

Clean Operation under sterile conditions where the GI tract,

GU tract and respiratory tract are not breached, e.g. varicose vein surgery, hernia repair. The risk of postoperative wound infection is less than 5%.

Clean/contaminated Operation performed under sterile conditions where the GI tract, GU tract or respiratory tract are opened with minimal contamination, e.g. cholecystectomy, partial gastrectomy. The risk of postoperative wound infection is about 10%.

Contaminated Operation performed where contamination is inevitable, e.g. perforated appendicitis, faecal peritonitis. The risk of postoperative wound infection is greater than 50%.

Prophylactic antibiotics (→ also below)

Clean wounds Prophylactic antibiotics are not required unless infection has an added risk, e.g. immunosuppressed patient, diabetic, insertion of prosthesis, e.g. vascular graft or hip replacement.

Clean/contaminated Prophylactic antibiotics are indicated. They should be given intravenously either with the premedication or on induction of anaesthesia, e.g. for cholecystectomy.

Contaminated Antibiotics are given as therapy, not prophylaxis.

ANTIBIOTICS IN SURGERY

Antibiotics are never a substitute for sound surgical technique. Pus, dead tissue and slough need removing. Antibiotics should be used carefully and only with positive indications. Prolonged or inappropriate use of antibiotics may encourage resistant strains of organisms to emerge. Except in straightforward cases, advice of a microbiologist should be sought.

PRINCIPLES OF ANTIBIOTIC THERAPY

Selection of antibiotic

The decision to prescribe antibiotics is usually clinical and is based initially on a 'best-guess' policy, i.e. based on experience of that particular condition, what the organism is likely to be, and to what it is most likely to be sensitive. The following sequence of events usually occurs:

1. A decision is made on clinical grounds that an infection exists.
2. Based on signs, symptoms and clinical experience, a guess is made at the likely infecting organism.

3. The appropriate specimens are taken for microbiological examination, i.e. culture and sensitivity testing.
4. The cheapest and most effective drug or combination of drugs effective against the suspected organism is given.
5. The clinical response to treatment is monitored.
6. The antibiotic treatment is altered, if necessary, in response to laboratory reports of culture and sensitivities.

Occasionally the response of the infection to an apparently appropriate antibiotic is poor. Possible causes for this include:

- failure to drain pus, excise necrotic tissue or remove foreign bodies
- failure of the drug to reach the tissues in therapeutic concentrations, e.g. ischaemic limbs
- organism isolated is not the one responsible for the infection
- after prolonged antibiotic therapy, new organisms develop
- inadequate dosage or inappropriate route of administration.

Route of administration

Antibiotics should be given i.v. in severe infections in seriously ill patients. Some antibiotics, e.g. gentamicin, can only be given by the parenteral route. When the patient improves and the GI tract is functioning satisfactorily, drugs may be given orally.

> It is best to avoid the intramuscular route if possible as it is uncomfortable for the patient and in shocked patients absorption would be inadequate.

Duration of therapy

This depends on the individual's response and laboratory tests. For most infections which show an appropriate response to treatment after 48 hours, a suitable 'course' should be for 5–7 days. A clinical cure is the most appropriate response but this should be taken in conjunction with microbiological data.

Dosage

The dosage may need to be modified in renal and liver disease.

SPECIFIC ANTIBIOTICS AND ANTIMICROBIALS

This section deals with antibiotics particularly as they are used in the surgical patient. The list is not meant to be comprehensive.

Penicillins

Benzylpenicillin It is active against streptococci, pneumococci, clostridia, *Neisseria gonorrhoea*, *N. meningitidis*. Few staphylococci are now sensitive. The main surgical indications are for the prophylaxis of gas gangrene and tetanus and for streptococcal wound infections. It is given parenterally, either i.v. or i.m.

Phenoxymethylpenicillin (penicillin V) This is given orally. It may follow a course of i.v. benzylpenicillin to complete a course of treatment. It is used prophylactically following splenectomy to prevent pneumococcal septicaemia especially in children where it is used long term. May also be used for prophylaxis in patients with rheumatic heart disease.

Flucloxacillin This is given orally, i.m. or i.v. for penicillin-resistant *Staphylococcus aureus*. Used as an adjunct to drainage of abscesses especially in diabetics or immunosuppressed patients.

Amoxycillin and ampicillin This is given orally, i.m. or i.v. Used in surgical wards largely for chest infections or UTIs. Many staphylococci and coliforms produce ß-lactamase and are therefore resistant. Active against *Streptococcus faecalis* and *Haemophilus influenzae*.

Co-amoxyclav (augmentin) It contains amoxycillin and potassium clavulanate. Given orally or i.v. The clavulanate is inhibitory to ß-lactamase and extends the spectrum of amoxycillin. Active against coliforms, staphylococci and bacteroides. It is also useful in surgery for prophylaxis in bowel, hepatobiliary and GU surgery.

Piperacillin This is given i.m. or i.v. Active against bacteroides, coliforms, *Klebsiella*, and *Pseudomonas aeruginosa*. Often used in combination with an aminoglycoside for life-threatening infections.

Imipenem This is administered i.v. Broad spectrum active against Gram-positive and Gram-negative aerobes and anaerobes. ß-lactamase inhibitor. Use for life-threatening infections.

Cautions With all penicillins, care should be taken to check for previous sensitivity. Caution should be exercised in asthmatics and other history of allergic conditions. Hypersensitivity is usually manifested by urticarial rash although anaphylaxis may occur. Cross-sensitivity occurs between different penicillins. Most penicillins are relatively non-toxic and therefore large doses can be given. Caution must be exercised in patients with renal and/or cardiac failure as injectable forms contain K^+ and Na^+ salts. Rarely convulsions may occur after giving high doses i.v. or by intrathecal injection.

Cephalosporins

These drugs are assigned to three generations. Specific examples of each generation in surgical usage will be described below.

Cephradine First-generation cephalosporin. Given orally, i.m. or i.v. In practice it is most commonly used orally. Active against a wide range of Gram-positive and Gram-negative organisms including *Escherichia coli*, *Klebsiella*, *Proteus* and *Staph. aureus* (unless methicillin-resistant). It is not active against *Strep. faecalis*, *P. aeruginosa* and bacteroides. Second-line drug useful for treatment of UTIs, respiratory infections, skin, and soft tissue infections.

Cefuroxime A second-generation cephalosporin. Given orally, i.m. or i.v. In practice it is most commonly used i.v. Broad spectrum against Gram-positive and Gram-negative organisms. It is only moderately active against bacteroides and not at all against pseudomonas. Widely used in prophylaxis especially in combination with metronidazole in colorectal and biliary tract surgery.

Cefotaxime and ceftazidime Third-generation cephalosporins. Used i.m. or i.v. Broad spectrum similar to second-generation drugs but are also active against pseudomonas. They are normally reserved for use in serious sepsis due to susceptible aerobic Gram-negative bacilli.

> ***Cautions*** About 10% of people who are hypersensitive to penicillin are also hypersensitive to cephalosporins. Rashes and fever may occur. Dose reduction is required in renal failure. Mild transient rises in liver enzymes may occur.

Sulphonamides and trimethoprim

Co-trimoxazole (sulphamethoxazole + trimethoprim: 5:1) May be given orally, i.m. or i.v. Used for treatment of UTIs and respiratory infections. Active against Gram-positive and Gram-negative organisms. *P. aeruginosa* is resistant. Used for salmonella septicaemia and pneumocystis pneumonia.

> ***Cautions*** Nausea, vomiting, rashes, mouth ulcers may occur. Leukopenia and thrombocytopenia may occur occasionally.

Trimethoprim Given orally or i.v. (slow infusion). Used for UTIs and respiratory infections.

Cautions Avoid in pregnancy. Nausea, vomiting, rashes, stomatitis and marrow suppression may occur. Potentiates action of warfarin and phenytoin.

Macrolides

Erythromycin Given orally or i.v. (slow infusion). Use in surgery is limited. Usually used as a second-line drug in patients sensitive to penicillin. Active against streptococci, staphylococci, clostridia, campylobacter. Used for skin and soft tissue infections and respiratory tract infections. Valuable in atypical pneumonia, Legionnaire's disease and *Campylobacter* enteritis.

Cautions The chief side-effect when given orally is diarrhoea. When given i.v. phlebitis at the site of the infusion is a common side-effect. It may potentiate warfarin and cyclosporin.

Aminoglycosides

These are the first-choice drugs for severe Gram-negative infections, usually given in combination with a ß-lactamase antibiotic. The most commonly used are gentamicin and amikacin.

Gentamicin Given i.m. or more usually i.v. Active against coliforms, *P. aeruginosa*, staphylococci. Streptococci and anaerobes are resistant.

Amikacin Reserved for life-threatening infections with gentamicin-resistant organisms with proven amikacin sensitivity.

Cautions The major side-effects are ototoxicity (vertigo or deafness) and nephrotoxicity. Therapeutic levels depend on renal function. Serum levels must be monitored. Accurate monitoring of levels is essential with patients with impaired renal function, and patients on long-term therapy.

Quinolones

Ciprofloxacin Given orally or i.v. Broad spectrum against Gram-negative bacteria including *P. aeruginosa*, staphylococci. Anaerobes are resistant. Uses in surgery include urinary tract infections especially catheter related, prostatitis, and skin and soft tissue infections with *P. aeruginosa*. Also useful for chest infections especially due to Gram-negative organisms.

> **Cautions** Side-effects include nausea, diarrhoea and vomiting. CNS side-effects include anxiety, nervousness, insomnia and rarely convulsions. Ciprofloxacin potentiates warfarin.

Other antibiotics and antimicrobials

Metronidazole Widely used in surgery both prophylactically and therapeutically. Given orally, i.v. or rectally. Active against anaerobic bacteria, e.g. bacteroides, clostridia. Also active against protozoa – *Entamoeba histolytica* and *Giardia lamblia*. Used for intraperitoneal sepsis and gynaecological sepsis. Used prophylactically in appendicitis against wound infection (usually given rectally) and in colorectal surgery (i.v. with induction of anaesthesia). Also given for giardiasis, intestinal amoebiasis and amoebic liver abscess.

> **Cautions** Side-effects include anorexia, sore tongue, and unpleasant metallic taste. It potentiates warfarin.

Tetracycline Of limited use in surgery. May be used in chronic bronchitis, non-specific urethritis and atypical pneumonia.

Fusidic acid Used for penicillin-resistant staphylococcal infections and osteomyelitis. Tissue concentration is good. Given orally or i.v.

Vancomycin Given orally or i.v. Active against staphylococci (including methicillin-resistant strains), streptococci and clostridia. Used for severe infections. Recently, use has increased because of intraperitoneal administration in CAPD peritonitis.

Teicoplanin Teicoplanin is a bactericidal glycopeptide active against both aerobic and anaerobic Gram-positive bacteria. It is usually administered i.v. It is active against *Staph. aureus* and coagulase-positive staphylococci (sensitive or resistant to methicillin), streptococci, enterococci, *Listeria monocytogenes*, micrococci and Gram-positive anaerobes including *Clostridium difficile*. Teicoplanin is clinically related to vancomycin, with similar activity and toxicity.

> **Cautions** Side-effects include phlebitis when given i.v., ototoxicity and nephrotoxicity. Serum levels should be monitored to control dosage.

PROPHYLACTIC ANTIBIOTICS

Despite aseptic techniques, some operations carry a high risk of postoperative wound infection, bacteraemia or septicaemia. Administration of antibiotics in the perioperative period will reduce the risks.

Indications for prophylactic antibiotics

These include:

- implantation of foreign bodies, e.g. cardiac prosthetic valves, artificial joints, prosthetic vascular grafts
- patients with pre-existing cardiac disease who are undergoing surgical procedures including dental procedures, e.g. patients with mitral valve disease as prophylaxis against SBE
- organ transplantation
- immunosuppressed patients
- diabetics
- amputations especially for ischaemia or crush injuries where there is dead muscle; risk of gas gangrene is high especially in contaminated wounds; penicillin is the antibiotic of choice
- compound fractures and penetrating wounds
- surgical incisions where there is a high risk of bacterial contamination, i.e. clean contaminated wounds.

Most prophylactic antibiotics are given to prevent wound infection. In some cases, they are given prior to instrumental procedures in potentially infected sites, e.g. when performing cystoscopy, when they are given to prevent septicaemia. Any patients with congenital heart disease, rheumatic heart disease, or prosthetic valve should be given antibiotics before an elective procedure which may result in bacteraemia. Procedures include dental procedures (including scaling and polishing), GU instrumentation, GI endoscopy, respiratory tract instrumentation and open surgery. In most cases, one dose is given preoperatively either orally if under LA (1 hour preoperatively) or i.v. if under GA, and then 1–4 doses postoperatively. The aim is to achieve therapeutic levels at the time of surgery. Table 5.1 (pp. 92–93) shows some indications for prophylactic antibiotics, the likely organism involved and a recommended prophylactic regimen.

SURGICAL INFECTIONS

Cellulitis

A spreading inflammation of connective tissue. It is usually subcutaneous and caused by ß-haemolytic streptococci. This organism produces hyaluronidase and streptokinase which

Table 5.1
Prophylactic antibiotics

Clinical situation	Likely organism(s)	Prophylactic regimen
Appendicectomy	Anaerobes	Metronidazole (single dose PR 1 h preop.)
Biliary tract surgery	Coliforms	Cephalosporin (i.v. immediately preop. and for 24 h postop.)
Colorectal surgery	Coliforms Anaerobes	Metronidazole + cephalosporin or gentamicin (i.v. immediately preop. and for up to 48 h postop.)
GU Surgery Instrumentation	Coliforms	Gentamicin (single i.v. dose pre-procedure)
Open surgery		Cephalosporin (i.v. immediately preop. and for 24–48 h postop.) or gentamicin (single i.v. dose immediately preop.)
Insertion of prosthetic joints	*Staph. aureus* *Staph. epidermidis*	Fluxcloxacillin (i.v. immediately preop. and 24–48 h postop.)
Amputation of limb	*C. perfringens*	Penicillin (i.v. immediately preop. and for 24 h postop.)
Vascular surgery with prosthetic graft	*Staph. aureus* *Staph. epidermidis* Coliforms	Cephalosporin (i.v. immediately preop. and for 24 h postop.)
Prevention of tetanus in contaminated wound (+ immuno-prophylaxis)	*C. tetanus*	Penicillin (i.v. or i.m. on presentation)

Table 5.1
Prophylactic antibiotics *(contd)*

Clinical situation	Likely organism(s)	Prophylactic regimen
Prophylaxis of endocarditis:		
• Minor dental procedure under LA	Oral streptococci	Amoxycillin (single oral dose 1 h preop. Clindamycin if allergic)
• Major dental procedure under GA		Low risk: amoxycillin (oral dose 4 h preop. and one dose postop.) High risk: amoxycillin & gentamicin (i.m. or i.v. immediately preop. Vancomycin if allergic)

dissolve the ground substance of connective tissue and fibrin respectively allowing the inflammation to spread.

Symptoms and signs Redness, oedema, and localized tenderness. A scratch, insect bite, ulcer or surgical wound may be apparent. There is usually fever and malaise. Lymphangitis or lymphadenitis may be present.

Investigations • WBC • Blood cultures.

Treatment The usual organism is a streptococcus which is usually sensitive to penicillin. Immobilization and elevation of a limb may be required. Occasionally an abscess with thin watery pus forms and requires drainage.

Erysipelas is an uncommon skin infection which is caused by a streptococcus (Group A). The condition is usually encountered on the scalp, face and neck. Pain and redness of the skin are apparent, the margin being well demarcated and raised above the normal skin. Pyrexia and malaise usually accompany the local signs. Treatment is with penicillin.

Lymphangitis and lymphadenitis

Lymphangitis is a non-suppurative infection of lymphatic vessels that drain an area of cellulitis. Lymphadenitis is infection of the regional lymph nodes as a result of infection in the areas which they drain. It usually, but not always, results from cellulitis and lymphangitis. Occasionally the nodes suppurate and form an abscess.

Symptoms and signs Lymphangitis produces red tender streaks in the line of lymphatics extending from the area of cellulitis towards the regional lymph nodes. Lymphadenitis is represented by enlarged tender regional lymph nodes. Occasionally the overlying skin is red and the glands may be fluctuant.

Investigations • WBC • Blood cultures.

Treatment If accompanying cellulitis, treat with penicillin. Lymphadenitis may follow various types of infection in the sites drained by the nodes. Treatment depends upon isolation of the infecting organism.

Furuncle (→ Ch. 7)

Carbuncle (→ Ch. 7)

Hidradenitis suppurative (→ Ch. 7)

Necrotizing fasciitis

This is a rapidly progressive bacterial infection caused by a mixture of organisms which spreads along fascial planes. It causes vascular thrombosis resulting in necrosis of the tissues involved. Organisms involved include microaerophilic streptococci, staphylococci, coliforms and anaerobes. It may result from a small puncture wound, surgical incision or penetrating trauma of a hollow viscus.

Symptoms and signs Redness, oedema, tenderness, haemorrhagic bullae, crepitus, skin necrosis and discharge. The patient is febrile and toxic.

Investigations • WBC • Blood culture • Swabs • Radiograph may show gas in tissues.

Treatment Remove all infected and dead tissue. The tissue is usually oedematous, grey and smells. The subcutaneous fat and fascia are involved. Muscle is viable. Specimens are taken for culture. Treatment is usually with penicillin and gentamicin intravenously and antibiotics are changed according to culture and sensitivities. The wound is inspected regularly and any further necrotic tissue excised. Mortality rate is about 25% in extensive cases. Necrotizing fasciitis of the scrotum is known as Fournier's gangrene.

Gas gangrene

Myositis and cellulitis caused by *Clostridium perfringens*, an anaerobic, spore-forming and gas-producing organism. The organism is found in soil and faeces. It is an infection associated with deep, penetrating, contaminated wounds usually involving an extremity and rarely is seen as a complication of amputation of an ischaemic limb. It may involve the abdominal wall following penetrating trauma of, or surgery to, the GI tract.

Symptoms and signs Acute onset 6 hours to 3 days after injury. Severe pain at site of injury. The tissues are swollen, and brownish, serous, malodorous fluid may drain from the wound. Patchy necrosis and crepitus occur. The patient is toxic and may be confused or delirious. The temperature is not always elevated.

Investigations • WBC • Bilirubin raised because of haemolysis • Gram-stain of discharge shows Gram-positive bacilli • Radiograph shows gas in tissues.

Treatment

Prophylactic Adequate debridement of wound at time of initial injury. All contused and dead tissue should be removed and the wound thoroughly irrigated and left open. Prophylactic penicillin should be given to all patients with contaminated wounds and to patients with ischaemic limbs undergoing amputations.

Therapeutic Radical debridement of all necrotic tissue is mandatory. If the muscle of a limb is involved, amputation will be necessary. This should be done at a level where the muscle bleeds and contracts when cut. Large doses of penicillin should be given intravenously. Hyperbaric oxygen may be given to counteract the anaerobic environment. Its value, however, is unproven. Anti-gas gangrene serum either prophylactically or therapeutically is of unproven value. The main treatment is urgent and radical debridement with amputation if necessary.

Tetanus

This is a rare condition in the UK owing to widespread immunization. It is caused by *C. tetani*, an anaerobic Gram-positive bacillus which produces a neurotoxin. It is found in soil and faeces. The neurotoxin enters peripheral nerves and travels to the spinal cord where it blocks inhibitory activity of spinal reflexes resulting in the characteristic features of the disease. The disease follows the implantation of spores into deep, devitalized tissues.

Symptoms and signs

History of injury This may be as minor as the prick of rose thorn. The incubation period is 1–30 days. Muscle spasm usually occurs first at the site of inoculation and is followed by trismus resulting in the typical risus sardonicus (lock-jaw). Stiffness in the neck, back and abdomen follow together with generalized spasms which may cause asphyxia. The muscles remain in spasm between convulsions. Opisthotonos (arching of the back and neck due to spasm) may occur. This stage is followed by convulsions which are extremely painful and during which the patient is conscious. Death may occur from asphyxia due to involvement of respiratory muscles or from inhalation of vomit with aspiration pneumonia.

Differential diagnosis
- Strychnine poisoning: the muscles are flaccid between convulsions.
- Tetany: usually carpopedal spasm and does not affect the trunk.
- Epilepsy.
- Meningitis: there is usually only neck stiffness but convulsions may occur.
- Hysteria.

Treatment

Prophylactic
- Active immunization with tetanus toxoid. All children should be immunized and this is repeated at 6 weeks and 6 months after the initial dose. Booster doses should be given at 5-yearly intervals. All patients attending an A&E department with new trauma, however mild, should have a booster unless one has been given within the previous year.
- Contaminated and penetrating wounds should be debrided and prophylactic penicillin administered. A tetanus toxoid booster dose should be given to the previously immunized patient. Those not previously immunized should be given human antitetanus immunoglobulin.

Therapeutic
1. Isolate the patient in a quiet darkened room. Give diazepam or chlorpromazine. In severe cases, the patient will need to be paralysed and ventilated. Feeding should be given via a fine-bore nasogastric tube. Ventilation may need to be continued for up to 4 weeks. A trial period of weaning off relaxants without recurrence of spasm will indicate when ventilation is no longer required. Tracheostomy may be required.

→

2. Administer penicillin, tetanus toxoid, and human anti-tetanus immunoglobulin.
3. Excise and drain any contaminated wound.
4. Regular physiotherapy will be required during the recovery period.

Prognosis The mortality rate is inversely proportional to the length of the incubation period. If spasm occurs within 5 days of the time of injury, the prognosis is poor. The mortality rate is also directly proportional to the severity of the symptoms.

INFECTION AND THE SURGEON

The surgeon, as indeed any medical, nursing, or paramedical personnel, is at risk from three main viral infections: HIV, hepatitis B, hepatitis C.

HIV

Infection with HIV is permanent and it is likely that all carriers will eventually develop AIDS. Surgical personnel are a high risk. Infection with HIV results from the passage of infected body fluid (usually blood) from one person to another. Needle-stick injuries and scalpel injuries are possible sources of infection. In the general population, HIV may be transmitted by unprotected anal, vaginal, and oral intercourse, sharing needles in drug abuse, and infected blood products (e.g. as happened in the past with haemophiliacs).

Risk categories

The following are at risk of becoming HIV positive: homosexuals or bisexual males, prostitutes (male and female), intravenous drug abusers, haemophiliacs who were treated before routine testing became available and sexual partners of the above categories.

Prevention of HIV

Care at operation needs to be exercised with patients who are known to have AIDS or be HIV positive. Patients with anorectal disease related to homosexuality, haemophiliacs and sexual partners and children of the above should be treated with appropriate caution.

Counselling is required and consent must be obtained for HIV testing. If a patient refuses and is suspected of being HIV positive, then precautions must be taken with nursing care and any invasive procedures from simple venepuncture to major surgery.

HEPATITIS B

Infection is largely blood borne. It may be transmitted by blood transfusion, syringe and needle sharing in drug addicts, sexual intercourse with an infected partner or homosexual practices. Antigen carriage is a risk for hospital staff especially those in 'high-risk' areas, e.g. theatre staff. Dialysis units are often quoted as being a 'high-risk' area, but following outbreaks many years ago, all staff and patients are tested for HBsAg.

Hepatitis vaccine is offered to all high-risk health workers. These categories involve surgeons, theatre nurses, pathology staff, accident and emergency staff, staff in liver transplant units, workers in residential units for the mentally handicapped, staff of GI units, and staff of infectious and communicable disease units.

HEPATITIS C

Hepatitis C (HCV) is present in blood and spreads in the same way as HBV by blood transfusion, intravenous drug abuse, and from mother to infant. Sexual transmission is uncommon. The incubation period is 2–4 months, at which stage a mild disease occurs in about 1:10 individuals. Carriers are a source of infection. About 50% of infected patients develop chronic active hepatitis, and 20% progress to cirrhosis. Infection is also associated with liver cancer.

PRECAUTIONS FOR THE CARE OF KNOWN AND SUSPECTED HIV, HBV AND HCV CARRIERS

- All personnel involved in patient care should be aware of the problem.
- Protection from contaminated body fluids.
- Correct disposal of contaminated fluids, dressings.
- Theatre:
  - The patient should be marked as a category III on the operating list indicating that there is a risk factor present. Under no circumstances should the actual disease causing the risk be placed upon the operating list.
  - Only absolutely necessary personnel should be in theatre. There should be no spectators.
  - Remove all but essential equipment.
  - Disposable scrub suit, footwear, gowns, and drapes.

- Plastic aprons, two pairs of gloves, visors to prevent splashing in the eyes.
- Operation: no-touch technique if possible, meticulous attention to haemostasis. Stapling devices rather than needles if possible.
- All disposable equipment should be removed in specifically marked containers.
- The theatre should be thoroughly cleansed with dilute bleach solution.
- Recovery staff must be aware of the risk also.

Accidental injury to staff

HBV-positive patient Let the stab site or laceration bleed. Wash well with soap and water. Fill in accident form. Report to occupational health. If not immunized (which is extremely unlikely), start course of vaccine. Administer hyperimmune serum.

HIV Let it bleed. Wash with antiseptic and water. Report to Occupational Health. Blood tests may be required in future to check for HIV.

6

Management of malignant disease

Patients with malignant disease form a major part of the workload of a surgical unit. The total number of patients with malignant disease is rising owing to increased life expectancy. Where possible, the aims should be to prevent malignancy, e.g. cessation of smoking in the prevention of lung cancer, and the avoidance of excessive ultraviolet light in the prevention of skin cancer. Screening programmes should be instituted to make earlier diagnoses of the common forms of cancer and hopefully maximize the cure rate.

SCREENING

This is the examination of an asymptomatic population at risk of a particular condition, with a view to early diagnosis and consequent increase in cure rate. It must be demonstrated that early diagnosis and treatment do increase the cure rate and also that the cost of screening large populations is justified by the yield.

Examples of screening programmes being carried out at present are:

- cervical smears for cervical carcinoma
- mammography for carcinoma of the breast
- faecal occult bloods for carcinoma of the colon.

PREMALIGNANT CONDITIONS

It is important that these conditions are recognized and appropriate action taken.

Examples of premalignant conditions include:

- *Skin*: actinic keratoses, Bowen's disease, erythroplasia of Queyrat (penis).
- *GI tract*: leukoplakia (mouth and tongue), Plummer–Vinson syndrome, Barrett's oesophagus, villous adenoma, familial polyposis coli, ulcerative colitis, Crohn's disease.
- *GU tract*: leukoplakia of the bladder, bilharzia.

GENERAL SYMPTOMS AND SIGNS OF MALIGNANT DISEASE

These may relate to the primary tumour, metastases, or generalized systemic manifestations.

They may be broadly classified as follows:

Palpable swelling This is usually painless unless invading other structures. Common examples include the palpable masses of the primary tumour in carcinoma of the breast, carcinoma of the thyroid, carcinoma of the caecum.

Obstruction Examples include dysphagia in carcinoma of the oesophagus, obstructive jaundice in carcinoma of head of pancreas, large bowel obstruction in carcinoma of the colon, vomiting in gastric outlet obstruction from carcinoma of the gastric antrum.

Bleeding

- Overt: haemoptysis, haematemesis, haematuria, rectal bleeding.
- Occult: carcinoma of the stomach or carcinoma of the caecum. Anaemia occurs.

Symptoms due to compression or invasion of local structures SVC obstruction with bronchial carcinoma; back pain with retroperitoneal invasion with pancreatic cancer; invasion of nerves, e.g. facial paralysis with carcinoma of the parotid gland, recurrent laryngeal nerve palsy with anaplastic carcinoma of the thyroid.

Metastases

- Enlarged lymph nodes: may be discrete or hard, irregular and matted.
- Hepatomegaly: primary in stomach, colon, bronchus, or breast.
- Jaundice: from nodes in the porta hepatis, with primary in the stomach, pancreas, or colon.
- Ascites: ovarian or any GI malignancy.
- Abdominal mass due to omental secondaries – often in association with ascites.
- Pathological fractures from bony metastases, e.g. breast, bronchus, thyroid, prostate, kidney.
- Pleural effusion, e.g. from breast cancer.
- Fits, confusion, personality change from cerebral metastases, e.g. breast, bronchus, malignant melanoma.

Generalized manifestations Examples include cachexia, PUO (lymphoma, hypernephroma), hypertrophic pulmonary osteoarthropathy (carcinoma of the bronchus), thrombophlebitis migrans (carcinoma of the pancreas), neuropathies and myopathies (carcinoma of the bronchus), endocrine manifestations, e.g. ADH or ACTH production in bronchial carcinoma.

Asymptomatic incidental findings Axillary lymphadenopathy on routine examination, e.g. with small impalpable carcinoma of the breast. Silent pulmonary primary or metastases on routine CXR.

DIAGNOSTIC PROCEDURES

Biopsy This is mandatory, and may be carried out in a variety of ways:

- Fine-needle aspiration using a 22G needle: smear produced on slide; read by experienced histopathologist.
- Needle biopsy, e.g. trucut: core of tissue removed for histological examination.
- Incisional biopsy: removes a small accessible piece of the lesion for histological examination.
- Excisional biopsy: the complete removal of a discrete lesion without a wide margin and without it being considered curative of the malignancy.
- Staging laparotomy: used for Hodgkin's disease: largely superseded by CT scanning.

Imaging (e.g. ultrasound, CT or MRI) This is used for confirming a suspected diagnosis and assessing spread. A negative study does not exclude microscopic disease.

STAGING OF CANCER

The extent of the malignancy of a tumour may be established clinically to provide an indication of the prognosis and to act as a guide for the type of treatment. It is also necessary for comparing the efficacies of different treatments in clinical trials. Three methods may be used, i.e. clinical, pathological, and histological. Pathological staging is very subjective and there is a degree of observer variation. The tumour may be described as well differentiated, moderately differentiated or undifferentiated.

CLINICAL STAGING

An example of this is the Manchester classification of carcinoma of the breast (→ Ch. 10). This is based purely on clinical findings but is somewhat imprecise.

CLINICAL AND PATHOLOGICAL STAGING

The TNM classification is recommended by the International Union Against Cancer. This method uses both clinical and laboratory results to grade the tumour. The clinician assesses three factors:

- extent of the tumour (T)

- node status (N)
- presence of metastases (M).

See Chapter 10 for application of TNM classification to breast cancer.

A method that is based on pathological staging only is Dukes' classification for colorectal carcinoma (→ Ch. 14).

TUMOUR MARKERS

These are substances present in the body in a concentration which is related to the presence of a tumour. They are rarely sufficiently specific to be of diagnostic value. The tumour marker may be a substance which is secreted into the blood or other body fluid or expressed at the cell's surface by malignant cells in larger quantities than that of their normal counterparts. Detection is by measuring the concentration of the marker in the body fluids, usually by immunoassay, although some markers may be detected in histological sections by immunohistochemistry. The main value of tumour markers is in following the course of a malignant disease and monitoring the response to treatment and hence determining the prognosis. They may also be used for tumour localization and antibody-directed therapy. The following are examples of tumour markers in common use.

α-fetoprotein (AFP) This is raised in primary hepatocellular carcinoma and is valuable in monitoring the response to treatment. It is usually raised in testicular teratoma and is valuable in monitoring metastases and the response to treatment.

Carcinoembryonic antigen (CEA) Although not of diagnostic value, it may be useful in following the progression of GI cancer.

Human chorionic gonadotrophin (HCG) This is one of the first tumour markers to be recognized. It is raised in choriocarcinoma and hydatidiform moles. β-HCG is a valuable tumour marker for testicular cancers.

Prostatic acid phosphatase (PAP) This can be measured separately from total acid phosphatase. It is not specific enough for screening but it is valuable in following the response to treatment. It has largely been superseded by PSA.

Prostate-specific antigen (PSA) This is the most useful marker in prostatic cancer. It is organ specific and is elevated in a higher proportion of patients than PAP.

TREATMENT OF CANCER

Major treatments are surgical excision, radiotherapy, chemotherapy and hormonal manipulation.

SURGERY

Curative

The ideal operation for cancer is the one that completely eradicates the tumour. This may require wide excision of the tumour together with removal of the lymph nodes in continuity with the tumour. Often, when the tumour is explored, it is found that it cannot be removed. On some occasions, the tumour is operable, i.e. the primary tumour can be removed but tumour remains behind, in which case it is incurable.

Palliative

When operating on a tumour it may be discovered that it is impossible to remove the primary lesion. However, a palliative operation may be carried out, e.g. bypassing an obstructing tumour in the GI tract to prevent the symptoms of intestinal obstruction.

Occasionally, operations are undertaken purely for palliative reasons when it is known that it will be impossible to remove the primary tumour, e.g. for bleeding, pain, obstruction. Occasionally, surgery is used to 'debulk' a tumour. This is often the case in extensive ovarian malignancy where removal of the greater mass of tumour will improve the efficacy of subsequent chemotherapy.

RADIOTHERAPY

Delivery of radiotherapy

Radiotherapy can be delivered to the site of a tumour in three ways.

External beam radiation This method is the most commonly used form of radiotherapy for skin and deeper tumours. For deep lesions it is possible to concentrate the beam deep to the skin, thus avoiding the severe skin lesions which previously were a side-effect of radiotherapy.

Implantation radiotherapy (e.g. intracavitary or intralesional) The source of irradiation may be placed within a cavity, e.g. in the vagina for irradiation of the cervix or directly into the lesion, e.g. iridium-192 (^{192}Ir) wires in carcinoma of the tongue.

Systemic irradiation ^{131}I can be administered orally for follicular and papillary carcinoma of the thyroid gland. Experimentally, radioisotopes can be directed at cancer cells by attaching them to tumour-specific antibodies.

Use of radiotherapy

Radiotherapy can be used in three ways:

- radiotherapy with a view to cure (radical radiotherapy)
- adjuvant radiotherapy
- palliative.

Radical applications

- Basal cell and squamous cell carcinoma of the skin.
- Some head and neck tumours and laryngeal tumours.
- Hodgkin's disease.
- Lymph node metastases of a testicular seminoma following orchidectomy.

Adjuvant radiotherapy This is aimed at clinically undetectable metastases due to spread locally or into the regional lymph nodes, e.g. carcinoma of the breast giving radiotherapy to the scar, axillary nodes, supraclavicular nodes and internal mammary nodes.

Palliative radiotherapy

- Bony metastases – pain relief is often dramatic.
- Cerebral metastases.
- Ulcerating or fungating breast cancer – controls oozing and bleeding and allows skin healing.
- Lung cancer to prevent cough and haemoptysis.

The complications of radiotherapy are shown in Table 6.1.

CHEMOTHERAPY

Chemotherapeutic agents destroy tumour cells in a variety of different ways. Most tumours are treated by a combination of cytotoxic drugs, the combinations being chosen so that their toxic effects on any particular organ are minimized. The most appropriate combinations have usually been established by clinical trials based on initial empiricism. Drugs are usually given in short courses with a period of rest between courses to allow recovery of the normal tissues. The response of tumours to chemotherapy is very variable. Some are highly sensitive while others are insensitive.

Highly sensitive tumours in which there are prospects of a cure include Hodgkin's disease, testicular teratoma, childhood leukaemias, osteogenic sarcoma (lung secondaries).

Moderately sensitive tumours where palliation is the aim include ovarian tumours, breast cancer, and bronchial carcinoma.

Table 6.1
Complications of radiotherapy

General	Tiredness, malaise
Skin	Rashes, moist desquamation
Blood vessels	Endarteritis obliterans. Impairs blood supply. Progresses for many years after treatment. Many of the effects on other systems may have endarteritis obliterans as a precipitating cause
Healing	This is delayed, e.g. failure of skin grafts, anastomotic breakdown, intestinal fistulae.
Renal tract	Frequency, cystitis
GI tract	Nausea, vomiting, anorexia. Irradiation proctitis (after irradiation of the cervix), causes rectal bleeding and tenesmus. Small bowel irradiation may give rise to intestinal fistulae and strictures
Head and neck	Xerostomia (dry mouth). Epiphora (red-watery eye) due to damage to tear duct

Apart from oral and intravenous administration, cytotoxic agents may be directly administered into a tumour, e.g. 5-fluorouracil for liver metastases and close intra-arterial injection in malignant melanoma; instillation into the bladder for superficial bladder tumours.

Side-effects

Chemotherapy is not only toxic to malignant cells but also to normal body cells especially those with a high turnover rate, e.g. bone marrow and GI epithelium. Many side-effects are extremely unpleasant and should be carefully explained to, and discussed with, the patient prior to starting the course. (For side-effects → Table 6.2.)

HORMONAL MANIPULATION

This is applicable to carcinoma of the breast and carcinoma of

Table 6.2
Side-effects of chemotherapy

Non-specific	Nausea, vomiting, metallic taste, general malaise
GI tract	Oral ulceration, diarrhoea
Reproductive system	Loss of libido, sterility, mutagenesis
Bone marrow	Bone marrow suppression with anaemia, thrombocytopenia, (bleeding), leukopenia (infection)
Immune system	Immunosuppression. Opportunistic infections, e.g. candidiasis, and *Pneumocystis carinii*
Skin	Rashes, ulceration, hair loss (regrows after course is stopped)
Urinary tract	Cystitis (cyclophosphamide), gout due to massive tumour destruction, leads to hyperuricaemia which may lead to renal failure – prevented with allopurinol
Oncogenesis	20-fold increase in incidence of other malignancies

the prostate. Removal of the source of hormones or blocking their effect may inhibit tumour growth.

Breast

Oophorectomy may prolong the disease-free interval prior to recurrence. It has no effect on long-term survival rates. However, it is useful where there are widespread metastases in that it may relieve pain in about 50% of cases. Tamoxifen, an anti-oestrogen, is useful as an adjuvant to primary surgical treatment. It may also be given for recurrent or metastatic disease. In the past, adrenalectomy and hypophysectomy have also been used, the aim being to eliminate all sex hormones. These methods are rarely used since the introduction of tamoxifen.

Prostate

The only aetiological factor here is hormone dependence, i.e.

dependence on testosterone. Subcapsular orchidectomy is the preferred treatment when metastases are present. Other treatments include cyproterone acetate, which inhibits androgens.

TERMINAL CARE

Most patients with disseminated malignancy deteriorate until they reach a terminal phase. This phase is often accompanied by many unpleasant symptoms which are difficult to control. Support should not only be medical but should be emotional, psychological and spiritual. Initially, it may be possible to manage the patient at home with the support of family, friends, Macmillan nurse and family doctor. Eventually hospitalization may be required for terminal care. Patients may be best managed in a hospice where all expertise is available to support the patients and their relatives.

PRINCIPLES OF TERMINAL CARE

1. Assess prognosis.
2. Discuss prognosis with patient and relatives.
3. Inform the family doctor of the situation and encourage regular visits.
4. Ensure all support that the patient may need to remain at home as long as possible, e.g. commodes, home help, district nurse, Macmillan nurse.
5. Anticipate problems and try to prevent them, e.g. nausea, constipation, pain.
6. Regular review of medication to make sure pain relief is adequate and nausea and vomiting are well controlled.
7. Arrange appropriate hospital, or preferably hospice, accommodation when required.

TREATMENT OF SYMPTOMS

Pain

Regular opiates are needed to prevent 'breakthrough' pain. Suitable analgesics include MST tablets, morphine elixir, subcutaneous morphine, PCA via pump and spinal opioids; local blocks may help. In addition, steroids and chlorpromazine may be helpful. The correct dose of analgesic is that which relieves the pain. Opiate dependency and respiratory depression are irrelevant in the dying patient.

Nausea and vomiting

Anti-emetics should be given, e.g. metoclopramide, domperidone, prochlorperazine. Ondansetron is an expensive but very effective anti-emetic. If there is a mechanical reason for the nausea and vomiting it may be difficult to control. If possible, a tube gastrostomy carried out under local anaesthetic may help. It allows the patient to swallow a suitable liquidized diet which will then drain through the gastrostomy tube without subsequent vomiting.

Constipation

Regular laxatives and enemas may be required.

Dysphagia

A stent may be already in situ. Tasty liquidized food is helpful.

Mouth care

Careful attention to oral hygiene may prevent problems. 'Swish and swallow' nystatin may prevent candidiasis. If ulcers develop they may be treated with local anaesthetic gel and metronidazole gel.

Cough

This may be treated with morphine or codeine.

Insomnia

Treat with chlorpromazine or benzodiazepines.

7
Skin

Skin lesions that involve the surgeon are usually lumps, ulcers, or pigmented lesions. Many skin lesions can be diagnosed on history and clinical examination alone. In some cases biopsy will be necessary to confirm the diagnosis. It must be remembered that skin lesions may be a manifestation of systemic disease. A classification of 'surgical' skin lesions is shown in Table 7.1.

PRINCIPLES OF MANAGEMENT OF 'SURGICAL' SKIN LESIONS

- Simple excision for straightforward clinically diagnosed lesions, e.g. skin tags, sebaceous cysts.

Table 7.1
'Surgical' skin lesions

Benign	
Epidermis	Pedunculated papilloma, wart, seborrhoeic keratosis, keratoacanthoma
Dermis	Pyogenic granuloma, fibrous histiocytoma, keloid
Appendages	Furuncle, carbuncle, hidradenitis suppurativa, sebaceous cyst, dermoid cyst, pilonidal sinus
Subcutaneous	Lipoma, neurofibroma
Melanotic	Intradermal naevus, blue naevus, compound naevus, juvenile naevus
Vascular	Campbell de Morgan spots, port wine stain, strawberry naevus, spider naevi, glomus tumour
Premalignant	
Epidermis	Actinic (solar) keratosis, Bowen's disease, erythroplasia of Queyrat (penis)
Malignant	
Epidermis	Basal cell carcinoma, squamous cell carcinoma
Dermis	Kaposi's sarcoma, secondary deposits
Appendages	Sebaceous carcinoma (rare), sweat gland carcinoma (rare)
Subcutaneous	Liposarcoma, neurofibrosarcoma
Melanotic	Malignant melanoma
Vascular	Angiosarcoma (rare)

- Excision biopsy if risk of malignancy, e.g. small pigmented lesions where change may have occurred recently.
- Incisional biopsy, e.g. for ulcers which have failed to heal and there is need to exclude malignancy or vasculitis.
- Wide excision with or without skin grafting, e.g. for malignant melanoma.
- Radiotherapy for basal cell carcinoma as an alternative to surgery especially in sites where skin preservation is important (eyelid).
- Remember that skin lesions may be a manifestation of systemic disease.

BENIGN LESIONS

EPIDERMIS

Pedunculated papillomas (skin tags)

These small polypoid lesions occur in adults, most frequently on the trunk, neck, axilla and groin. They may catch on clothes and bleed, and are often cosmetically unacceptable. They are removed by excision under local anaesthetic. Small skin tags may be treated by tying a fine ligature around the base which leads to necrosis.

Warts (verrucae vulgaris)

These are caused by papovavirus, and usually occur in the second decade of life. They are common on fingers, hands and soles of feet (verrucae plantaris). Plantar warts may be very painful. Resolution of warts may occur spontaneously. Treatment may be by curettage, freezing with liquid nitrogen or application of keratolytic agents, e.g. podophyllin.

Seborrhoeic keratoses

These are found in elderly patients, and are often multiple, well-demarcated raised lesions with varying degrees of pigmentation. It may be difficult to differentiate from malignant melanoma if deeply pigmented. Treatment is to leave alone or treat by surgical excision or curettage.

Keratoacanthoma

This is a nodular lesion with a central crater containing a keratin ‘plug’. They progress rapidly in 2 weeks to 2 months. Probably of viral aetiology, they often show spontaneous regression. Occasionally, they are difficult to distinguish from squamous cell carcinomas. Treatment is by excision biopsy unless the lesion is obviously regressing.

DERMIS

Pyogenic granuloma

This is a dark red nodule of exuberant granulation tissue and polymorphs. There is rapid initial growth often at the site of trauma. Occasionally the surface may ulcerate and then must be distinguished from amelanotic melanoma. Treatment is by excision.

Fibrous histiocytoma

This is a well-circumscribed deep reddish brown tumour. On inspection it may be mistaken for a malignant melanoma. However, palpation reveals hard consistency due to the dense fibrous stroma. Treatment is by excision.

Keloid

This involves excessive deposition of collagen beyond and above the wound itself and is covered by normal epithelium. It must be distinguished from a hypertrophic scar in which the wound becomes broad and raised; the latter usually settles within 6 months. Keloid may increase after 6 months. Black Africans and the young are particularly affected. It may follow burns. Treatment is by injection of triamcinolone into the scar or by applying steroid-impregnated tape. Excision of a keloid scar should be avoided as it merely makes the keloid worse.

SKIN APPENDAGES

Boil (furuncle)

This is an infection in a hair follicle usually caused by *Staphylococcus aureus*. It can occur in any part of the body but is more common in the head, neck, axilla and groins. Diabetes, immunosuppression and general debility are predisposing conditions. Multiple boils (furunculosis) are common in diabetics. Any patient presenting with boils should have the urine tested for sugar.

Usually they are self-limiting and heal when pus has discharged. Antibiotics should be avoided except in the following situations:

- 'dangerous' areas of the face, i.e. between the orbit and angle of the mouth where venous drainage is into the cavernous sinus; cavernous sinus thrombosis may occur
- multiple boils with surrounding cellulitis in diabetics and immunosuppressed patients where septicaemia is a risk.

Carbuncle

An infection which dissects through the dermis and subcutaneous tissues to form connecting channels, some of which open to the surface. There is considerable induration and pus discharges through the sinuses. The back of the neck is a common site. Treatment is with antistaphylococcal antibiotics, e.g. flucloxacillin, with desloughing and adequate drainage of the abscesses if necessary.

Hidradenitis suppurativa

A chronic indolent disease of skin and subcutaneous tissue in apocrine gland-bearing areas, e.g. axilla, groin, perineum and perianal areas. The involved area is indurated, fibrotic and inflamed with sinuses draining pus. *Staph. aureus* is the usual organism grown but occasionally coliforms may be cultured. Differential diagnosis includes furunculosis, carbuncle, cellulitis or in the perianal area complex fistula-in-ano. Biopsy confirms the diagnosis. Treatment is initially by antibiotics. Abscesses are incised and drained. Advanced cases may need wide excision and grafting. Severe perianal disease may require a diverting colostomy prior to skin grafting.

Sebaceous cysts

These are common on the scalp, face, neck, back and are soft or firm and spherical. They contain cheesy sebaceous material which may become infected and discharge. They are attached to the skin and a punctum is usually seen at the point of attachment. Treatment is by excision under local anaesthetic.

Dermoid cysts

These may be congenital or acquired.

Congenital They are formed in intrauterine life when skin dermatomes fuse and present at birth or a few years after. They are most common in head and neck, e.g. outer end of eyebrow (external angular dermoid). Treatment is by excision.

Acquired These are implantation dermoids. A piece of skin is forcibly implanted into the dermis as a result of trauma. They are common on fingers. Treatment is by excision.

Pilonidal sinus

This chronic infection in the sinus is caused by penetration of hairs into skin and subcutaneous tissues. Infection leads to pilonidal abscesses. The sinus leads to a cavity filled with hair and granulation tissue. Common sites include posteriorly in the midline over the sacrococcygeal area and natal cleft (usually hirsute males with sedentary occupations); between the fingers in hairdressers; occasionally umbilicus, axilla and nipple.

Differential diagnosis includes perianal fistulae, hidradenitis suppurativa, simple boils. Treatment includes:

- deroofing the track, removing the hairs and packing; the surrounding skin should be shaved until the sinuses have healed
- injection of the sinuses with methylene blue, followed by wide excision of all tracts until no dye is seen and either packing or primary suture carried out under GA
- for pilonidal abscesses, incising, curetting and packing.

SUBCUTANEOUS TISSUES

Lipoma

This is a common, benign tumour of fatty tissue which is soft, lobulated and pseudofluctuant and the overlying skin appears normal. It is slow growing. Treatment is by excision. Multiple lipomas may occur. These need to be distinguished from neurofibromata by biopsy of at least one lesion. Occasionally, there may be multiple tender lipomas on the trunk (Dercum's disease). Treatment of lipoma is by excision which is curative. Liposarcomatous change may rarely occur in a benign lipoma.

Neurofibroma

These are benign tumours arising from the connective tissue element of peripheral nerves. They are often multiple and may be asymptomatic, but if closely related to the nerve the patient may get paraesthesia in the distribution of the nerve. Biopsy of one lesion may confirm the diagnosis. If neurofibromata are multiple, congenital and familial, the condition is known as von Recklinghausen's disease. Occasionally malignant change to neurofibroscarcoma occurs.

PREMALIGNANT LESIONS

Actinic (solar) keratoses

These are rough scaly epidermal lesions on sites of exposure to the sun. 10–20% undergo malignant change. The diagnosis is confirmed by biopsy and then the lesion is excised. Topical chemotherapy with 5-fluorouracil cream has been used in patients with multiple lesions.

Bowen's disease

Intraepidermal squamous cell carcinoma (carcinoma-in-situ). A well-defined erythematous plaque with occasional crusting, it occurs in the fourth to sixth decade and may be associated with the presence of internal malignancy. Diagnosis is confirmed by a biopsy. Treatment is by curettage, excision, grafting or topical 5-fluorouracil. Intraepidermal carcinoma may occur on the glans penis and is then called erythroplasia of Queyrat and appears as a reddish brown velvety plaque.

MALIGNANT LESIONS

EPIDERMIS

Basal cell carcinoma (rodent ulcer)

It is common in the middle-aged and elderly. Locally invasive; it rarely if ever metastasizes. Frequently found on skin exposed to sunlight, the commonest area is the face above a line drawn from the angle of the mouth to the lobe of the ear. It starts as a nodule which ulcerates and develops rolled edges with a pearly appearance and local telangiectasia. Differential diagnosis includes seborrhoeic keratoses and malignant melanoma. Treatment includes surgical excision or radiotherapy. Cure rate is high when treated early and adequately.

Squamous cell carcinoma

This may grow rapidly. It metastasizes via lymphatics and rarely via the bloodstream. Exposure to sunlight may be a causative factor. It can also develop in areas of Bowen's disease and erythroplasia of Queyrat. Other causative factors include chemical burns, chronic ulcers (e.g. Marjolin's ulcer, i.e. malignant change in a chronic venous ulcer), irradiation dermatitis.

It starts as a lump which ulcerates with bleeding and discharge. The edge of the ulcer is characteristically raised and everted. Local lymph nodes may be involved. Differential diagnosis includes keratoacanthoma, basal cell carcinoma, amelanotic malignant melanoma, pyogenic granuloma, traumatized seborrhoeic wart. Diagnosis is confirmed by biopsy. Treatment is by wide excision or radiotherapy. Block dissection of regional lymph nodes is required if these are affected.

DERMIS

Kaposi's sarcoma

These are raised purplish nodules. Initially they are usually single, but gradually multiple nodules occur and may ulcerate. It is the commonest tumour to develop in patients with AIDS. 90% are in male subjects. The solitary nodule should be excised. Local radiotherapy or cytotoxic therapy is useful for multiple lesions.

Metastatic carcinoma

Small, hard, painless, skin nodules may occur. Skin secondaries are commonest with cancer of the breast, lung and bowel. In most patients, the primary will be obvious or will already have been treated. Ulceration of the secondaries may occur. Biopsy confirms the diagnosis. Treatment is given that is appropriate for metastatic disease for that particular tumour, e.g. tamoxifen in carcinoma of the breast.

Others

Malignant change may take place in neurofibromas and lipomas giving rise to neurofibroscarcoma and liposcarcoma. Other soft tissue sarcomas may also arise in this area and are treated by wide excision.

MELANOTIC LESIONS

BENIGN LESIONS

Intradermal naevus (→ Fig. 7.1)

This is the commonest variety. It is light or dark in colour, flat or raised. A hairy mole is of this variety. It may be found in all

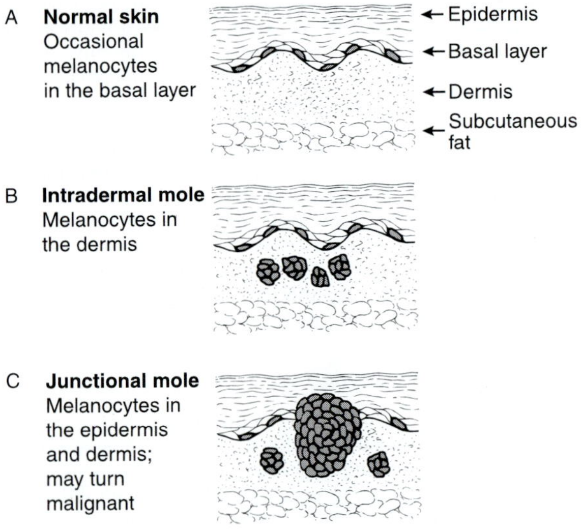

Fig. 7.1 Pathological varieties of naevus (mole)

situations except the palm of the hand and sole of the foot and never turns malignant. A blue naevus is merely an intradermal naevus lying deep in the dermal layer.

Junctional naevus (→ Fig. 7.1)

They develop at or before puberty and can occur anywhere including the palm of the hand and the sole of the foot. Melanocytes are seen both in the dermis and epidermis at the junctional region between the two. Only a small percentage of these turn malignant but that is still enough to provide the vast majority of malignant melanomas.

Compound naevus

This shows both intradermal and junctional features and is indistinguishable clinically from the intradermal naevus. It does, however, have malignant potential.

Juvenile naevus

This is a rapidly growing pigmented lesion that appears in children before puberty. It increases in size rapidly but rarely gets to greater than a centimetre. It is entirely benign. The junctional activity regresses at puberty. Microscopically it may resemble a malignant melanoma. Treatment is excisional biopsy.

MALIGNANT MELANOMA

About 3000 cases of malignant melanoma occur annually in the UK. They may occur anywhere on the skin, but especially on the leg, sole of the foot, head and neck, and nail beds (subungual melanoma). Rarely, spontaneous regression occurs. When disease is confined to the primary site, 5-year survival approaches 80%. With lymph node metastases the figure falls to 30%, and with distant metastases, the patients rarely survive 1 year. The majority of malignant melanomas probably arise in pre-existing junctional naevi.

Signs of malignant change in a mole

These include:

- change in size
- change in colour with deepening pigmentation
- bleeding or ulceration
- itching
- inflammatory ‘halo’
- satellite nodules
- palpable regional lymph nodes.

Classification

Lentigo maligna melanoma Appears on exposed surfaces, in those aged 65–70 years. It is a large flat, freckle-like lesion (3–5 cm) with differing degrees of pigmentation.

Superficial spreading melanoma Smaller than lentigo maligna melanoma (2–3 cm), it has an irregular border and differing degrees of pigmentation. Found at age 50–60 years.

Nodular melanoma Found at age 30–60 years. Initially it is the smallest of the three types. Elevated and uniformly black, it usually has rapid growth with dermal invasion. It may not show pigmentation, i.e. amelanotic melanoma, and may require special histochemical tests to confirm diagnosis. The prognosis is particularly poor with the nodular form.

Spread of melanoma occurs by local growth and infiltration. Lymphatic spread occurs early. Bloodstream spread occurs to almost any organ, particularly the liver, brain and lung.

Treatment

1. Confirm the diagnosis. Occasionally a malignant melanoma is clinically obvious but lesions may need to be confirmed by excisional or incisional biopsy.
2. Check the depth of invasion on histology. Breslow's method involves measuring the depth of invasion in millimetres from the basal layer of the epidermis. A depth of invasion of less than 0.76 mm carries a good prognosis; invasion greater than 1.5 mm carries a high risk of metastases and a poor prognosis. Treatment is by excision down to the deep fascia with a wide margin of normal tissue. For deep lesions on the Breslow classification, a 5-cm clearance may be necessary.
3. Block dissection of lymph nodes if clinically involved.
4. Cytotoxic drugs may be given either parenterally or by isolated limb perfusion.
5. Radiotherapy and immunotherapy have been used but are strictly palliative.

Prognosis Favourable factors include early diagnosis, a depth of penetration of less than 0.76 mm, and superficial spreading melanoma. Unfavourable factors include late presentation, a depth of penetration of greater than 1.5 mm, nodular melanoma, trunk and scalp lesions, lymph node and distant metastases. If the disease is confined to the primary site and has a penetration of less than 1.5 mm, then a 5-year survival of 80% may be expected. With lymph node metastases this is reduced to 30% and with distant metastases patients rarely survive for 1 year.

LESIONS OF VASCULAR ORIGIN

Campbell de Morgan spots

These are small bright red spots containing capillaries and connective tissue. They are rare before the age of 40 and increase with age. They are of no serious significance. Patients should be reassured and the lesions left alone.

Angiomas

Port wine stains These are flush with the skin and occur on the face, lips and buccal mucosa. They remain unchanged during life and are reddish blue in colour. If the lesion is small, surgical excision may be attempted. Larger lesions are cosmetically distressing. Sclerosing agents and argon lasers have been used. Advice on the use of cosmetic preparations may be the most appropriate. These lesions may be seen in association with Sturge–Weber syndrome, i.e. facial angioma associated with intracranial angioma which may cause focal epileptic fits. Similar lesions may be seen in the Klippel–Trenaunay syndrome.

Strawberry naevi They occur in early childhood and are red, soft, compressible fleshy lesions found on the head and neck. Parents can be reassured that the lesion will eventually regress spontaneously.

Spider naevi Small red lesion consisting of a central arteriole and radiating capillaries. Pressure on the central arteriole with a pin head causes the lesion to blanch. They occur on upper trunk, face and neck and are a sign of chronic liver disease. Occasionally a few appear in pregnancy.

Glomus tumour Glomus bodies occur in the subcutaneous tissues of the limbs especially the fingers, toes and nail bed. They are small arteriovenous communications associated with muscle and nerve (angioneuromyoma). Clinically, they are small, raised, bluish-red lesions. They are painful and exquisitely tender if pressed. Treatment is by surgical excision.

DISORDERS OF THE NAILS

Ingrowing toenail (IGTN)

A common condition, it usually appears on the great toe, particularly the lateral side. Caused by a combination of tight shoes and paring the nail downwards into the nail fold rather than cutting it transversely. The sharp edge of nail then grows into the nail fold producing ulceration, infection, and granulation tissue.

Treatment

Non-infected Give advice on correct cutting of nails, i.e. transversely. Avoid tight, pointed shoes. Tuck a pledget of cotton wool soaked in mild antiseptic under the corner of the nail to lift it out of the soft tissue. Soak feet in warm water regularly.

Infected With mild infection it may be possible to adopt the above regimen in addition to the administration of anti-staphylococcal antibiotics. If this fails carry out the following:

- Simple nail avulsion with curettage of infected granulation tissue under local anaesthetic. Antistaphylococcal antibiotics should be administered.
- Wedge excision. Lateral or medial nail and nail bed are removed together with granulation tissue and germinal matrix. Liquefied phenol may be applied to the germinal matrix to ensure complete removal.
- Zadik's procedure. This is reserved for recurrent IGTN. The nail is avulsed and the germinal matrix completely excised after raising a skin flap to expose it. To ensure complete removal of the germinal matrix liquefied phenol is applied after protecting the skin. The nails should not regrow after this procedure.

Complications Recurrence may occur. This is common after simple avulsion. Spikes of nail may occasionally regrow after a Zadik's procedure. Infection may occur and it is appropriate to give a course of antistaphylococcal antibiotics prophylactically. Osteomyelitis and septic arthritis may occur after Zadik's procedure.

Onychogryphosis

This is a 'rams horn' deformity of the toe nail. The nail thickens and curls over the end of the toe as it grows. Common in the elderly, it may follow trauma to the nail in the younger patient. It can be treated by either cutting the nail with bone forceps or grinding the nail down. Avulsion is always followed by recurrence. Zadik's operation is curative.

Nail bed lesions

Haematoma There is a history of trauma, e.g. trapping, or dropping a heavy object on the nail. Very painful. A haematoma is evacuated by piercing the nail with a red-hot paper clip. Small haematomas following trivial injury may closely simulate subungual melanoma. Haematomas grow out with growth of the nail. If there is any doubt, biopsy should be carried out.

Melanoma Subungual malignant melanoma is not uncommon. The lesion does not grow out with the nail. Biopsy is necessary. If the diagnosis is confirmed, amputation of the digit is required.

Subungual exostosis This nearly always affects the great toe. It occurs in adolescents and young adults. It lifts the overlying nail and causes deformity. Diagnosis is confirmed by radiograph. Treatment is to remove the nail and excise the underlying bony nodule.

Glomus tumour See above under lesions of vascular origin.

8

Head and neck

The majority of head and neck problems seen in a surgical clinic are usually lumps. Often it is difficult for the family doctor to decide whether the lump lies in the field of the general surgeon, ENT surgeon, dental surgeon or dermatologist. The conditions described in this chapter are those which one may expect to see in a general surgical clinic. The student is referred to a book on ENT surgery for those conditions affecting the nose, pharynx and larynx.

SCALP SWELLINGS

These include sebaceous cysts, lipomas, papillomas, squamous cell and basal cell carcinomas and melanoma (→ Ch. 7). Other swellings of the scalp include the following.

Cephalhaematoma

This is a subperiosteal haematoma. It occurs following birth trauma or direct injury in babies. The haematoma occurs beneath the periosteum and is limited by the suture lines. It usually resolves spontaneously.

Ivory osteoma

Osteoma of the outer table of skull is a smooth hard swelling, and skin moves over it freely. It is confirmed by radiograph. It is asymptomatic. It should be left or excised if it enlarges.

Cock's peculiar tumour

This is a suppurating sebaceous cyst with granulation tissue. It may be mistaken for a squamous cell carcinoma.

FACIAL SWELLINGS

These include boils, sebaceous cysts, dermoid cysts, squamous cell carcinoma, basal cell carcinoma, malignant melanoma (→ Ch. 7).

CONDITIONS OF THE LIPS, ORAL CAVITY AND TONGUE

STOMATITIS

Stomatitis is a general term used to describe inflammation of the

Table 8.1
Causes of stomatitis

Local	Ill-fitting dentures Sharp teeth Smoking Local ulceration Infections, e.g. herpes simplex, candida, Vincent's angina Trauma, e.g. chemical, thermal, irradiation
General	Haematological: • leukaemia • agranulocytosis • anaemia Vitamin deficiency B and C Debilitating illness: • cancer • tuberculosis • following major surgery Drugs, e.g. septrin, phenytoin

lining of part, or the whole, of the mouth. (For causes of stomatitis → Table 8.1.)

Symptoms of stomatitis

A sore dry mouth; mastication is painful. There may be painful cracking at the corners of the mouth.

Specific causes

Candida stomatitis It is found in children and adults with debilitating disease, those on immunosuppressive drugs, and those with AIDS. It is also found in diabetics.

Symptoms and signs Clinically small red patches appear which are then covered by a white membrane.

Investigations • FBC • Blood sugar • Oral swab • HIV test (if suspected and only after counselling).

Treatment Nystatin mouth washes.

Vincent's angina (acute ulcerative gingivitis) It is caused by *Borrelia vincenti* (a spirochaete), and *Fusobacterium fusiformis*, which are Gram-negative anaerobes.

Symptoms and signs Swollen, painful, inflamed gingiva. Ulcers develop which may spread to the tonsils and buccal mucosa. Other signs are bleeding, halitosis, cervical lymphadenopathy.

Investigations • Mouth swab.

Treatment Penicillin, metronidazole.

Angular stomatitis (cheilosis) Inflamed fissures at the corner of the mouth. The common cause is dribbling saliva at the corners of the mouth. It may occur in school-age children who lick the corners of the mouth. Treatment is aimed at adequate diet, improving oral hygiene, and local application of Vaseline.

General principles of management

History Smoking, drugs, hot spicy foods, dentures, antibiotics.

Examination Check dentures, check for sharp teeth, check general oral hygiene. Examine clinically for other signs of vitamin deficiency or haematological disease.

Investigations • Hb • FBC • ESR • Blood sugar • CXR • VDRL • Mouth swab with film for fungus and culture and sensitivity for bacteria.

Treatment Treatment is that of the underlying disease.

ULCERS

Traumatic Caused by a sharp tooth or ill-fitting dentures. They heal rapidly when the causative agent is removed.

Aphthous A small white deep painful ulcer, it may be solitary or multiple and heals spontaneously. Pain is relieved by local anaesthetic gel.

Herpes simplex Multiple small painful ulcers of mouth or lips, they usually appear in debilitated patients. They may also appear as part of AIDS. Treat with topical acyclovir cream, oral or intravenous acyclovir.

Syphilitic These are rarely seen. Chancre in primary, 'snail track' in secondary, and gumma in tertiary syphilis.

Tuberculous These are rare, and usually found on the tongue. Painful ulcers with undermined edges, they are associated with advanced pulmonary tuberculosis.

Malignant (See below.)

LEUKOPLAKIA

Leukoplakia may occur anywhere within the mouth but is common on the tongue. Areas affected by it appear thickened, white and may show cracks and fissures. Unlike candida it cannot be rubbed off. It is a premalignant condition.

ORAL CANCER

Squamous cell carcinoma may present as a lump or ulcer on the lips, in the mouth, or on the tongue. It spreads via the lymphatics to glands in the neck. It is usually a disease of the elderly and more common in males.

Predisposing factors

The six 'S's': smoking, syphilis, sharp tooth, spirits, spices, sepsis. These agents may predispose to chronic superficial glossitis which results ultimately in leukoplakia, which then results in malignant change with frank carcinoma. Exposure to sunlight may predispose to carcinoma of the lip.

Carcinoma of the lip

Symptoms and signs An ulcer which does not heal in those aged 60 years and above. More common in men than women. Preceded by leukoplakia, it may occur in pipe smokers. A non-tender ulcerative lesion, it may be associated with lymphadenopathy.

Investigations • Excision or incisional biopsy depending on size.

Treatment Wide excision. Block dissection of neck if nodes involved. Radiotherapy.

Carcinoma of the tongue

Although it is more common in males, the incidence has been decreasing over the past 25 years. The incidence is stable in females but the overall incidence remains higher in the male. Most frequently it appears on the lateral margins of the anterior two-thirds of the tongue as a small warty growth, ulcer, or indurated fissured area. Initially painless it becomes painful when secondary infection occurs or invasion is deep into the tongue. Pain may be referred to the ear, being referred from the lingual branch of the trigeminal nerve which supplies the tongue to the ear via the auriculotemporal nerve. If the tumour is extensive and is on the posterior one-third of the tongue, swallowing and speaking may be difficult.

Investigations • Biopsy, incisional or excisional depending on size of tumour.

Treatment

- Small tumours less than 1 cm can be treated by simple excision or radiotherapy.
- Larger lesions may be treated with radiotherapy or more extensive surgery, e.g. subtotal glossectomy and block dissection of neck. Occasionally this may require removal of part of the mandible with major plastic reconstruction.

Carcinoma of the floor of the mouth

Often these are extensive ulcerating tumours which may invade the floor of the mouth and extend into the root of the tongue and the gums. Spread to regional lymph nodes occurs early.

Investigations • Biopsy • CT scan.

Treatment Extensive surgery with block dissection of the neck and plastic reconstruction. Radiotherapy may be the most appropriate treatment in some cases and can be given by either external beam or implants.

Prognosis For small cancers of the lips, 5-year survival rates of 90% have been reported. However, overall carcinoma of the lip has a 5-year survival of over 60%. Tumours of the tongue and floor of the mouth have a poorer survival, being about 30% at 5 years.

CYSTIC LESIONS OF THE LIPS AND MOUTH

Mucous retention cyst

These occur on the inner surface of the lips and anywhere in the mouth where there are mucus-secreting glands. Obstruction to the duct causes the cyst.

Symptoms and signs Painless cystic lesion. Pinkish grey. Transilluminates.

Treatment Excision or it may burst spontaneously.

Ranula

A large mucus retention cyst of the floor of the mouth, it looks like a frog's belly (ranula is Latin for frog). It occurs in children and young adults.

Symptoms and signs A swelling in floor of mouth between symphysis menti and the tongue in the midline. Soft, fluctuant, transilluminates, bluish in colour.

Treatment Complete excision or marsupialization.

Sublingual dermoid

Although congenital, these are rarely noticed before the age of 10. Usually midline, it results from inclusion of the ectoderm during fusion of mandibular processes.

Symptoms and signs Swelling in floor of mouth. Usually painless. May present as 'double chin' if below mylohyoid. In the latter case it may be mistaken for a thyroglossal cyst.

Treatment Excision.

LUMPS IN THE NECK

A convenient classification of these is superficial, lymph nodes and deep swellings (→ Table 8.2).

Table 8.2
Lumps in the neck

Superficial	Sebaceous cyst Lipoma Dermoid cyst Abscess
Lymph nodes	
Deep	
Anterior triangle	Move on swallowing: • thyroid • thyroglossal cyst • lymph node Do not move on swallowing: • salivary glands • branchial cyst • carotid body tumour • carotid aneurysm • sternomastoid 'tumour'
Posterior triangle	Cervical rib Subclavian artery aneurysm Pharyngeal pouch Cystic hygroma

SUPERFICIAL

Superficial lumps include sebaceous cysts, lipomas, dermoids and infective lesions, e.g. boils and abscesses. A common site for lipomas is in the midline posteriorly at the level of the collar line (→ Ch. 7).

LYMPH NODES

The majority of swellings in the neck especially in children are likely to be lymph nodes. The lymph nodes of the head and neck are basically arranged in two circles; an outer superficial one including submental, submandibular, preauricular, and occipital nodes; and an inner one surrounding the trachea and oesophagus and including the paratracheal and retropharyngeal nodes. Both the superficial and deep groups drain into a chain of deep cervical lymph nodes which surround the internal jugular vein. Lymph from there drains into the thoracic duct on the left and into the right lymphatic duct. The causes of cervical lymphadenopathy are shown in Table 8.3.

Investigation of cervical lymphadenopathy

Clinical examination. Look for local lesions, e.g. scalp, face, neck, mouth, tonsil. A full general examination of chest, breast,

Table 8.3
Causes of cervical lymphadenopathy

Infection	Local lesions on head and neck Upper respiratory tract infection Tonsillitis Glandular fever Toxoplasmosis Tuberculosis HIV Cat-scratch disease
Maligancy	Primary: • lymphoma • lymphosarcoma • leukaemia Secondary: almost anywhere in the body, e.g. breast, lung, testis
Sarcoidosis	

abdomen, testes and lower limb is required. Check for axillary and inguinal lymphadenopathy. Check for hepatosplenomegaly.

- Hb, FBC, ESR, Paul–Bunnell, *Toxoplasma* screen, viral antibodies, HIV.
- CXR.
- Laryngoscopy and examination of postnasal space.
- Possibly Kveim test for sarcoid if other clinical features of sarcoidosis.
- Lymph node biopsy or FNAC.

DEEP SWELLINGS OF THE ANTERIOR TRIANGLE

SWELLINGS THAT MOVE ON SWALLOWING

Thyroid

Swellings of the thyroid gland are dealt with in Chapter 11.

Thyroglossal cyst

This is an embryological remnant of the thyroid and may present as a fluctuant swelling in the midline of the neck. It may occur anywhere along the line of thyroid descent but is most common just above the body of hyoid bone and attached to it.

Symptoms and signs Usually a painless, cystic swelling in the midline of the neck which moves on swallowing. It also moves on protrusion of the tongue. Occasionally may become infected, with pain, tenderness, and increased swelling.

Treatment This is by excision.

Lymph node

Occasionally a lymph node may be attached to thyroid isthmus and this will move on swallowing.

SWELLINGS THAT DO NOT MOVE ON SWALLOWING

Salivary glands: inflammatory

The parotid gland is included here although only a part of the gland extends into the neck under normal conditions. In pathological conditions it may present with the swelling largely in the neck. The causes of swellings of the salivary glands are shown in Table 8.4.

Acute sialadenitis This is most common in the parotid gland and is due to epidemic viral parotitis of mumps. It is bilateral. Occasionally sialadenitis of both parotids and submandibular

Table 8.4
Swellings of the salivary glands

Inflammatory and infective	Acute sialadenitis, e.g. mumps parotitis Chronic sialadenitis, e.g. calculus, duct stenosis
Neoplastic	Benign: • adenolymphoma • pleomorphic adenoma Malignant: • adenocarcinoma
Autoimmune	Mikulicz's syndrome Sjögren's syndrome

glands can be caused by poor oral hygiene, dehydration or duct obstruction by stone or stenosis. Acute bacterial sialadenitis is often unilateral.

Symptoms and signs Sudden onset of pain and swelling over salivary glands. Made worse by eating. General malaise. Examination reveals redness, tenderness and swelling in the region of the gland.

Treatment Viral parotitis – treat symptomatically with analgesics. Acute bacterial sialadenitis is treated by antibiotics, e.g. flucloxacillin. If an abscess forms, drainage is required. Recurrent parotitis should be investigated by sialography to exclude sialectasis and areas of duct stenosis.

Chronic sialadenitis This is usually due to calculus in the duct or duct stenosis. Salivary calculi are composed of calcium or magnesium phosphate and are usually radio-opaque.

Symptoms and signs Pain and swelling of the affected gland occur on eating and drinking. The swelling can be reproduced in clinic by putting lemon juice on the tongue. If the stone becomes impacted, the gland remains swollen. Infection and abscess formation may ensue. Inspect the duct orifice. In the case of submandibular calculi, the swelling may be seen in the duct in the floor of the mouth. Feel along the duct with a gloved finger in the floor of the mouth, palpating bimanually from the outside with the other hand. The calculus may be felt.

Investigations • Plain radiograph • 'Floor of mouth' view for submandibular calculi • If no stone is seen arrange sialogram.

Treatment

- Stone in the submandibular duct may be removed by incising directly over the stone into the duct in the floor of the mouth. The stone is extracted leaving the duct marsupialized.
- With duct stenosis, a ductoplasty (widening of the duct orifice) is carried out.
- For the stones in the gland itself, total (submandibular) or partial (parotid) removal of the gland is indicated.

Salivary glands: tumours

Salivary gland tumours are rare. 85% arise in the parotid gland. Of these, the majority are benign and are usually pleomorphic adenomas.

Adenolymphoma (Warthin's tumour) This is a cystic tumour which contains epithelial and lymphoid elements. It is benign.

Symptoms and signs Middle and old age. More common in males. Slow-growing, painless swelling over angle of jaw. It is soft and well defined.

Treatment Surgical excision. Recurrence is rare.

Pleomorphic adenoma 90% occur in the parotid. The old name of 'mixed parotid' tumour arose from the histological appearances of mixed element, i.e. epithelial, fibrous, myxomatous and 'pseudocartilaginous'. The latter was, in fact, mucus. They are slow growing and may enlarge over many years. The tumour sends processes into the surrounding parotid tissue thus explaining why shelling out (enucleation) of these lesions may leave tumour behind with a high recurrence rate. After many years (10–30 years of slow growth), some pleomorphic adenomas develop into invasive malignant tumours.

Symptoms and signs Early and middle adult life. Painless swelling on side of face. Slow growing. Examination reveals a non-tender, diffuse swelling in the angle between the mandible and mastoid process. It may extend down into the neck and forward on to the cheek overlying masseter. Test the integrity of the facial nerve. Diagnosis is made on clinical history and examination.

Differential diagnosis Parotitis, sebaceous cyst, lipoma, pre-auricular lymph node, tumour of ramus of mandible.

Treatment Superficial parotidectomy, i.e. removal of the gland superficial to the facial nerve. Enucleation is associated with a high incidence of recurrence.

Complications Facial nerve palsy either temporary or permanent. Salivary fistula – usually dries up spontaneously. Frey's syndrome, i.e. facial flushing and sweating on eating, occurs in areas supplied by auriculotemporal nerve.

The patient should be warned of these complications, especially the facial nerve palsy, prior to informed consent being obtained.

Carcinoma Usually affects parotid and may arise in a pleomorphic adenoma. The gland becomes hard, irregular and painful. Facial nerve palsy may develop. Treatment is by radical parotidectomy with sacrifice of the facial nerve. Block dissection of the neck may be required. Radiotherapy is of limited value. The prognosis is poor.

Salivary glands: autoimmune

This is a slow painless enlargement of salivary glands. The glandular tissue is invaded by lymphocytes.

Mikulicz's syndrome This causes symmetrical enlargement of the salivary glands, both parotid and submandibular. There is involvement of lacrimal glands and a dry mouth (xerostomia).

Sjögren's syndrome This has the same symptoms as Mikulicz's disease but in addition has keratoconjunctivitis sicca (dry eyes) and seronegative arthritis.

Treatment No treatment may be required but steroids may help. Dry eyes may be treated with hypromellose drops (artificial tears).

Branchial cyst

This is a remnant of the second branchial cleft. It may be associated with a sinus or fistula.

Symptoms and signs It appears in early adult life, usually with soft swelling but consistency varies with tension in the cyst and some may be firm. It occurs at the level of the junction of the upper third and lower two-thirds of sternomastoid, appearing from under the anterior border of that muscle. It may be associated with the branchial sinus which opens over the anterior border of sternomastoid at the junction of the middle and the lower thirds of that muscle. The sinus may extend up between the internal and external carotid arteries and open as a fistula into the side wall of the pharynx.

Differential diagnosis of a branchial cyst This is a lymph node. Diagnosis can be confirmed by aspirating the cyst and examining the fluid under the microscope when cholesterol crystals will be seen.

Treatment Surgical excision of cyst, sinus or fistula tract.

Carotid body tumour

This is a chemodectoma; a slow-growing tumour which arises from the carotid body at the carotid bifurcation. It is usually benign but rarely becomes malignant. Pathologically, it is described as a 'potato' tumour because of the shape and consistency when it is cut.

Symptoms and signs Age 40–60 years. Painless, slow-growing lump with transmitted pulsation. May be associated with fainting attacks from pressure on the carotid sinus.

Investigations • CT scan • Angiography: shows a tumour blush at carotid bifurcation with splaying of the bifurcation (this investigation has largely been superseded by CT scanning).

Treatment Surgical excision. Large tumours may require carotoid bypass grafting.

Carotid aneurysm

A true aneurysm is extremely rare. A false aneurysm may arise following penetrating trauma of the neck. A tortuous carotid artery appearing from under the anterior border of sternomastoid may give the impression of an aneurysm. Careful examination will reveal the tortuosity and lack of an expansile area.

Sternomastoid 'tumour'

This is a swelling of the middle third of sternomastoid in neonates. It consists of oedematous and infarcted muscle.

Symptoms and signs Neonates. Difficult birth, e.g. breach or forceps. Lump or torticollis. Pain on attempting to strain neck. Head becomes turned to opposite side and tilted towards shoulder on side of lesion.

Treatment Sternomastoid tenotomy.

DEEP SWELLINGS OF THE POSTERIOR TRIANGLE

Cervical rib

This may cause neurological or vascular symptoms in the arm (→ Ch. 15). It is often asymptomatic. Occasionally the rib is palpable.

Symptoms and signs Vascular symptoms, e.g. Raynaud's phenomenon or venous thrombosis in the arm. Neurological symptoms, e.g. wasting of the small muscles of the hand (T1 myotome). Paraesthesia on the inner upper aspect of the arm in the dermatomal distribution of T1. May be a palpable lump in the supraclavicular fossa.

Diagnosis • CXR to include thoracic inlet • Count the ribs – if there are 13 there is a cervical rib.

Treatment Excise the rib if causing symptoms.

Subclavian artery aneurysm

This is often just a poststenotic dilatation distal to a cervical rib. True aneurysms are rare. Treatment is by excision if symptomatic.

Pharyngeal pouch

This is a pulsion diverticulum of the pharynx occurring between the thyropharyngeus and cricopharyngeus muscles of the inferior constrictor, i.e. through Killian's dehiscence. The swelling is thought to be due to formation of a high-pressure area at Killian's dehiscence because of incoordination of the contraction of the two parts of the inferior constrictor of the pharynx.

Symptoms and signs Middle or old age. Regurgitation of food on lying down. May develop aspiration pneumonia. Dysphagia due to pouch pressing on oesophagus. Swelling presents behind sternomastoid below the level of the thyroid cartilage. May gurgle on palpation. Halitosis.

Diagnosis • Barium swallow. *Never* endoscopy. The pouch may be perforated if the endoscope passes into it.

Treatment Excision of the pouch with cricopharyngeal myotomy to prevent the incoordination of muscle contraction.

Cystic hygroma

This is a collection of dilated lymphatic sacs which occur near the right lymphatic duct or thoracic duct in the lower part of the posterior triangle. They probably arise because of failure of the lymph channels to connect with main lymphatic drainage.

Symptoms and signs Swelling in the lower part of the posterior triangle present at birth or occurring in the first few years of life. Soft, lobulated, fluctuant, compressible and brilliantly transilluminable.

Treatment Surgical excision. Cyst walls are gossamer thin and rupture easily. Difficult to excise completely and therefore risk of recurrence.

9 Thorax

HEART AND GREAT VESSELS

PRINCIPLES OF CARDIAC SURGERY

Surgery for heart disease has advanced to a point where safe and effective treatment can be offered for most conditions. Assessment of patients has become more refined with the development of special diagnostic techniques, e.g. echocardiography, scintigraphy, cardiac catheterization and cine-angiography. Improvements in diagnostic techniques, anaesthesia, surgical techniques and postoperative management have led to better results with lower mortality rates and a reduction in complications.

Indications for surgery

- Failed medical treatment.
- The mortality and morbidity of a surgical procedure is less than that of the condition.

Contraindications for surgery

Correction of a defect alone is contraindicated in the presence of the following:

- irreparable myocardial damage
- pulmonary vascular resistance equal to systemic vascular resistance
- irreversible failure of other organs, e.g. kidneys and lungs.

However, it is now possible to correct these problems with multiple organ transplants and the above are only contraindications to repair of the defect alone.

Preoperative preparation

- Accurate diagnosis. This requires not only a full examination but a variety of investigations including CXR, ECG, echocardiography, dopplers, cardiac catheterization, MRI, radionuclide scanning, pulmonary function tests.
- Psychological preparation, especially for intensive care.
- Control of cardiac failure with drugs.
- Correction of anaemia.
- Correction of electrolyte imbalance.
- Correction of nutritional deficiencies.
- Chest physiotherapy, bronchodilators, antibiotics, stop smoking.

Surgery

Most open-heart surgery is carried out via a median sternotomy incision. The heart is opened and a bloodless field provided by cardiopulmonary bypass. Closed mitral valvotomy used to be carried out via a left thoracotomy; the operation is rarely performed nowadays. A left posterolateral thoracotomy is used for ligation of a patent ductus arteriosus.

Cardiopulmonary bypass The heart and lungs are excluded from the circulation, being replaced by a pump and a bubble or membrane oxygenator. Venous blood returning to the heart is diverted, through tubes inserted into the right atrium, to a blood oxygenator where oxygen is bubbled through it. The blood then passes through a defoaming section and is collected in an arterial reservoir. A roller pump is used to return oxygenated blood to the patient through a cannula placed in the ascending aorta which is cross clamped below its point of entry. A small amount of blood returning to the LA from the bronchial arteries via the pulmonary veins is sucked out by additional suckers, defoamed and returned to the oxygenator. When the aorta is occluded the myocardium becomes ischaemic. Two methods are available to preserve the myocardium:

- intermittent or continuous coronary perfusion
- depression of myocardial metabolism.

The former consists of cannulation of either of the coronary ostia and infusion of blood or intermittent release of the aortic cross clamp. Reduction of myocardial metabolism is accomplished by cooling the heart with a 'cardioplegic' solution at 4°C infused into the coronary arteries, which arrests the heart in diastole. Aortic occlusion is tolerated for 2–3 hours using cold 'cardioplegic' solution. After closure of the cardiac incisions, the heart is allowed to fill up with blood, air is removed from the heart, the aorta unclamped, the heart restarted and bypass discontinued.

Postoperative complications

Low cardiac output This may result from haemorrhage, cardiac failure, tamponade, pulmonary hypertension, or cardiac arrhythmias.

Respiratory failure This may be due to pulmonary oedema or atelectasis giving rise to hypoxia. Pain from the surgical incision reducing respiratory effort may be contributory.

Renal failure Due to ATN resulting from renal hypoperfusion. Dialysis may be required.

Jaundice Usually a result of transfusions or haemolysis occurring as a result of cardiopulmonary bypass. Occasionally, liver failure occurs because of low cardiac output.

Cerebral damage May be due to anoxia, air embolism, thrombus or fat embolism. Cerebral oedema may occur.

Postoperative treatment

Maintenance of cardiac output Ensure adequate filling pressure of ventricles (preload). Maintain adequate CVP. Ensure myocardial contractility – inotropes. Maintain heart rate around 100/minute. Use isoprenaline or pacing wires inserted at surgery. Reduce peripheral resistance (afterload) with vasodilators, e.g. GTN. Metabolic acidosis may occur and is an indication of poor perfusion. Aortic balloon pumping may be used to reduce cardiac afterload. Haemorrhage and tamponade require urgent re-exploration. Pulmonary hypertension may respond to prostacyclin. Arrhythmias require drugs, cardioversion or pacing.

Prevention of respiratory problems Optimize cardiac output. Use positive pressure ventilation, diuretics, pain relief, physiotherapy.

Maintenance of urine output Optimize cardiac output, diuretics, e.g. frusemide, renal dose of dopamine.

Prevention of cerebral problems Maintain normal BP. Reduce CO_2 by positive pressure ventilation, avoid hyperpyrexia, give dexamethasone.

CONGENITAL HEART DISEASE

This occurs with an incidence of 8 : 1000 live births. Aetiological factors include maternal rubella, Down's syndrome and maternal drugs, e.g. warfarin and phenytoin.

The following lesions are most commonly encountered (in order of decreasing frequency): VSD, ASD, PDA, pulmonary stenosis, aortic stenosis, tetralogy of Fallot, coarctation of the aorta and transposition of the great vessels. Congenital heart disease may be classified as cyanotic (significant R to L shunt) or acyanotic (L to R or no shunt). The reader is referred to a textbook of medicine for the symptoms, signs and investigations of these conditions. The treatment and prognosis are indicated below.

ACYANOTIC

Ventricular septal defect (VSD)

Small defects may close spontaneously but surgery is indicated for large defects, cardiac failure, increased pulmonary vascular resistance and patients with pulmonary blood flow one and half times greater than systemic flow. The defect is closed with a prosthetic patch using cardiopulmonary bypass. Mortality and morbidity depend on the preoperative state of the patient and degree of pulmonary vascular resistance. An uncomplicated VSD has an operative mortality of less then 5%.

Atrial septal defect (ASD)

Surgery is indicated if pulmonary flow is one and half times systemic. The defect is closed with a patch. Ideally the operation should be carried out before a child goes to school. Mortality is less than 1% but increases in the presence of pulmonary vascular resistance.

Patent ductus arteriosus (PDA)

At birth the pulmonary vascular resistance decreases markedly as the lungs inflate and the ductus arteriosus closes within a few days. Failure of closure may occur in premature babies, hypoxia or maternal rubella. In premature babies a prostaglandin synthetase inhibitor, e.g. indomethacin, may promote closure. All persistent ducts should be closed to prevent infective endocarditis. The ductus is doubly ligated via a left thoracotomy. Endovascular techniques are now in common use. Mortality is less than 0.5%.

Coarctation of the aorta

There are two types, i.e. adult and infantile. In the adult form the aorta is narrow in the region of the ligamentum arteriosum just beyond the origin of the left subclavian artery. Proximal hypertension and LV overload occur. Surgical correction is required and the ideal age is 7–15 years. Operative procedures include resection with end-to-end anastomosis. If the gap is too large, a woven Dacron graft is inserted. Complications include residual hypertension, spinal cord ischaemia during surgery, recurrent laryngeal nerve palsy, and mesenteric ‘arteritis’ due to increased pulse pressure. Without surgery the majority of patients are dead before the age of 40. Death occurs from aortic rupture, infective endocarditis, LV failure, cerebral haemorrhage. The operative mortality is about 5%.

The infantile form is rare and usually preductal. It may be associated with other cardiac defects in 60% of infants. Operative mortality is high, reaching 70% for surgery in the first 3 months of life.

Coarctation is commonly now treated by angioplasty in small children.

Congenital valve disease in children

Aortic stenosis or pulmonary stenosis may occur. Treatment is by balloon dilatation during cardiac catheterization or occasionally by open surgery.

CYANOTIC

Congenital cyanotic heart disease is uncommon. The two common forms are the tetralogy of Fallot and transposition of the great vessels. Cyanosis may also occur where the L-to-R shunt of a VSD reverses owing to pulmonary hypertension (Eisenmenger complex).

Tetralogy of Fallot

This consists of a VSD, overriding aorta, pulmonary stenosis and RV hypertrophy. Treatment involves total correction after the age of 2 years. This involves reconstruction of the RV outflow tract and closure of the VSD. Nearly all children are corrected by a one-stop procedure and early correction in infancy is now the procedure of choice. Very rarely an aortopulmonary shunt is used for palliative purposes in the first instance. A Blalock–Taussig shunt is the most common. The subclavian artery is divided on one side and anastomosed to the ipsilateral pulmonary artery to improve pulmonary blood flow. The shunt is closed and the defects corrected between the ages of 3 and 5 years. There should be no mortality associated with the shunt operation. However, the quality of cardiopulmonary bypass in children has now improved considerably such that one can expect to get good results with a one-stop procedure.

Transposition of the great vessels

The aorta arises from the RV and the pulmonary artery from the LV. Survival is dependent on coexisting defects, e.g. PDA, VSD, ASD, which permit mixing of the two circulations. Treatment initially involves cardiac catheterization and balloon atrial septostomy to enlarge the foramen ovale into an ASD, thus allowing adequate intracardiac mixing of blood. This allows the child to thrive. Definitive surgical correction is then undertaken. This involves an 'arterial switch' where the aorta and PA are transected and reanastomosed, aorta to LV and PA to RV. This operation has to be done in the first 2 weeks of life before the LV decreases in size. Alternatively interatrial repair can be undertaken at 6 months. A 'baffle' made of pericardium is created in the atrium to direct caval blood behind the baffle to the mitral valve and LV and PA, with the pulmonary venous return channelled in front of the baffle to the tricuspid valve, RV and aorta. Operative mortality is about 10%.

ACQUIRED VALVULAR HEART DISEASE

This is limited to the aortic, mitral and occasionally tricuspid valves. The pulmonary valve is rarely affected. The valve may be narrowed (stenosis) or rendered incompetent (regurgitation), or both may occur. Except for mitral stenosis and tricuspid incompetence, surgical treatment of acquired valvular disease requires valve replacement. Some types of mitral stenosis may be treated by closed mitral valvotomy while tricuspid incompetence may be treated by valvoplasty.

Types of valve

Mechanical valves These include:

Ball valve The Starr–Edwards is a metal cage with a silastic ball. It is durable for long periods (up to 25 years).

Disc valve The Bjork–Shiley is a tilting disc valve.

Both types require lifelong anticoagulation with its attendant risks. There remains a small risk of thrombosis and embolism. Failure is sudden.

Tissue valves These are usually porcine heterografts. They are mounted on a frame with a sewing ring. The embolic rate is very low and therefore anticoagulants are not required. They lack long-term durability with up to 30% failure rate at 10 years. They fail gradually. Free aortic homograft is still a major choice and antibiotic-preserved fresh homografts may also be used.

Human cryopreserved allograft valves Usually aortic valve inserted without a frame. Anticoagulants are not required and the graft is cheap.

Complication of artificial valves

- Thromboses with valve dysfunction or embolism.
- Failure – calcification and rupture with tissue valves; mechanical breakage with prosthetic valves.
- Bacterial endocarditis.
- Obstruction – tissue growth on to valve ring.
- Paravalvular leakage.
- Haemolysis.

ISCHAEMIC HEART DISEASE

This is the commonest cause of death in the UK. Coronary artery disease is four times more common in men than in women although the incidence in women is increasing. It accounts for one-third of all male deaths and one-quarter of all female deaths.

Aetiology Male sex, smoking, family history, hypertension, hyperlipidaemia, diabetes, obesity, myxoedema.

Symptoms and signs Angina, MI, CCF. Sudden death. Often nothing to find on examination. Occasionally xanthelasma. Cholesterol nodules. Arcus senilis. Stigmata of diabetes. Peripheral vascular disease.

Investigations • Hb • FBC • Lipid profile • CXR – occasionally cardiomegaly • ECG: may be normal at rest in up to 75% of patients; S–T depression with angina. Exercise ECG may be necessary to confirm diagnosis • Echocardiogram: LV hypertrophy, ejection fraction, areas of infarction • Cardiac catheterization and coronary angiography – contrast medium is injected into each coronary artery and views recorded by cinephotography – the site and severity of disease is assessed • LV function is assessed by ventriculography and intracardiac pressures.

Treatment

Conservative Stop smoking. Dietary restrictions. Exercise, correct hyperlipidaemia, control anaemia, control diabetes. Avoid stress. Vasodilators, e.g. nitroglycerine spray; β-blockers, e.g. propranolol. Calcium antagonists, e.g. nifedipine, diltiazem. Aspirin.

Percutaneous transluminal coronary angioplasty (PTCA) This is indicated with localized proximal incomplete blocks causing angina unresponsive to medical treatment. A balloon is inserted under radiographic control and the stenosis dilated. There is a 5% risk of infarction and a mortality of less than 1%.

Coronary artery bypass graft (CABG) Surgery is indicated when there is intractable or unstable angina; triple vessel disease with depressed ventricular function, and left main stem stenosis. A reverse segment of saphenous vein is anastomosed between the aorta and the coronary artery distal to the obstruction. Total arterial revascularization is increasingly common. Both right and left internal mammary arteries are →

used as well as the radial artery as an arterial replacement. The gastroepiploic artery is being used to anastomose to the right posterior descending. The results are good when left ventricular function is normal, with a mortality of approximately 1%. At 1 year, 85% of patients have complete freedom from angina. This reduces to 50% at 10 years. About 5% of patients suffer perioperative MI.

Surgery for complications of myocardial infarction (MI)

Ventricular aneurysm The prognosis without surgery is poor with less than 20% of patients surviving 5 years. Death is due to LVF or MI. Rupture is rare but fatal. Surgery is required for excision of the aneurysm. This is carried out on cardiopulmonary bypass with CABG if appropriate.

Mitral regurgitation Infarct involves the papillary muscles. Treatment is by valve replacement with CABG if appropriate.

Ruptured intraventricular septum This carries a high mortality rate. Early operative repair is advisable but the perioperative mortality rate is high. The defect is repaired with a Dacron patch.

PERICARDITIS

This is inflammation of the parietal and visceral layers of the pericardium. It may occur as an isolated lesion or as part of a systemic disease. Causes include idiopathic (probably viral), tuberculosis, bacterial (staphylococcus, streptococcus or haemophilus septicaemia), rheumatic fever, collagen diseases, uraemia, traumatic, neoplastic (direct invasion from bronchial carcinoma), postpericardiotomy syndrome, MI.

Symptoms and signs Sharp precordial pain. Radiates to shoulders and neck. Malaise. Fever. Pericardial friction rub. Diminished heart sounds if effusion. If tamponade – tachycardia, hypotension, raised JVP, pulsus paradoxus.

Investigations • Hb • FBC • WCC elevated • ESR raised • U&Es: uraemia • Blood culture • CXR: globular heart if effusion • ECG: S–T elevation • Echocardiogram: exudates may show bright echoes on pericardium – pericardial effusion • Diagnostic aspiration • Biopsy.

Treatment This is of the underlying cause or of complications.

COMPLICATIONS OF PERICARDITIS

Cardiac tamponade

A pericardial effusion as small as 100 ml may produce symptomatic tamponade if it occurs rapidly, while larger amounts may be well tolerated if it accumulates slowly. Rapid development of an effusion interferes with diastolic filling and results in reduced cardiac output. The fluid may be blood (trauma, ruptured ventricular aneurysm) or inflammatory exudate (any pericarditis).

Symptoms and signs Tachycardia, hypotension, raised JVP with systolic descent, pulsus paradoxus, reduced heart sounds.

Treatment Urgent when signs of peripheral circulatory failure. Tamponade is treated by pericardiocentesis with a wide-bore needle inserted under xiphoid process. Samples are sent for bacteriological and cytological examination unless the cause is clearly traumatic. Persistence or recurrence of symptoms is an indication for surgery. The pericardium is opened via a left anterior thoracotomy. A drain is inserted. If the cause is traumatic, a coexistent laceration of the heart may require suture.

Constrictive pericarditis

The rigid pericardial sac limits ventricular filling. Aetiological factors include TB, renal failure, post-cardiac surgery.

Symptoms and signs Dyspnoea, fatigue, oedema, abdominal swelling. Raised JVP which rises with inspiration (Kussmaul's sign), tachycardia, reduced pulse volume, ascites, hepatomegaly.

Investigations • ECG: low voltage, T inversion • CXR: may be calcified pericardium • Echocardiogram: thick and calcified pericardium.

Treatment Surgical removal of thickened pericardium.

THORACIC AORTA

Aneurysms

Aneurysms of the thoracic aorta may be true (fusiform, saccular), false or dissecting. Causes include arteriosclerosis, syphilis, previous aortic dissection, trauma and cystic medial necrosis.

Symptoms and signs Asymptomatic. Found on routine CXR. In ascending aorta it may be associated with valvular incompetence, hoarseness may be due to pressure on the recurrent laryngeal nerve, back pain may be due to vertebral erosion, dysphagia may be due to pressure on the oesophagus and dyspnoea may be due to phrenic nerve involvement. Rarely pain is due to erosion of the sternum.

Investigations • VDRL: syphilis • CXR: mediastinal widening • CT scan.

Treatment Indications for surgery include rupture, documented enlargement, pain, aortic incompetence. Aneurysms of the ascending aorta and arch require a prosthetic graft replacement on cardiopulmonary bypass. Replacement of the aortic valves and reimplantation of the coronary arteries may be necessary. Aneurysms of the descending aorta are repaired using left heart bypass, replacing the aorta with a prosthetic graft. The most serious complication of repair of descending thoracic aortic aneurysms is paraplegia occurring in about 5% of patients.

Aortic dissection

In aortic dissection, blood breaks through the intima and creates a false passage through the media. This may rupture back into the main lumen leaving an aorta with a double lumen and the patient may survive. In other cases, rupture with exsanguination may occur, or occlusion of the normal lumen may occur with obstruction to the blood flow through the major branches. As dissection advances, occlusion of side branches may occur, e.g. carotid (hemiplegia), spinal branches (paraplegia), renal arteries (anuria and renal failure), visceral arteries (ischaemic bowel). The aneurysm may rupture back into the pericardium with cardiac tamponade and death. Aetiological factors include arteriosclerosis, hypertension, Marfan's syndrome and cystic medial necrosis.

Symptoms and signs Sudden excruciating chest pain radiating to the back. May be difficult to distinguish from MI. Shock. Signs of cardiac tamponade. Hypotension. Disparity of pulses or BP in extremities. MI may occur if disease extends proximally.

Investigations • ECG may exclude MI • CXR: mediastinal widening, pleural effusion if rupture • CT • MRI • Thoracic aortogram will show extent of dissection with site of intimal tear.

Treatment

Medical Control hypertension, e.g. nitrates, alpha blockers. May prevent further dissection. Obtain CT, MRI or angiogram when BP controlled.

→

Surgical If the ascending aorta is involved, surgery is undertaken immediately because of the high risk of rupture and fatal cardiac tamponade. The ascending aorta is replaced with a tube graft with or without aortic valve replacement. The principle of the operation is to replace the segment of aorta up to where the blood has entered the false channel and to reapproximate the layers of aorta at the distal suture line. Blood now enters the true lumen, decompressing the false channel and restoring blood flow through the branches. If the dissection is distal to the left subclavian artery, medical or surgical treatment may be undertaken. Surgery is indicated for rupture, failure to control BP, compromise of blood flow to kidneys and other abdominal organs. Paraplegia may occur because of compromise of blood flow to the spinal cord.

Prognosis Operative mortality is 10–20%. Some patients do not reach hospital alive. If medical therapy is undertaken, patients need regular follow-up with adequate control of BP.

THORACIC TRAUMA

Thoracic trauma accounts for 25% of deaths from trauma. Injuries may be open or closed. Open injuries are the result of penetrating trauma from knives or gunshot wounds. Closed injuries follow blunt trauma and deceleration. The commonest cause of closed injuries is road traffic accidents. Only about 25% of chest injuries require open surgical intervention.

Open injuries

There may be catastrophic bleeding from penetration of the heart or great vessels. Haemothorax, pneumothorax, cardiac tamponade and visceral damage with mediastinitis may occur.

Closed injuries

Rib fractures, pneumothorax, haemothorax, flail chest, aortic injury, myocardial contusion, ruptured diaphragm, ruptured oesophagus, pulmonary contusion and haemorrhage.

Symptoms and signs Shock, cyanosis, dyspnoea, pain. Hypotension, peripheral vasoconstriction, cyanosis, pulsus paradoxus, diminished heart sound, tracheal deviation, tension pneumothorax. Reduced breath sounds. Altered percussion note. Tenderness over ribs.

Investigations • FBC: cross-match • CXR: widened mediastinum, pneumothorax, fractured ribs, fractured sternum, pleural fluid (haemothorax), mediastinal or subcutaneous emphysema, enlarged cardiac outline, ruptured diaphragm • Aortography • Water-soluble contrast swallow • Peritoneal lavage • ECG.

Treatment This may be required before any investigations are carried out.

1. Establish airway, breathing and circulation.
2. If dyspnoea, tracheal deviation and absent breath sounds over lungs fields, insert chest drain or wide-bore needle immediately.
3. Examine for other injuries as well as chest injuries.
4. Cover or close sucking chest wounds.
5. Radiographs should be carried out when the patient is stable.

Management of specific complications of thoracic trauma

Pneumothorax (→ Fig. 9.1)

Open sucking wounds Air is sucked into the pleural cavity during inspiration. This causes a to-and-fro movement of the mediastinum during respiration and leads to respiratory embarrassment. The open wound must be sealed immediately by application of Vaseline gauze dressings. Surgical closure is carried out as soon as possible. A chest drain should be inserted meanwhile.

Closed pneumothorax This results from an air leak from lung, tracheobronchial tree or oesophagus. It may occur from open or closed trauma.

Simple pneumothorax May be associated with haemothorax. If the pneumothorax is small (less than 10%) on CXR, it may be reassessed later by repeat CXR. If larger, a chest drain connected to an underwater seal should be inserted.

Tension pneumothorax This may cause sudden death. Chest pain, dyspnoea, cyanosis occur. Hypotension results from vena cava distortion when the mediastinum is pushed over, decreasing venous return to the heart. There is tracheal deviation to the opposite side and absent ipsilateral breath sounds. Immediate life-saving treatment is by inserting a wide-bore i.v. cannula to decompress the pleural cavity if a chest drain is not immediately available. The wide-bore needle should be replaced by a chest drain connected to an underwater seal.

Flail chest This is due to blunt chest trauma causing multiple rib fractures, anteriorly and posteriorly, which isolate a segment

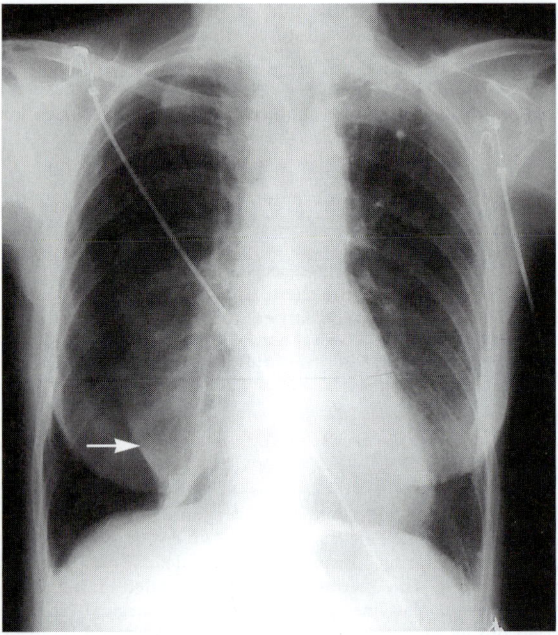

Fig. 9.1 A pneumothorax is visible on the right side. Note the absence of lung marking at the periphery. The lung edge is visible (arrow).

of the chest wall. The classical description is that the isolated segment moves in and out with respiration in a paradoxical fashion. There is usually associated pulmonary contusion and pneumothorax. If there is no pneumothorax or haemothorax, then the intrapleural pressure remains negative and the flail segment moves inwards as the intrapleural negative pressure increases during inspiration and outwards during expiration. Although paradoxical movement is an important physical sign, it has probably in the past received undue emphasis in the management of flail chest. Often the chest does not move paradoxically because the patient does not allow it to do so because it hurts so much. Treatment involves endotracheal intubation, intermittent positive pressure ventilation and drainage of the pleural cavity with underwater seal. If the flail segment does not settle within 10 days, tracheostomy and rib cage fixation may be required.

Simple rib fractures These may be very painful and inhibit breathing and coughing, leading to chest infection especially in the elderly. Pain is best relieved by intercostal nerve blocks with a long-acting local anaesthetic. Strapping of the chest wall is a method which affords some comfort but inhibits chest wall movement and may predispose to pulmonary complications. The practice has largely been abandoned.

Cardiac trauma This may cause damage to the following:

- the myocardium with infarction
- valves with development of symptoms of valvular incompetence
- conducting mechanisms with heart block and arrhythmias.

Lacerations will cause cardiac tamponade. Initial treatment is conservative unless there is cardiac tamponade, in which case needle aspiration or open thoracotomy is required.

PLEURA AND LUNGS

PLEURAL EFFUSION

This is fluid in the pleural space and may be:

- serous effusion, either a transudate (protein concentration less than 30 g/l) or an exudate (protein concentration greater than 30 g/l)
- pus: an empyema
- blood: haemothorax
- chyle: chylothorax.

(For causes → Table 9.1.)

Symptoms and signs Pleuritic chest pain, breathlessness, signs of CCF, peripheral oedema. Ipsilateral reduced expansion, dullness to percussion, absent breath sounds.

Investigations • CXR: dense shadow over a lung field with concave upper limit (→ Fig. 9.2). If the upper border is horizontal then a pneumothorax is also present • Diagnostic aspiration – assess protein content • Culture and sensitivity • TB culture • Cytology for malignant cells • Pleural biopsy.

Table 9.1
Causes of pleural effusions

Transudate	Congestive cardiac failure Renal failure (nephrotic syndrome) Hepatic failure (hypoproteinaemia)
Exudate	Infection: • pneumonia • tuberculosis • empyema • subphrenic abscess
Malignancy	Primary (mesothelioma) Secondary
Other	Pulmonary embolus (with infarction) Pancreatitis Haemothorax Connective tissue disease

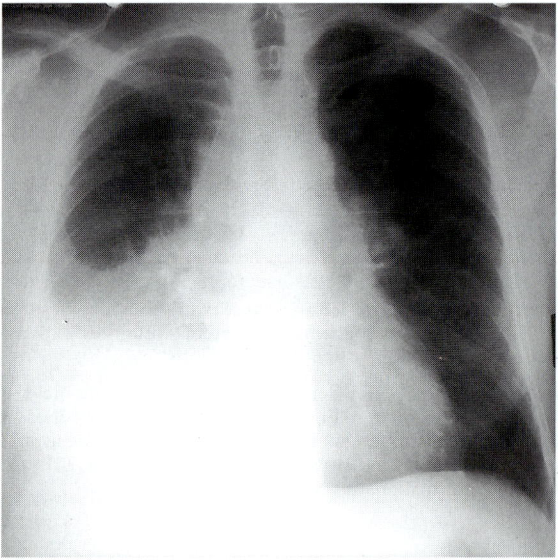

Fig. 9.2 A right-sided pleural effusion. Note the dense shadow and the concave upper limit of the effusion.

Treatment It is of the underlying cause. Large effusions need drainage but not more than 1 litre should be removed at one sitting. In malignant effusions, chemical pleurodesis by instilling a substance into the pleural cavity after drainage. Talc is the most effective with tetracycline the second most effective and bleomycin occasionally used but less effective. Decortication of the pleura is effective in the control of effusions.

TUMOURS OF THE PLEURA

Primary tumours of the pleura are increasing in incidence. The commonest pleural neoplasm is mesothelioma. Mesothelioma occurs in people with a history of exposure to asbestos. The disease is exceptionally rare in those who have not been exposed. It is most common in males between 40 and 50. Symptoms include malaise, weakness, cough, dyspnoea, weight loss and fever. Radiograph shows pleural fluid and thickening. Diagnosis is established by cytology or pleural biopsy. Radiotherapy or chemotherapy are palliative. Neoplasms of the pleura may also be due to secondary spread from other tumours, e.g. bronchus, breast.

PULMONARY INFECTIONS

Bronchiectasis

This is a complication of repeated pulmonary infection where the respiratory pathways are permanently damaged and dilated. It usually affects the lower lobes. The dilated bronchi harbour infected sputum which is expectorated, often in large amounts. Common pathogens include haemophilus and pseudomonas. Causes of bronchiectasis includes cystic fibrosis, Kartagener's syndrome (bronchiectasis, sinusitis, dextrocardia), whooping cough, measles, tuberculosis, inhalation of foreign bodies, pneumonia.

Symptoms and signs Repeated chest infections, chronic cough, copious purulent sputum. Haemoptysis, malaise, clubbing. Rhonchi, coarse crepitations.

Investigations • CXR: cystic shadows (possibly with fluid levels), areas of fibrosis, 'tram lines' due to bronchial oedema • Sputum culture • Lung function tests • Sweat test (cystic fibrosis) • Thin section CT scan • Differential perfusion scan – to define non-functioning lung tissue.

Treatment Physiotherapy with postural drainage. Antibiotics. Bronchodilators. Surgery for localized disease.

Complications Recurrent chest infections, haemoptysis (massive haemoptysis may occur), metastatic cerebral abscess. Rarely pneumothorax may occur.

Lung abscess

The causes are bronchial obstruction due to carcinoma, inhalation pneumonitis, inhaled foreign body especially lung abscess in a child, septic embolus, infected pulmonary infarct, transdiaphragmatic extension of subphrenic abscess. Other causes include: infected cyst; secondary to pneumonia, bronchiectasis or TB; immunosuppression; blood-borne, e.g. staphylococcal septicaemia; fungal.

Symptoms and signs Obviously ill. Purulent sputum. Haemoptysis. Fever. Rigors. Pleuritic pain. Pyrexial. Clubbing. Reduced breath sounds, dullness to percussion, bronchial breathing, signs of pleural effusion, metastatic abscesses, e.g. cerebral.

Investigations • FBC • CXR: consolidation early in disease. Later cavitation and fluid level • Bronchoscopy to exclude foreign body and carcinoma • Sputum culture and sensitivity • Ultrasound scan to confirm and may be aspirated under ultrasound control.

Treatment This is of the underlying cause. Postural drainage and antibiotics. A great majority of cases resolve on medical treatment. Surgery is only required where medical treatment fails or there is a need for treatment of an underlying cause, e.g. removal of bronchial carcinoma.

Tuberculosis

The reader is referred to a textbook of medicine. Surgery is little required in this condition at the present time since anti-tuberculosis therapy is effective in most cases. However, the incidence of TB is increasing and new cases are being seen associated with AIDS. Surgery is required for some of the complications of TB, e.g. bronchopleural fistula, persistent open cavities with positive sputum, bronchiectasis, haemorrhage and destroyed lung. Of historical interest are the operations of thoracoplasty and phrenic nerve crush. Patients who have had these procedures are occasionally seen (usually in finals!). The procedures are designed to collapse the chest wall and the diaphragm on to the lungs, deflating and 'resting' the lungs while healing occurs.

LUNG TUMOURS

Bronchial carcinoma

This is the commonest cancer in males in the UK accounting for approximately 50 000 deaths per year. It is the second commonest in females. 75% of all lung cancers are related to smoking. Other aetiological factors include chronic exposure to asbestos, nickel, arsenic, petroleum products and radioactive materials. Four histological types are described:

- adenocarcinoma (30–45%)
- squamous cell carcinoma (25–40%)
- small cell (oat cell) carcinoma (15–25%)
- undifferentiated large cell carcinoma (rarest).

Symptoms and signs

Primary The tumour may be asymptomatic and seen on routine CXR. Cough, haemoptysis, dyspnoea, chest pain, wheeze, hoarseness, recurrent chest infections, dysphagia.

Complications

- Thoracic: pleural effusion, recurrent laryngeal nerve palsy (hoarseness), SVC obstruction, Horner's syndrome (ptosis, meiosis, enophthalmos, anhidrosis) especially with Pancoast's tumour (invasive cancer of apex of lung).
- Metastatic: cachexia, malaise; brain (headaches, fits, personality change); bone (pathological fractures); liver (jaundice); adrenal (Addison's disease).
- Non-metastatic, extrapulmonary: ADH, ACTH secretion, hypercalcaemia, myasthenic neuropathy, hypertrophic pulmonary osteoarthropathy, thrombophlebitis migrans, gynaecomastia, clubbing.

Investigations • FBC • ESR • LFTs • Calcium • CXR: PA and lateral (→ Fig. 9.3), mass, raised diaphragm with involvement of phrenic nerve, pleural effusion • Sputum cytology for malignant cells • Bronchoscopy and biopsy or brushings • Bronchoscopic biopsy is best for central lesions, percutaneous biopsy for peripheral lesions. Biopsy will confirm histological type • Pleural tap if effusion present, cytological examination for malignant cells • CT scan: local spread and invasion • Brain scan and liver scan for metastases • Mediastinoscopy • Lymph node biopsy • Bone scan.

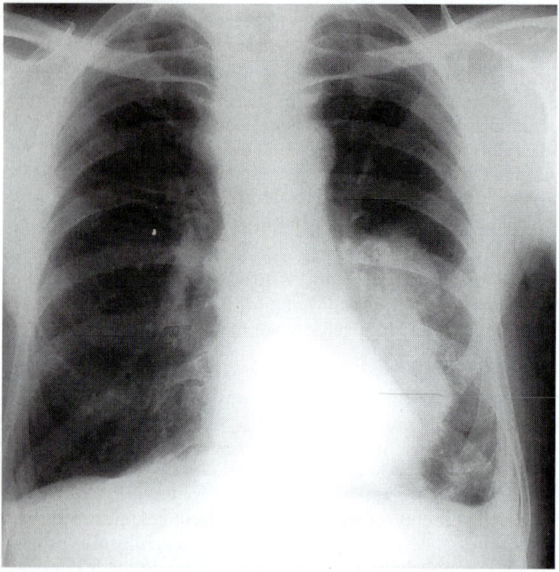

Fig. 9.3 A large bronchial carcinoma in the left lung.

Treatment Surgery offers the only hope of cure. Depends on histological type. Non-small cell tumours, if small and localized (especially if occurring peripherally), may be resected. Larger ones may respond to radiotherapy. Small cell tumours have almost always disseminated at presentation. Combination chemotherapy and radiotherapy prolong survival in small cell tumours. Squamous cell carcinoma is radiosensitive. Most patients are incurable at presentation. Symptomatic relief is the aim. Radiotherapy is appropriate for a bronchial obstruction with lung collapse, SVC obstruction, bone pain and haemoptysis. Endobronchial and SVC stenting procedures may be carried out. SVC obstruction treated by stenting has a success rate of 90% with insertion of a stent via the right femoral vein. Extensive endoluminal disobliteration can be carried out using a cryoprobe/laser and endoluminal brachytherapy.

Surgical treatment involves lobectomy or pneumonectomy and is the only potential cure. Careful selection of patients is required and operability should be assessed by bronchoscopy, CT scan, radioisotope bone scan and ultrasound scan (liver). Contraindications to surgery include distant metastases, SVC obstruction, malignant pleural effusion, recurrent laryngeal nerve and phrenic nerve involvement.

Prognosis About 35% survive 5 years after lobectomy and 25% after pneumonectomy. Since 75% are not candidates for surgery, the overall survival for 5 years is about 5–10%. Prognosis ultimately depends on the cell type and stage of the disease at the time of diagnosis. Small cell carcinoma has the worst prognosis.

Metastatic lung tumours

Metastatic tumours are common in the lung, which in some cases may be the only site of metastases. Secondaries may be from adenocarcinoma (breast, kidney, bowel), sarcoma (bone) or malignant melanoma. Rarely, single or multiple metastatic lung tumours may be removed as part of the treatment. The primary tumour must be controlled and no metastases should be present elsewhere (CT scan, ultrasound scan, bone scan). The best results are obtained with tumours for which there is effective chemotherapy. The best example is the surgical treatment of pulmonary metastases in patients with osteogenic sarcoma.

Solitary pulmonary nodules (coin lesions)

These are well-circumscribed peripheral nodules seen on routine CXRs of patients who are usually asymptomatic. The lesions may be infective, granulomatous, or neoplastic. About 10% are malignant.

Symptoms and signs Usually asymptomatic. Smokers. Cough, haemoptysis, weight loss, hypertrophic osteoarthropathy. Beware of the overlying skin lesions seen on radiograph.

Investigations • Picked up on CXR: concentric or heavy calcification suggests benign lesion. Documented absence of growth over 1 year suggests benign lesion • Sputum cytology and culture • CT scan to exclude multiple lesions.

Treatment Surgical excision if malignancy cannot be excluded.

MEDIASTINUM

Mediastinal masses may be found incidentally on routine CXR or may be symptomatic. A lateral CXR and CT scan may be required to localize the mass and indicate its aetiology.

Certain lesions are more likely to occur in characteristic mediastinal sites:

- superior mediastinum: retrosternal goitre
- anterior mediastinum: dermoid cysts, teratoma, pericardial cysts, bronchogenic cysts, diaphragmatic hernia (foramen of Morgagni), thymoma

- posterior mediastinum: neurogenic tumours, e.g. dumbbell tumours of neurofibroma, paravertebral mass, e.g. TB abscess, phaeochromocytoma, diaphragmatic hernia, achalasia, hiatus hernia.

In addition to the above, aneurysms and lymph nodes may be apparent in any site. Causes of lymph node enlargement include secondary deposits, sarcoid, lymphoma and TB.

Symptoms and signs Asymptomatic, cervical lymphadenopathy, SVC obstruction, hoarseness (left recurrent laryngeal nerve palsy), Horner's syndrome.

Investigations • FBC (blood dyscrasias) • ESR • Sputum culture • Kveim test (sarcoid) • Thyroid scan • CT scan • Bronchoscopy • Oesophagoscopy • Barium swallow • Needle biopsy under CT control • Angiography (vascular lesions) • Mediastinoscopy.

Treatment Surgery may be required. Median sternotomy may be required to confirm the diagnosis and for appropriate treatment.

10 Breast

Breast problems constitute about 15% of all new referrals to a surgical outpatients'. Whatever the presenting symptoms, the patient fears she may have breast cancer. A rapid, efficient and sympathetic approach paying attention to psychological and emotional problems is required in dealing with breast disease.

SYMPTOMS OF BREAST DISEASE

Patients with breast disease present with either a lump, discharge from the nipple, pain in the breast, abnormality of the nipple, or a change in size of the breast (→ Table 10.1).

Table 10.1
Presentation of breast disease

Breast lump	Carcinoma, cyst, localized area of fibroadenosis, fibroadenoma, breast abscess, fat necrosis, duct ectasia, lipoma, galactocele, phylloides tumour, cyst of Montgomery's glands, sebaceous cyst
Pain in the breast	Cyclical and non-cyclical breast pain Carcinoma (85% are painless) Duct ectasia (pain behind the nipple) Infection: • puerperal mastitis • breast abscess Fat necrosis Costochondritis (Tietze's disease) Mondor's disease (superficial thrombophlebitis of veins of the chest wall)
Nipple discharge	Bloodstained (intraduct carcinoma, intraduct papilloma, Paget's disease) Serous (early pregnancy) Yellowish, brown or dark green (benign nodularity) Thick and creamy (duct ectasia) Purulent (rarely in association with breast abscess) Milky (late pregnancy, post-lactation, prolactinoma)

Table 10.1
Presentation of breast disease (*contd*)

Nipple abnormalities	Retraction (congenital, duct ectasia, carcinoma) Inflammation (eczema, Paget's disease) Destruction (Paget's disease) Mamillary fistula
Breast enlargement	Benign hyperplasia, pregnancy, cancer, giant fibroadenoma, phylloides tumour, elephantiasis.

History Take note of the following: the duration of symptoms, parity, age at menopause, age at menarche, breast feeding, contraceptive pill and HRT and family history of breast cancer.

Examination

- Observe with patient sitting inclined at 45°, e.g. symmetry, masses, peau d'orange, skin dimpling, nipple retraction.
- Observe with hands raised above head, e.g. obvious skin dimpling/asymmetry.
- Examination of the nipples, e.g. nipple retraction, Paget's disease, expression of blood from a duct.
- Palpate each quadrant and the axillary tail with the flat of the hand. With the patient in the akimbo position pressing hand on hip, test for deep fixation.
- Palpate axilla. Mobile or fixed nodes.
- Palpate supraclavicular fossa.
- General examination for distant metastases, e.g. chest – pleural effusion; hepatomegaly – liver metastases.

Investigations • FNAC: a negative result does not exclude carcinoma • Mammography: 95% accurate. Unreliable under the age of 35 years because of the density of breast • Core biopsy.

BENIGN BREAST DISEASE

This presents as: breast nodularity; fibroadenoma; duct ectasia; fat necrosis; intraduct papilloma; breast abscess; related conditions such as Tietze's disease or Mondor's disease.

Benign nodularity/breast pain

This occurs between 20 and 45 years and settles after the menopause. It probably results from an abnormal response of the breast to changes in the hormonal environment. The terms fibroadenosis and cystic hyperplasia describe the pathological condition well. There is exaggeration of the fibrotic element, i.e. fibrosis, the epithelial element undergoes hyperplasia, i.e. adenosis, and there is a tendency to cyst formation. The condition may be extremely painful, especially premenstrually, hence the terms cyclical mastitis or cyclical mastalgia.

Symptoms and signs Cyclical breast pain worse before period. Intermittent breast masses or areas of thickening with no discrete mass. Discrete mass, i.e. cysts, may be noticed by patient. Examination reveals nodular breasts with multiple thickened areas (usually upper and outer quadrant) which are usually tender. Lesions change in number and size during menstrual cycle. If condition is suspected, examination should be repeated at different stages of the menstrual cycle.

Investigations • Mammography to exclude carcinoma • USS – fibroadenoma, cyst – ultrasound-guided FNAC and core biopsy • Aspiration may be diagnostic and therapeutic for a cyst.

Treatment

This condition may be exceptionally painful and cause severe distress to the patient. Keeping a breast pain chart to document severity and symptoms in relation to menstrual cycle is important. An explanation of the condition and treatment options should be clearly and sympathetically made. 90% of patients require no further treatment.

- Firm supporting bra to 'rest' the breast. This should be worn day and night when the patient is symptomatic.
- Evening primrose oil.
- Danazol is given for severe symptoms. Androgenic side-effects need to be explained to the patient. About 50% of patients cannot tolerate danazol.
- Rarely, some patients are so severely troubled they become suicidal. Subcutaneous mastectomy with implants has been used in extreme cases.
- The condition occasionally responds to hypnotherapy and acupuncture.
- If there is a dominant mass, this should be aspirated for cytology.

Fibroadenoma

This occurs at age 15–35 years.

Symptoms and signs Very mobile breast lump noted by patient. Non-tender. On examination there is a mobile, discrete, smooth, firm and rubbery swelling in the breast. It slips under the examining fingers, hence its name breast 'mouse'.

Treatment Excisional biopsy if there is any doubt about the diagnosis. In young women in their teens it is reasonable to observe. However, if observation is carried out FNA or core biopsy should be undertaken.

Duct ectasia (periductal mastitis)

This occurs chiefly in the fifth decade. The aetiology is obscure but is associated with dilatation of the ducts behind the nipple and a periductal inflammatory reaction rich in plasma cells. The condition is sometimes called plasma cell mastitis.

Symptoms and signs Pain and periareolar erythema. Nipple discharge may be either thick and creamy or greenish brown. There may be a periareolar tender mass. The nipple may become retracted when healing occurs by fibrosis. Occasionally infection occurs with periareolar abscess formation.

Differential diagnosis Carcinoma of the breast with nipple retraction.

Investigations • Mammogram: opaque mass of dilated ducts and skin indentation may be apparent.

Treatment

- If infection is present aspiration should be carried out and antibiotics given.
- If an abscess is present surgical drainage may be required.
- A mammillary fistula may occur as a complication. If it does it should be laid open.
- With severe discharge or recurrent sepsis the nipple ducts should be excised (mammadochectomy). The ducts are excised through a circumareolar incision preserving the nipple.

Fat necrosis

This is due to trauma with rupture of fat cells and a consequent inflammatory reaction which may become calcified.

Symptoms and signs There may be a history of trauma, often minor. The partner's teeth may be an aetiological factor and patients may be embarrassed to explain this possible cause. The lump may have decreased in size before the patient is seen in clinic. In the early phases, the lump is tender. In the later phases it is hard and irregular and tethered to the skin.

Investigations • FNAC • Mammography to distinguish it from carcinoma of the breast. • Core biopsy.

Treatment Excision biopsy may be necessary ultimately to distinguish the condition from cancer of the breast.

Intraduct papilloma

The papilloma is usually in a solitary duct near the nipple in a young woman.

Symptoms and signs Blood-stained discharge from a single duct on to the nipple. Occasionally a small mass may be palpable. Usually, however, no mass is palpable. Pressure over a certain spot or the palpable mass will cause bleeding from a single duct orifice.

Investigations • Mammography may be required to exclude carcinoma.

Treatment If the duct orifice from which the bleeding is coming can be identified, microdochectomy is carried out. If not, excision of the major nipple ducts is necessary. Histological confirmation is required to exclude in situ or invasive cancer.

Breast abscess

This most commonly occurs following suppuration of acute mastitis in the lactating breast. The infecting organism is usually *Staphylococcus aureus*. The early phase of acute mastitis may settle with appropriate antistaphylococcal antibiotics.

Symptoms and signs Lactating breast. Patient generally unwell with painful, tender, red and warm swelling of breast. The swelling may become fluctuant and eventually the abscess points and discharges.

Treatment Incision and drainage. Often multiloculated and loculi need to be broken down. Occasionally abscesses occur in the glands of Montgomery and appear as a boil-like lesion and should be treated as for a boil. Periareolar abscesses may occur with duct ectasia.

Related conditions

Patients may occasionally present with apparent pain in the breast where the condition responsible for the pain is not within the breast.

Tietze's disease This is costochondritis and usually involves the second, third and fourth costal cartilages. The cause is unknown and radiographs are unhelpful. The condition is self-limiting although NSAIDs and infiltration with local anaesthetic and steroids may be helpful if the pain is severe.

Mondor's disease (superficial thrombophlebitis of the subcutaneous veins of the chest wall). The cause is unknown and the condition self-limiting. Recent reports have suggested a relationship with underlying carcinoma. The veins of the chest wall are felt as red, tender cords often extending on to the anterior axillary fold. The breast should be carefully palpated for underlying masses. Mammography is advised to exclude an underlying carcinoma. NSAIDs may help relieve symptoms.

CARCINOMA OF THE FEMALE BREAST

This is the most common malignancy in the female. About 13 000 women die annually in the UK from carcinoma of the breast. The incidence of the disease appears to be rising. The cause remains unknown. Although the 5-year survival rate has increased, the overall mortality has changed little in the past 25 years.

Risk factors

- Family history – first-degree relatives with early-onset disease.
- Contralateral breast carcinoma.
- Atypical hyperplasia on previous biopsy.
- Nulliparous women.
- Early menarche.

Symptoms and signs Symptoms include: painless lump in the breast; nipple retraction or discharge; skin dimpling; peau d'orange; breast asymmetry; erythema over skin or nipple; symptoms of metastases, e.g. bone pain, headache, breathlessness, jaundice. Examination may reveal: hard irregular mass, fixed to skin or fixed deeply; erythema; Paget's disease of nipple; peau d'orange; axillary glands mobile, fixed or matted; supraclavicular nodes palpable; signs of metastases – liver (jaundice, hepatomegaly, ascites), lung or pleural metastases (pleural effusion, consolidation), bone secondaries (bone tenderness or pathological fractures), brain secondaries (headache, fits, personality change, papilloedema).

Investigations • Hb: anaemia with marrow infiltration • LFTs: raised alkaline phosphatase with liver secondaries • Calcium: hypercalcaemia with advanced disease • Mammography (→ Fig. 10.1) • USS of breast • FNAC – if negative proceed to core biopsy; excision with frozen section (rarely performed, owing to accuracy of FNAC and core biopsy). • Bone scan • USS of liver • CT scan of brain.

Clinical staging Two forms are in wide use (→ Tables 10.2 and 10.3).

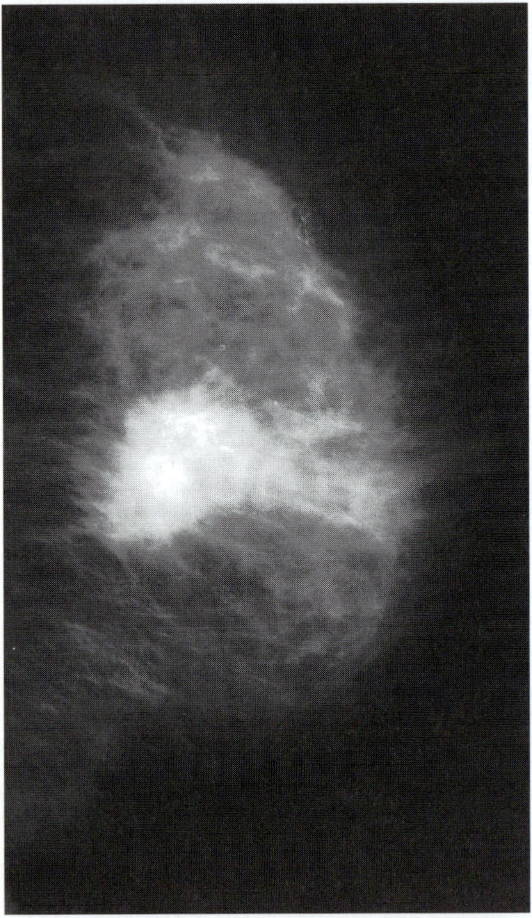

Fig. 10.1 A mammogram showing a carcinoma of the breast. There is a dense mass with microcalcification. Malignant microcalcification requires careful examination of the film with magnification: it does not reproduce well in photographs.

Table 10.2
Manchester classification (modified)

Stage I	Lump less than 5 cm; not fixed deeply
Stage II	As for stage I but mobile, ipsilateral axillary nodes
Stage III	Lump greater than 5 cm fixed to skin with fixed ipsilateral axillary nodes, or supraclavicular nodes, or peau d'orange, or arm oedema
Stage IV	Distant metastases

Table 10.3
TNM classification

Primary (T)	T1S – carcinoma in situ T0 – no primary tumour located T1 – tumour less than 2 cm T2 – tumour 2–5 cm T3 – tumour greater than 5 cm T4 – extension to chest wall
Nodes (N)	N0 – no nodal involvement N1 – mobile ipsilateral axillary nodes N2 – fixed ipsilateral axillary nodes N3 – ipsilateral supraclavicular nodes
Metastases (M)	M0 – no metastases M1 – distant metastases

Treatment Surgery to the breast ranges from wide local excision to mastectomy combined with adjuvant chemotherapy. Treatment options should be discussed with the patient. Preoperative counselling by the surgeon and a specially trained breast nurse should explain the treatment options and prepare the patient for treatment. Recent trends are to more conservative management of breast cancer.

Surgery for early breast cancer (T1, T2)

- Wide local excision: removal of the lump with a margin of normal breast tissue. This should be combined with axillary node sampling or axillary clearance according to local protocol.

→

- Simple mastectomy and axillary node sampling or axillary clearance.
- Modified radical mastectomy (Patey procedure): removal of the breast, pectoralis minor muscle and the axillary contents inferior to the axillary vein.

Patients with early breast cancer should be considered for systemic adjuvant treatment, i.e. tamoxifen and/or chemotherapy. Tamoxifen should be used in those who are oestrogen receptor +ve. Primary tamoxifen therapy without surgery may be used in elderly/unfit patients.

Surgery for advanced breast cancer (T3, T4)
- Locally advanced disease (no systemic disease) – neo-adjuvant therapy – chemotherapy/radiotherapy/surgery.
- Salvage mastectomy.

Palliation (Stage IV)
- Local palliation (e.g. radiotherapy for fungating lesions).
- Radiotherapy to localized bony metastases.
- Aspiration of pleural effusions and instillation of cytotoxic agents.
- Hormonal manipulation, e.g. tamoxifen.
- Chemotherapy.

Extensive surgery may be required for chest wall defects which require grafting with myocutaneous flaps, e.g. latissimus dorsi flaps.

Recurrent disease Local recurrent disease may be treated by radiotherapy if this has not been given to the area before. Systemic local disease may be treated by hormonal manipulation or chemotherapy.

Follow-up
- Routine self-examination of operation site and other breast.
- Follow-up is in accordance with local protocols but should be continued for 5 years and patients who are disease free then should be discharged.
- Mammography to contralateral breast every other year and to ipsilateral breast, if conserved, every year.

Prognosis
- Stage I: 80% 5-year survival.
- Stage II: 50% 5-year survival.
- Stage III: 15% 5-year survival.
- Stage IV: 5% 5-year survival.

Complications of mastectomy Wound seromas, lymphoedema of the arm, stiffness of the shoulder. The main problems are psychological and should be managed both preoperatively and postoperatively by expert counselling and support.

Breast reconstruction Many patients are well rehabilitated with a prosthesis. Others, however, wish breast reconstruction. This may be performed immediately at the time of the initial surgery or at a later date.

Breast screening This is based on the premise that early detection of breast cancer improves the prognosis. Current screening in the UK invites women in the 50–64 age group to have 2-view mammography every 3 years. Suspicious lesions on mammography that cannot be palpated require mammographic localization by inserting wires into the lesions in two planes. The area at the site of the wires is then excised. A specimen is re-radiographed to make sure the lesion has actually been removed. Histology is then undertaken. If malignant, appropriate treatment is undertaken.

OTHER CONDITIONS OF THE BREAST

Paget's disease of the nipple

Associated with an intraduct carcinoma of the breast, the tumour cells spreading within the epithelium on to the nipple.

Symptoms and signs Red, eczematous-like lesion of the nipple which eventually erodes the nipple. There may be an associated palpable mass in the breast.

Differential diagnosis Eczema of the nipple. However, the latter is usually bilateral, itchy, and does not destroy the nipple.

Investigations • Mammography • Biopsy confirms diagnosis.

Treatment Simple mastectomy. In the absence of a palpable mass in the breast, the prognosis is excellent.

Inflammatory carcinoma (mastitis carcinomatosa)

May occur in pregnancy or lactation and is the most aggressive of breast carcinoma.

Symptoms and signs Oedema, erythema, peau d'orange, generalized breast enlargement. Metastasizes widely and rapidly.

Diagnosis • Core biopsy.

Treatment Palliative. Radiotherapy, tamoxifen, chemotherapy.

Prognosis Less than 5% of patients survive 5 years.

Phylloides tumour

This is a rapidly growing highly cellular variant of a fibroadenoma. It rarely metastasizes, but it recurs locally after an inadequate incision. It should not be shelled out like a fibroadenoma but should be excised with a rim of normal breast tissue.

Pseudolipoma

This is a soft lobulated swelling of the breast which resembles a lipoma. It is caused by an underlying carcinoma causing retraction of the suspensory ligaments of the breast resulting in bunching of the fat between the skin, septae of the breast, and the carcinoma. Beware the diagnosis of lipoma of the breast especially in the older patient. Mammography is advised.

CONDITIONS OF THE MALE BREAST

Gynaecomastia

Gynaecomastia is benign hypertrophy of duct and connective tissue elements of the male breast. It may occur in the following instances:

- at birth (maternal oestrogens crossing placenta)
- at puberty, where it may be unilateral or bilateral (embarrassing to the patient; it may resolve or may need surgery)
- because of drugs (cimetidine, spironolactone, digoxin, methyldopa, oestrogens)
- because of liver failure
- association with testicular tumours.

Carcinoma

This is rare and usually occurs over the age of 50 years. It presents with a unilateral, hard, painless mass.

Treatment This is by mastectomy with or without axillary node clearance. Tamoxifen is given if oestrogen receptor +ve. The prognosis of male breast cancer is now thought to be identical to that of the female type when compared stage for stage, but the male tends to present with skin infiltration more often than the female and therefore is seen at a later stage. Orchidectomy is an option in advanced cases.

11

Endocrine surgery

THYROID

CONGENITAL

The embryological line of descent of the thyroid gland is from the foramen caecum of the tongue to its normal position in the neck. Occasionally it may descend lower and even to the superior mediastinum.

Lingual thyroid

This occurs at the foramen caecum of the tongue. It may be asymptomatic or interfere with speech or swallowing. A radioiodine scan should be performed to confirm the presence of thyroid tissue. Treatment is by suppression of TSH with thyroxine, but surgical excision should be considered if hormonal therapy is ineffective or the patient has obstructive symptoms.

Thyroglossal fistula

This is not congenital but follows rupture, or inadequate excision of a thyroglossal cyst. Recurrent inflammation occurs and the fistula intermittently discharges mucus. Treatment is by excision of the fistula and may require dissection as far as the foramen caecum of the tongue.

Thyroglossal cyst (→ Ch. 8)

EXAMINATION OF THYROID GLAND

Inspection should be carried out initially from the front. Confirm that there is a mass in the neck in the area of the thyroid gland and that it moves up on swallowing. Place a finger in the suprasternal notch and check that the trachea is central. Examine the thyroid from behind. Place the thumbs on the vertebra prominens and the fingers on the anterior part of the neck on either side. Allow the head to tilt forwards slightly to relax the neck muscles. Feel up and down in the area of the thyroid. Applying gentle pressure to one side of the neck over the thyroid facilitates examination of the contralateral lobe. Decide whether there is a single nodule, many nodules or whether there is diffuse enlargement of the thyroid gland. Give the patient a glass of water to swallow and check again that the gland moves up on swallowing. Palpate up and down the deep cervical chain of lymph nodes to check for lymphadenopathy. Percuss over the sternum to check for retrosternal extension. Auscultate over the gland. Very vascular toxic glands may have a systolic bruit.

SYMPTOMS OF THYROID DISEASE

Lump in the neck

- Smooth non-toxic enlargement of the gland. This is characteristic of a physiological goitre which may occur at puberty or in pregnancy.
- A nodular non-toxic enlargement of the gland. This is characteristic of multinodular goitre.
- A smooth toxic enlargement of the gland associated with Graves' disease.
- A rapid increase in the size of nodule associated with haemorrhage into a cyst, a rapidly growing carcinoma or thyroiditis which may be painful.
- A smooth firm enlargement of the gland (occasionally asymmetrical), usually in middle-aged females and often associated with hypothyroidism, e.g. Hashimoto's disease.
- A hard irregular goitre with infiltration of muscles and lymphadenopathy in the older patient, i.e. anaplastic carcinoma.
- A solitary nodule in a lobe of the thyroid gland. This may be due to a palpable dominant nodule in a multinodular goitre, a cyst, an adenoma or a carcinoma.

Hoarse voice This is due to pressure on and/or malignant infiltration of one or both recurrent laryngeal nerves.

Dysphagia This may occur with very large goitres.

Dyspnoea It is due to tracheal deviation or compression. Stridor may be apparent.

Pain This may occur with haemorrhage into a nodule, infiltration by anaplastic carcinoma, subacute thyroiditis or, occasionally, Hashimoto's disease.

Eye symptoms Staring or protruding eyes (exophthalmos), double vision, dry 'gritty' eyes, difficulty closing eyes. The latter may lead to pain due to corneal ulceration.

Thyrotoxicosis Palpitations, dyspnoea, nervousness, irritability, tremor of hands, sweating. Increased appetite with weight loss, diarrhoea. Preference for cold weather. Amenorrhoea. Pretibial myxoedema may be found in Graves' disease.

Myxoedema (hypothyroidism) Slowness of thought, speech and movement. Weight gain. Cold intolerance, tiredness, lethargy, constipation. Loss of hair. Change of voice (hoarseness). Carpal tunnel syndrome.

INVESTIGATION OF THYROID DYSFUNCTION

This can be euthyroid, hyperthyroid or hypothyroid. Measure TSH, free T4, T3. TSH is elevated in hypothyroidism. TSH is suppressed in thyrotoxicosis. Thyroid autoantibodies suggest immune aetiology of disease.

Plain radiograph of chest and thoracic inlet They may show tracheal displacement or compression. Retrosternal extension.

Ultrasound scan It establishes the size and shape of the gland and may indicate if nodules are single or multiple. It will also distinguish between cystic and solid lesions.

Radioisotope scans These will indicate if thyroid nodules are single or multiple, and whether they are over-functioning (e.g. 'hot' nodule) or non-functioning (e.g. 'cold' nodule). Diffuse homogeneous uptake occurs in the normal gland; diffuse overactivity with generalized but patchy uptake occurs with a multinodular goitre. A 'cold' nodule shows no uptake, e.g. tumour or cyst, while a 'hot' nodule demonstrates an overactive area and may be associated with thyrotoxicosis. A 'hot' nodule is rarely malignant but about 20% of cold nodules are malignant.

Fine needle aspiration This will distinguish between a solid lesion and a cyst. If the lesion is solid, cells are sent for cytological examination. This is a safe technique. Usually it is possible to discriminate benign from malignant disease, although some difficulties may be encountered. In particular, distinction between benign and malignant follicular adenomata can be difficult. Fine needle biopsy should be performed in the investigation of all thyroid nodules. Its reliability can be improved by carrying out the biopsy under ultrasound guidance.

GOITRE

A goitre is an enlargement of the thyroid gland. (For classification → Table 11.1.)

Simple hyperplastic goitre

Iodine deficiency is the commonest pathological cause. Physiological causes include puberty and pregnancy. Endemic goitres occur in childhood and are common in areas where the drinking water has a low iodine content. They are rare in the UK where iodide is added to table salt.

Table 11.1
Classification of goitres

Simple (non-toxic goitre)	Simple hyperplastic goitre Multinodular goitre
Toxic goitre	Diffuse goitre (Graves' disease) Toxic nodule Toxic multinodular goitre
Neoplastic goitre	Benign: • adenoma Malignant: • papillary • follicular • anaplastic • medullary
Inflammatory	De Quervain's thyroiditis Riedel's thyroiditis
Autoimmune	Hashimoto's thyroiditis

Symptoms and signs The patient is usually euthyroid. Usually a smooth goitre. Iodine deficiency types of goitre may become very large.

Investigations • Free T4 usually normal • TSH may be raised • CXR and thoracic inlet radiograph to exclude tracheal compression or deviation. • CT scan (→ Fig. 11.1) – retrosternal goitre, tracheal deviation/compression.

Treatment Addition of iodized salt to diet in areas where iodine deficiency occurs. Thyroxine orally daily to suppress TSH. Partial thyroidectomy is indicated only if the gland is very large and causing pressure effects.

Multinodular goitre

This is the commonest cause of goitre in the UK. The gland is enlarged and irregular. The condition develops spontaneously and also in simple colloid goitres. There are areas of hypoplasia and hyperplasia within the gland. The condition is more common in women. With large glands, tracheal deviation and compression may occur. Toxic change may occasionally occur with the symptoms of hyperthyroidism.

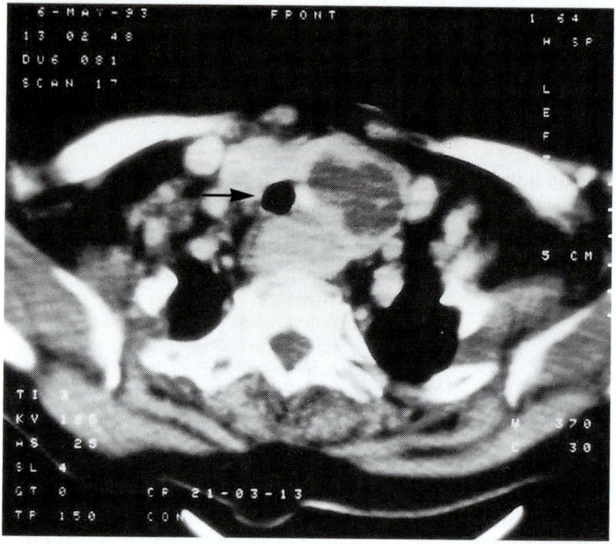

Fig. 11.1 A CT scan of the neck showing a goitre (large mass in the left lobe of the thyroid gland). The trachea (arrow) is slightly deviated to the right.

Symptoms and signs In endemic areas, nodular goitre appears at 15–30 years whilst sporadic ones occur later at 25–40 years. Smooth nodular gland. Occasionally only a solitary nodule is palpable. Dyspnoea, dysphagia may occur if the gland is very large. Pain may occur due to haemorrhage into a cyst.

Investigations • Free T4, TSH • An isotope scan will identify toxic nodules • Radiograph thoracic inlet.

Treatment If the patient is clinically euthyroid and the goitre is small, no treatment is required. If the gland is large and unsightly and causes symptoms of compression, or thyrotoxicosis occurs, partial thyroidectomy is indicated.

Toxic goitre

This may be a diffuse goitre (Graves' disease), toxic multinodular goitre, solitary toxic nodule. In Graves' disease, TSH receptor antibodies are present. In toxic multinodular goitre, several nodules in a non-toxic goitre begin to function independently of TSH stimulation. A solitary toxic nodule functions autonomously. Toxic goitre is six times more common in females.

Symptoms and signs Hyperthyroidism, tachycardia, palpitations, AF, tremor, increased tendon reflexes, exophthalmos, lid-lag. Occasionally bruit over gland. Pretibial myxoedema.

Investigations • Low TSH; T3 (↑); free T4 (↑) • Isotope scan may show 'hot' nodule.

Treatment

Antithyroid drugs Carbimazole 15 mg t.d.s. until euthyroid and then 5 mg t.d.s. for 12–18 months. About 50% of patients remain euthyroid when the drug is discontinued. Severely toxic patients may require β-blockers. Relapses, if they happen, usually occur within 2 years of stopping treatment. Hypothyroidism may develop. Side-effects of carbimazole include rashes and neutropenia. Patients must be warned to report any sore throat occurring especially in the initial stages of carbimazole treatment.

Radio-iodine ^{131}I is administered orally. It usually takes 8–12 weeks before the patient becomes euthyroid. Antithyroid drugs need to be taken until the symptoms settle. It is appropriate treatment for most patients with thyrotoxicosis, recurrent hyperthyroidism, and poor-risk patients. It should not be used in children and pregnant women because of potential radiation hazards. There is a high incidence of late myxoedema.

Surgery This is the treatment of choice for younger patients, children and patients with large goitres. The patient should be rendered euthyroid prior to surgery with antithyroid drugs. Blocking therapy with carbimazole, and replacing endogenous hormone production with thyroxine administration is optimum preparation for surgery. Propranolol may be needed if control is difficult to achieve or when urgent surgery may be indicated. Subtotal thyroidectomy is often the operation performed, but, increasingly, total thyroidectomy – particularly if a toxic multinodular goitre – is the preferred procedure. Thyroid lobectomy is the appropriate treatment for a solitary toxic nodule.

Prognosis Hypothyroidsim may occur after any of these treatments. The incidence is highest after radioactive iodine. After subtotal operations about 4% remain toxic and around 8–10% will become toxic again at a later time. ^{131}I treatment is then appropriate. About 4% become hypothyroid immediately and up to 20% may ultimately become hypothyroid. After subtotal operations lifelong monitoring of thyroid function is required.

Neoplastic goitre

Benign

Adenomas True follicular adenomas are encapsulated and usually greater than 2 cm on presentation. They are solid on ultrasound and 'cold' on isotope scans. FNAC will not distinguish them from follicular carcinoma. They must be excised in total and examined by the pathologist before confirming their benign nature. Lobectomy is adequate treatment with completion thyroidectomy if the nodule is a carcinoma over 1 cm in size.

Malignant The large majority are primary. Aetiological factors include exposure to ionizing radiation in childhood; endemic goitre may be associated with follicular carcinoma but the risk is small. There is also an association with breast disease and adenomatous colonic polyps. Evidence is emerging that some instances of papillary cancer may be associated with a family history of well-differentiated thyroid cancer. Family history is present in medullary carcinoma associated with MEN Type II. Metastatic carcinoma is very rare but may spread via the bloodstream from breast, lung, kidney and prostate. The main types of thyroid cancer are as follows.

Well differentiated (papillary and follicular)

- *Papillary (60%)* occurs at any age with a peak incidence in the third and fourth decades. Usually slow-growing nodule which may metastasize early to regional lymph nodes. They are often multicentric within the thyroid gland. The tumour is TSH dependent. The condition of 'lateral aberrant thyroid' more correctly represents secondary deposit of papillary carcinoma in lymph nodes.
- *Follicular carcinoma (20%)* has a peak incidence is in the 40–60 age group. Distant metastasis is normally to lung and bone. Occasionally the disease presents with bony secondaries.

Anaplastic carcinoma (5–8%) Occurs in old age. Usually rapidly growing and locally invasive with early spread via the lymphatics and bloodstream to lungs, bone and brain. Stridor, dysphagia, recurrent laryngeal nerve palsy may occur.

Medullary carcinoma (5%) May present at any age. Arises from parafollicular C cells. Secretes calcitonin. Presents with solitary nodule or mass and may spread to cervical nodes. It may be familial and associated with MEN. Identification of the ret-proto-oncogene on chromosome 10 is necessary. When present, family screening is indicated. Prophylactic thyroidectomy may be offered in positively screened individuals.

Lymphoma (5%) May be diagnosed on FNAC but usually on histopathology analysis after thyroidectomy. There is an increased incidence of lymphoma originating in the thyroid in Hashimoto's thyroiditis.

Symptoms and signs for malignant goitres Patients are usually euthyroid. Rarely is the tumour toxic. Well-differentiated thyroid cancer (i.e. papillary and follicular) usually presents with a thyroid nodule. Cervical nodes may be enlarged and there may be local discomfort in the neck. Bone pain may represent secondary disease and may be the presenting symptom. Cough may be due to lung metastases. Medullary carcinoma may be familial and associated with MEN. Anaplastic carcinoma occurs in the elderly. There will be a hard craggy mass which may be locally invasive with lymph node involvement. Stridor, dysphagia, pain, and hoarseness may occur.

Investigations • Ultrasound scan: solid nodule • Isotope scan: 'cold nodule' • FNAC • CXR: lung metastases • Skeletal radiographs if bone pain • Calcitonin levels if medullary carcinoma suspected • FNAC is the mainstay of preoperative investigation. When medullary cancer is present, evidence of other endocrine neoplasia must be sought; in particular, hyperparathyroidism and phaeochromocytoma must be identified or excluded.

Treatment

Well-differentiated (papillary/follicular) Total thyroidectomy and excision of all involved nodes. ^{123}I diagnostic scanning for secondary disease and ^{131}I ablation treatment. Life-long thyroxine treatment is required as (a) replacement therapy and (b) to achieve TSH suppression. Thyroglobulin estimations should be carried out 6-monthly as a marker of recurrent disease. Subsequent ^{131}I therapy may be used for secondary disease – although bony secondaries are best treated with external beam irradiation.

Anaplastic Surgery is rarely indicated. Response to radiotherapy is poor. Chemotherapy is usually ineffective. Surgical debulking to relieve pressure on the trachea and oesophagus may allow palliation.

Medullary Total thyroidectomy with removal of all affected lymph nodes. Follow-up includes regular calcitonin levels. Failure of reduction in calcitonin levels suggests residual →

tumour. Recurrence of high calcitonin levels suggests tumour recurrence. These should be sought and removed surgically. Inoperable tumours should be irradiated.

Lymphoma Treatment depends upon the type and is a matter for a specialist in lymphoma treatment.

Prognosis

Well-differentiated (papillary/follicular) Prognosis can be excellent. Around 9% of patients will die of the disease and 30% will need treatment for secondary disease. Adverse prognostic factors include increasing age (especially over 40) at first presentation, male gender and metastatic spread.

Anaplastic Poor prognosis. 1-year survival is less than 10%.

Medullary Without metastases the prognosis is excellent and cure may be expected. With metastases the 10-year survival is less than 50%.

INFLAMMATORY CONDITIONS OF THE THYROID

These are rare.

Subacute thyroiditis (de Quervain's)

This is a self-limiting condition associated with giant cells and granulomata. Symptoms include pain, swelling, enlarged tender thyroid, malaise, myalgia. The ESR is raised. Aspirin and steroids give symptomatic relief. The acute symptoms last 10–14 days.

Riedel's thyroiditis

This is a woody hard goitre which infiltrates into adjacent muscle. It may compress the trachea and may be associated with retroperitoneal fibrosis. It must be differentiated from anaplastic carcinoma. Surgery is necessary occasionally to confirm the diagnosis and to relieve pressure on the oesophagus and trachea.

Hashimoto's disease

An autoimmune disease, it causes diffuse lymphocytic infiltration of the thyroid gland with destruction of the functioning thyroid tissue. Eventually the patient becomes hypothyroid.

Symptoms and signs Occurs almost exclusively in females. Diffusely enlarged non-tender goitre. Symptoms and signs of hypothyroidism depending on stage of disease.

Investigations • TSH (↑) • May be low free T4 • Many patients are euthyroid • Antimicrosomal antibody titres and antithyroglobulin titres raised • Diagnosis confirmed by FNAC • Beware confusing this condition with lymphoma.

Treatment Surgery may be required for goitres causing severe pressure symptoms. Isthmusectomy may be appropriate.

THYROIDECTOMY

Indications

These are malignancy, thyrotoxicosis, tracheal compression, cosmetic for unsightly goitre.

Preoperative preparation

Thyrotoxic patients should be rendered euthyroid preoperatively. The vocal cords should be checked preoperatively. A very few patients may show an unsuspected vocal cord paralysis preoperatively. This is an important consideration in view of possible intraoperative recurrent laryngeal nerve damage. The patient should be warned of possible nerve damage. Permanent injury occurs in 1–2% of thyroidectomies but possibly as often as 10% in reexploration procedures. A warning should be given regarding hypocalcaemia which is usually a transient problem. It will be seen in about 30% of cases of total thyroidectomy with about 2% of patients still requiring replacement therapy at 3 months postoperatively.

Operations

The following operations are appropriate: solitary benign nodule requires lobectomy; cancer requires total thyroidectomy; thyrotoxicosis or large multinodular goitre requires subtotal or total thyroidectomy. Total thyroidectomy is increasingly the operation of choice.

Complications

Haemorrhage This may cause airways obstruction. Treatment is by opening the wound, evacuating the haematoma and securing haemostasis. This may need to be done on the ward. Instruments to remove clips or stitches must be within ready reach in the postoperative period.

Laryngeal oedema It may occur with or without compression from a haematoma. Stridor and respiratory distress occur. Intubation is required. The condition usually settles spontaneously.

Nerve damage

Recurrent laryngeal nerve Damage to this may be unilateral, bilateral, temporary, or permanent. Unilateral injury usually causes hoarseness. If this is due to neuropraxia, the voice returns to normal within 3 months. If damage is bilateral, airways obstruction occurs after extubation and repeating intubation or emergency tracheostomy is required. If injury is permanent, tracheostomy will be permanent. Laser arytenoidectomy to lateralize the vocal cords is an alternative.

Superior laryngeal nerve This may result in variable degrees of huskiness or weakness of the voice with change in volume and pitch. Singers, actors and others who rely on their voice professionally should be warned of this possible complication.

Thyroid storm (thyrotoxic crisis) Seen rarely nowadays, because of better preoperative preparation. Hypercatabolic state due to uncontrolled thyrotoxicosis usually in an inadequately prepared patient who is undergoing surgery for thyrotoxicosis. Symptoms include hyperpyrexia, confusion, restlessness, sweating, arrhythmias. Treatment includes propranolol, hydrocortisone and potassium iodide.

Hypocalcaemia Tetany may occur because of ischaemia, or removal, of the parathyroids. Usually occurs within 2–5 days postoperatively. Symptoms include circumoral paraesthesia with tingling of the extremities. Chvostek's sign (tap the facial nerve in front of the external auditory meatus – with hypocalcaemia the side of the face will twitch). In severe hypocalcaemia, painful carpopedal spasms and spasm of respiratory muscles may occur. Treatment is by slow infusion of 10 ml 10% calcium gluconate followed by oral calcium administration. Ionized calcium should be monitored to avoid symptoms developing. Usually calcium therapy is needed for a limited period of time – up to 3 months – but long-term management will require 1α vitamin D. This is also sometimes needed in the short term if hypocalcaemia is profound. Occasionally parathyroid recovery can be very slow – taking up to 2 years. Calcium levels must be monitored to avoid hypercalcaemia developing.

Wound infection This is rare.

Recurrent thyrotoxicosis

Hypothyroidism

Keloid scar

PARATHYROIDS

Hyperparathyroidism is the most common clinical disorder of the parathyroid glands. Ischaemia to the parathyroid glands may occur during thyroid surgery and result in hypoparathyroidism.

HYPERPARATHYROIDISM

Three types occur: primary, secondary and tertiary hyperparathyroidism.

Primary hyperparathyroidism

This may result from a parathyroid adenoma (85%), diffuse parathyroid hyperplasia (15%) and, rarely, from carcinoma of the parathyroid. Hyperparathyroidism is the commonest component of MEN I syndrome.

Symptoms and signs These are classically 'stones, bones, abdominal groans and moans'.

Stones Renal calculi occur in 5% of patients with hyperparathyroidism. All patients with renal calculi should have their serum calcium and phosphate checked.

Bones Osteitis fibrosa cystica. Bone pain and fractures may occur.

Abdominal groans Dyspepsia, constipation and peptic ulceration may occur; pancreatitis is a complication of hyperparathyroidism.

Moans Psychiatric manifestations may occur, e.g. confusion, depression, psychosis. However, many patients have non-specific symptoms, e.g. weakness, fatigue, lethargy, arthralgia, anorexia. Some patients are asymptomatic, hypercalcaemia being detected on routine screening performed for other reasons.

Investigations • Ca↑ (no tourniquet and correct for hypoalbuminaemia – ionized calcium preferred) • Phosphates usually↓ • PTH↑ • Increased urinary excretion of calcium (calcium-restricted diet) • Radiographs: skull may show characteristic 'ground glass' appearance • Abnormal sella turcica if MEN associated with pituitary tumour • Hands: subperiosteal resorption of bone (best seen on radial aspect of middle phalanges and tufts of terminal phalanges) • Abdomen: nephrocalcinosis • Preoperative localization of the problem:

- Ultrasonography.
- Technetium/thallium scanning. Thallium is taken up by thyroids and parathyroids while technetium is taken up only by the thyroid. Administer thallium and scan. Administer technetium and scan again. Subtract technetium image from thallium image. This will demonstrate parathyroids.
- Selective venous sampling and PTH assay from draining veins.
- CT or MRI.

Most tests, however, are neither sensitive nor specific enough. In general, localization is not carried out. An experienced surgeon is, however, essential. Sestamibi scanning is under evaluation and may be useful for localization. When the gland is not located at surgery, selective venous sampling of neck and mediastinal veins for PTH assay is indicated.

Differential diagnosis Need to exclude other causes of hypercalcaemia, e.g. malignancy, myeloma, sarcoidosis, milk–alkali syndrome. PTH is normal or low in these conditions.

Treatment Surgery is the treatment of choice. Some surgeons consider preoperative localization of the glands essential. All four glands should be identified at operation. Occasionally there are three, five or even six glands. A parathyroid adenoma is removed. If there is hyperplasia of all glands, total parathyroidectomy or $3\frac{1}{2}$ gland parathyroidectomy is performed. The residual $\frac{1}{2}$-gland should be marked with a surgical clip. The vogue for forearm reimplantation of the gland is now superseded. Patients having total parathyroidectomy can usually be managed on 1α vitamin D alone. When an adenoma cannot be found in the neck, or in the superior mediastinum explored through the neck – or when a hyperplastic gland is not identifiable – thoracotomy may be needed. This should only be done after the missing gland has been identified by venous sampling, isotope studies, or CT/MRI scanning. The missing gland may not be in the chest – it may be intrathyroidal. Parathyroidectomy is an operation for an experienced surgeon doing this type of surgery on a regular basis. Even so, an additional parathyroid gland may be overlooked and further surgery be required. Hypoparathyroidism may occur postoperatively.

Secondary hyperparathyroidism

This usually occurs in patients with chronic renal failure although it may be seen in any situation which results in low serum calcium. Hypocalcaemia results in stimulation of the parathyroids with resulting hyperplasia. Patients in CRF are unable to synthesize vitamin D and develop hypocalcaemia, hypophosphataemia, and impaired calcium absorption.

Symptoms and signs These are of CRF. Bone pain, pruritus, metastatic extravascular calcification.

Treatment Correct the underlying cause. In CRF, patients require aluminium hydroxide to reduce phosphate, vitamin D, calcium supplements and high-calcium dialysate. Surgery is required in patients refractory to medical treatment with bone pain, pruritus and metastatic calcification.

Tertiary hyperparathyroidism

Hyperparathyroidism persists in patients who have had successful renal transplants. The parathyroid hyperplasia of long-term renal disease becomes autonomous despite the return of calcium levels to normal. The symptoms are those of secondary hyperparathyroidism. Treatment is by subtotal parathyroidectomy.

ADRENAL GLAND

The adrenal glands consists of an outer cortex and an inner medulla. The adrenal cortex may overfunction because of hyperplasia or tumour. This may result in an overproduction of glucocorticoids (Cushing's syndrome) or mineralocorticoids (Conn's syndrome). The most common tumour of the adrenal medulla is a phaeochromocytoma which secretes adrenaline and noradrenaline. Adrenal insufficiency may be primary (Addison's disease) or due to tuberculosis, metastatic disease, adrenal haemorrhage or withdrawal after long-term steroid therapy.

ADRENAL CORTEX

Cushing's syndrome

This is the result of increased secretion of cortisol. Cushing's disease results from overproduction of ACTH by the pituitary resulting in bilateral adrenocortical hyperplasia. Cushing's syndrome refers to increased secretion of cortisol of any origin and includes adrenal adenoma, adrenal carcinoma, administration of exogenous corticosteroids, as well as ectopic ACTH secretion, e.g. oat cell bronchial carcinoma.

Symptoms and signs The presentation is variable. Any or all of the following may occur. Truncal obesity, buffalo hump, moon face, proximal myopathy of the limbs, skin striae, acne, hirsutism, capillary fragility with bruising, oedema, hypertension, osteoporosis, psychiatric disturbances, diabetes, peptic ulceration, pancreatitis, cataracts, skin pigmentation, avascular necrosis of bone.

Investigations • U&Es: hypokalaemia • Blood sugar↑ • CXR may show oat cell bronchial carcinoma • Plasma cortisol: the diurnal variation is lost • Low dose dexamethasone suppression test: give 2 mg of dexamethasone at 11 p.m. and check plasma cortisol at 8 a.m. Failure to suppress levels below 170 nmol/l suggests Cushing's • Urinary free cortisol is elevated in Cushing's syndrome • ACTH levels: high in pituitary-dependent cases, low or undetectable with adrenal tumour, may be very high with ectopic ACTH secretion • CT scan or MRI scan of adrenals and pituitary fossa.

Treatment If the symptoms are due to adenoma or carcinoma, the affected adrenal gland is removed. For bilateral hyperplasia, with ACTH suppression, bilateral adrenalectomy is indicated with permanent replacement steroid therapy. For pituitary tumours, hypophysectomy is required. This may be done by transphenoidal resection or an yttrium implant. For ectopic ACTH secretion the source should be excised if possible, e.g. pneumonectomy for oat cell carcinoma of the lung. In inoperable cases, radiotherapy may be useful. Bilateral adrenalectomy may be required to control the symptoms. Metyrapone, which inhibits cortisol production, may also be beneficial in cases not amenable to surgery.

Conn's syndrome (primary hyperaldosteronism)

There is excessive secretion of aldosterone independent of the renin–angiotensin mechanism. It is more common in females. The condition is usually due to a unilateral adenoma. Rarely, there are bilateral adenomas, carcinoma or bilateral hyperplasia. The primary type must be distinguished from secondary hyperaldosteronism where there is an increased plasma renin due to increased activity of the renin–angiotensin mechanism. This may occur in renal artery stenosis, cirrhosis, CCF or nephrotic syndrome.

Symptoms and signs May be asymptomatic. Hypertension, lethargy, fatigue, muscle weakness (due to hypokalaemia), polyuria, polydipsia.

Investigations • U&Es (hypokalaemia, alkalosis) • Plasma aldosterone raised (no diuretics) • Plasma renin levels low • CT scan will identify adenoma.

Treatment Unilateral adrenalectomy to remove adenoma. Preoperative preparation includes spironolactone daily for 4 weeks with potassium supplements. Bilateral adrenal hyperplasia responds to long-term spironolactone.

ADRENAL MEDULLA

Phaeochromocytoma

This is a catecholamine-producing tumour that arises from the chromaffin cells of the adrenal medulla or other sympathetic

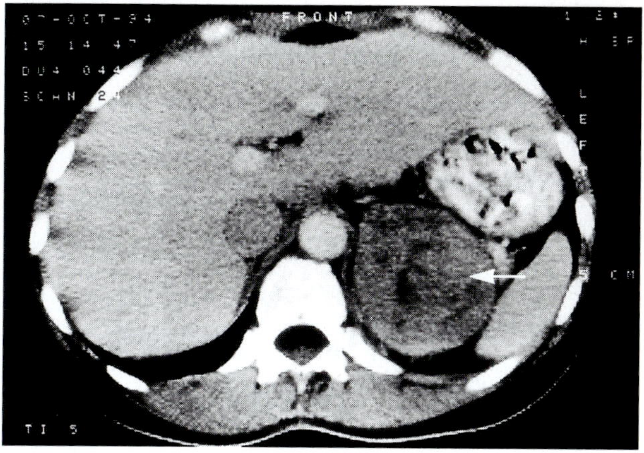

Fig. 11.2 An abdominal CT scan showing a large phaeochromocytoma (arrow) in the left adrenal gland.

nervous tissue, e.g. aortic paraganglia. 10% are malignant. 10% are associated with other conditions, e.g. MEN, von Recklinghausen's disease and von Hippel–Lindau disease.

Symptoms and signs Paroxysmal hypertension. Headaches, palpitations, sweating, pallor, dyspnoea, anxiety, chest pain, weakness.

Investigations • Blood sugar • 24-hour urine for VMA (spurious results occur with excess of tea, coffee, chocolates, bananas or vanilla extract) • CT scanning will locate 90% (→ Fig. 11.2) • ^{131}I-metaiodobenzylguanidine scanning.

Treatment Surgical excision. Preoperative stabilization required. α-adrenergic blockade with phenoxybenzamine and β-blockade with propranolol. Treatment should be given prior to surgery until symptoms are abolished. High dosage may need to be gradually introduced to block the adrenergic effects of the tumour. Any diabetogenic effect of the tumour should be controlled – often with insulin. Occasionally phaeochromocytomas can present acutely with cardiac arrhythmias, hypotensive episodes, encephalopathy and coma. Haemorrhagic rupture of the tumour may occur with shock. In these cases, α-adrenergic blockade with i.v. phentolamine followed by emergency surgery.

ADRENAL INSUFFICIENCY

This may be primary (Addison's disease) when adrenal destruction may be autoimmune, or due to sarcoidosis, tuberculosis, amyloidosis, secondary deposits, adrenal haemorrhage (anticoagulant therapy) or meningococcal septicaemia (Waterhouse–Friderichsen syndrome); or secondary due to pituitary disease or withdrawal of long-term steroid therapy. Bilateral adrenalectomy is an iatrogenic cause.

Symptoms and signs

Acute adrenal insufficiency Shock, nausea, vomiting, hyperpyrexia, rigors, abdominal pain, coma.

Chronic adrenal insufficiency Anorexia, lethargy, malaise, hypotension, weight loss, constipation, amenorrhoea, hyperpigmentation of skin.

Investigations • Check steroid therapy • Check BP • U&Es: $K^+\uparrow$, $Na^+\downarrow$, blood sugar↓, serum cortisol levels reduced with no response to synacthen test • ACTH levels high in Addison's disease and low in secondary causes • Adrenal antibody screen • CXR: may show TB • AXR: adrenal gland calcification in TB.

Treatment The acute case requires resuscitation with i.v. saline and hydrocortisone 100 mg i.v. 6-hourly. Clinical improvement is often dramatic. Chronic adrenal insufficiency is treated with oral hydrocortisone 20 mg mane and 10 mg nocte. Fludrocortisone as mineralocorticoid replacement (0.5–1.0 mg daily) is indicated in most patients. Fatigue, hypotension, and hyperkalaemia are signs of undertreatment. Hypertension, oedema, and hypokalaemia are signs of overtreatment. Patients on replacement therapy should be warned that increased doses are required at times of stress, e.g. surgery or an acute illness. Care should be taken in reducing steroids and discontinuing them in patients who have been under long-term therapy. In many patients, gradual withdrawal over weeks will allow endogenous steroid production to resume but in others, signs of insufficiency will appear.

MULTIPLE ENDOCRINE NEOPLASIA (MEN)

MEN syndromes are patterns of endocrine disease usually inherited as autosomal dominant traits.

MEN I

Manifestations are hyperparathyroidism, pancreatic tumours (insulinoma, gastrinomas) and pituitary tumours (prolactinoma).

Symptoms and signs Most patients present with symptoms related to peptic ulceration (gastrinoma) or to the pituitary tumour. The hyperparathyroidism is usually asymptomatic and is detected incidentally on checking Ca levels.

Treatment Directed at the tumours causing symptoms.

MEN IIa

Manifestations are medullary carcinoma of the thyroid, phaeochromocytoma and parathyroid hyperplasia.

Symptoms and signs Check relatives of patients with medullary carcinoma of the thyroid. Genetic screening for the ret-proto-oncogene in the patient. If latter is present family screening is necessary. If positive in the family, for example children, brothers, sisters (and their progeny), prophylactic thyroidectomy may be considered. Search should be made for all tumours in the syndrome prior to treatment.

Treatment If phaeochromocytoma is located, treat this first. Then deal with thyroid and parathyroid at the same operation.

MEN IIb

Manifestation are medullary carcinoma of the thyroid, phaeochromocytoma, multiple mucosal neuromas and marfanoid habitus.

Symptoms and signs Early appearance of marfanoid habitus and mucosal neuromas suggests diagnosis. It occurs in first and second decades. Other symptoms are as for Type IIa.

Treatment MEN IIb presents more aggressively than Type IIa and therefore prompt diagnosis and treatment are required.

12

Abdominal wall and hernia

HERNIAE

A hernia is an abnormal protrusion of a viscus or part of a viscus through an opening in the cavity in which it is normally contained. About 75% of all herniae occur at the groin.

Reducible hernia

This is one in which the contents of the sac reduce spontaneously or can be pushed back manually.

Irreducible hernia

This is one whose contents cannot be returned to the peritoneal cavity either because there are adhesions between the sac and contents or because of the narrow neck of the sac.

Irreducible herniae may be:

Incarcerated There are adhesions between the sac and the contents, but there is no obstruction or interference with blood supply. The hernia simply will not reduce.

Obstructed A hollow viscus is trapped within the sac and obstruction occurs. The blood supply remains intact. This is a common cause of small bowel obstruction.

Strangulated The arterial blood supply to the contents of the sac is compromised such that unless surgical relief is undertaken the contents of the sac will become gangrenous.

GENERAL DESCRIPTION OF A HERNIA (→ Fig. 12.1)

Defect This is in the abdominal wall, e.g. at the deep inguinal ring or femoral ring; or a defect in a surgical incision (incisional hernia).

Sac This has a neck which may be very narrow, a body and a fundus.

Contents of the sac May be omentum, bowel, ovary, etc.

CLASSIFICATION OF HERNIAE

Congenital

A congenital hernia develops in a peritoneal sac, which gives rise to a hernia in infancy, or provides a potential channel for one to form in later life, e.g. patent processus vaginalis in indirect inguinal hernia, or failure of closure of the umbilicus orifice in umbilical hernia. These sacs represent persistent embryological channels.

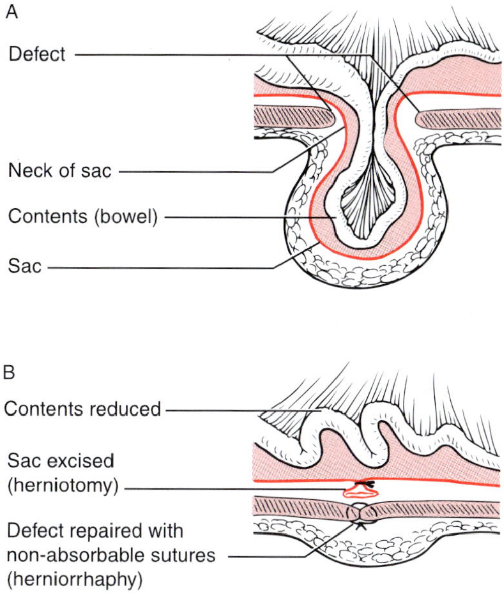

Fig. 12.1 **A.** General description of a hernia. **B.** Principles of repair.

Acquired

Aetiological factors

- Loss of tissue strength and elasticity, e.g. direct inguinal hernia in the older patient.
- Surgical trauma, e.g. incisional hernia.
- Enlargement of a foramen, e.g. enlarged oesophageal hiatus allowing development of a hiatus hernia.
- Nerve damage with consequent weakening of muscles, e.g. development of inguinal hernia after appendicectomy owing to damage to the ilioinguinal nerve.

If a potential weakness is present then the following factors may predispose to hernia formation by increasing intra-abdominal pressure. These include:

- heavy lifting or carrying
- coughing, e.g. asthma, COPD
- constipation
- benign prostatic hypertrophy
- pregnancy

- obesity
- ascites
- CAPD – may unmask persistent processus vaginalis with CAPD fluid filling a potential hernial sac and presenting as scrotal oedema.

TYPES OF HERNIA

Inguinal hernia

This is the most common form of hernia. There are two types:

Indirect A peritoneal sac protrudes through the deep inguinal ring, passes down the inguinal canal, and may extend as far as the upper pole of the testis. The defect is congenital and is due to a persistent processus vaginalis. It is more common in males. It may appear in infancy or early adult life. In infants there is often an associated hydrocele and undescended testis.

Direct This is acquired. The defect occurs in the abdominal wall, in Hesselbach's triangle (bounded by the inguinal ligament inferiorly, the inferior epigastric artery laterally and the lateral border of rectus muscle medially). It is due to a weakness of the transversalis fascia in the posterior wall of the inguinal canal. It is often bilateral and occurs in the older patient and may be associated with obesity, cough, constipation, prostatism.

Both types may occur and straddle the inferior epigastric artery, the so-called 'pantaloon' hernia.

Symptoms and signs Often none. Occasionally aching or dragging sensation in the groin. Some patients relate the development of the hernia to an episode of straining or lifting. Some patients can push the hernia back. A painful, tense, tender lump which will not reduce indicates incipient strangulation until proved otherwise. Examine the patient standing. A hernia that descends into the scrotum is likely to be indirect. A diffuse bulge medially over the canal is likely to be direct. Locate the pubic tubercle. If the hernia is above and medial to this it is an inguinal hernia, if it is below and lateral, it is a femoral hernia. Test for a cough impulse. Lay the patient down and reduce the hernia. Apply pressure over the deep inguinal ring, i.e. 1 cm above the midpoint of the inguinal ligament. Ask the patient to cough. If the hernia appears medial to the point of pressure, it is likely to be direct. If no hernia appears, release the pressure and again get the patient to cough. If it appears, it is likely to be indirect. For smaller herniae it is possible to distinguish between direct and indirect by invaginating the scrotum with the little finger into the inguinal canal. Get the patient to cough. If the hernia is indirect the impulse hits the tip of the finger; if direct it hits the pulp. The difference, in fact, is academic since both will be carefully looked for at surgery.

Treatment

Uncomplicated Elective herniotomy (i.e. excision of sac) in children. Herniotomy and herniorrhaphy (repair of the defect) in adults. There are two accepted methods of repair of inguinal hernia:

1. Lichtenstein repair – this is a tension-free mesh repair using polypropylene mesh
2. Shouldice repair – this is a double-breasted repair of the transversalis fascia followed by suturing of the conjoint tendon to the inguinal ligament with non-absorbable sutures.

Trusses may be used if surgery is contraindicated. A spring-loaded pad is applied to the defect after the hernia has been reduced. The patient should apply it after lying down and reducing the hernia. They are uncomfortable and unhygienic. Indications for a truss are rare.

Obstructed and strangulated herniae These require emergency surgery, with resection of bowel if necessary followed by surgical repair.

Complications Recurrence may occur but should be less than 2%. Other complications include infection, ilioinguinal nerve entrapment, and testicular ischaemia. Testicular ischaemia is rare after initial repair but occurs with a higher incidence after repair of recurrent herniae, possibly owing to cord damage.

Femoral hernia

The defect is in the transversalis fascia overlying the femoral ring at the entry to the femoral canal. The hernia passes through the femoral canal and presents in the groin, below and lateral to the pubic tubercle. It is more common in females and carries a higher risk of strangulation. Femoral herniae are often of the Richter type.

Symptoms and signs A lump occurs below and lateral to the pubic tubercle. It may be reducible. It may not be noticed until it becomes tender and painful. This type of hernia should be carefully sought in the obese patient who presents with signs of intestinal obstruction without an obvious cause.

Treatment Surgical repair. An incision is made directly over the swelling. The sac is opened and the contents reduced and the sac removed. The defect is repaired by inserting non-absorbable sutures between the inguinal ligament and the pectineal ligament thus closing the femoral canal. If the hernia

→

is strangulated or obstructed, a separate abdominal incision will be required to deal with the bowel. There is no place for a truss in the treatment of femoral hernia. It may, in fact, be dangerous by compressing the contents of an incompletely emptied sac against the pubic bone. This is one reason why it is necessary to distinguish accurately between inguinal and femoral herniae. Recurrence rate following surgery should be less than 3%.

Umbilical hernia

This occurs in children because of incomplete closure of the umbilical orifice. The majority close spontaneously during the first year of life. It is more common in black children. Surgical repair should only be carried out if the hernia has not disappeared by the age of 3 and the fascial defect is greater than 1.5 cm in diameter.

Paraumbilical hernia

It occurs just above or just below the umbilicus, and is more common in females. Predisposing factors include multiple pregnancies and obesity. The neck of the sac is usually narrow and therefore there is a high risk of strangulation. The most common content is omentum followed by transverse colon and small intestine. Treatment is by excision of the sac and a two-layer overlapping repair (Mayo repair).

Epigastric hernia

This is usually a small protrusion through the linea alba in the upper part of the abdomen. Often the hernia consists of extraperitoneal fat only, but it may contain omentum or small bowel. It may be extremely painful, probably because of trapping and ischaemia of extraperitoneal fat. Treatment is by simple suture of the defect with non-absorbable sutures.

Incisional hernia

This occurs through a defect in the scar of a previous abdominal incision.

Aetiology

- Age. Wound healing is poor in the older patient.
- General debility, e.g. carcinomatosis, cirrhosis.
- Obesity.
- Postoperative wound infection.
- Postoperative wound haematoma.
- Raised intra-abdominal pressure postoperatively, e.g. coughing, straining, constipation, ileus.
- Steroid therapy.

- Type of incision. Midline vertical wounds have a higher incidence than transverse incisions. Incisional hernia is exceptionally rare through a Pfannenstiel incision.
- Poor suturing technique. Rarely does a suture break.

Symptoms and signs May occur up to 5 years postoperatively. A swelling protrudes through the wound. Many are large and involve the whole incision and consequently the neck of the sac is wide and the risk of strangulation rare. If the defect is small there is a greater risk of strangulation.

Treatment

Small herniae These may be repaired with interrupted non-absorbable sutures.

Large herniae These may be very unsightly and noticeable through the clothes. If the patient is unfit for surgery, a corset may be worn. Surgical repair should otherwise be undertaken. The old scar should be excised and normal rectus sheath identified. The edges may then be approximated with non-absorbable sutures. Often to get an adequate repair the hernia is repaired in two layers overlapping. Very large defects may need interposition of foreign material, e.g. polypropylene mesh (Marlex) or ePTFE sheet. The recurrence rate is high, being 10–20%.

Richter's hernia (→ Fig. 12.2)

Part of the circumference of the bowel becomes trapped in the defect. This is usually the antimesenteric border of the small bowel. A strangulated Richter's hernia may reduce spontaneously leaving a segment of bowel with a gangrenous area which may subsequently perforate with resulting peritonitis.

Spigelian hernia

This is a hernia through the linea semilunaris at the lateral border

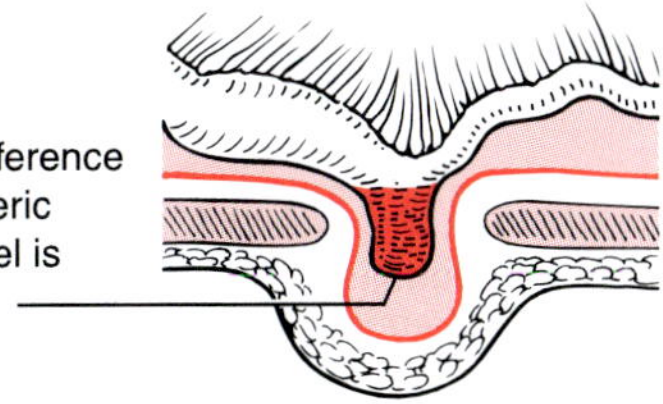

Fig. 12.2 Richter's hernia.

of the rectus sheath. It occurs at a point a hand's breadth above the pubic symphysis at the level of the linea semicircularis (arcuate line of Douglas). This is the point at which the posterior rectus sheath becomes deficient and all aponeuroses of the abdominal muscles pass in front of the rectus muscle. Surgical repair is required.

Littre's hernia
This is a hernia that contains a Meckel's diverticulum in the sac.

Sliding hernia (hernia-en-glissade → Fig. 12.3)
The posterior parietal peritoneum 'slides' on the underlying tissue; therefore, the posterior wall of the sac is formed, not of peritoneum alone, but of sigmoid colon on the left and caecum on the right. These herniae occur in older patients especially males with obesity and weak musculature. Diagnosis is made at surgery. Care needs to be taken when excising the sac.

Obturator hernia
This hernia occurs through the obturator foramen. It is commoner in elderly females. The diagnosis is usually made via a laparotomy for intestinal obstruction. It is difficult to feel the hernia as it occurs in the groin deep to pectineus. The hernia may cause pressure on the obturator nerve at the obturator foramen causing referred pain down the medial side of the thigh, especially if the hernia is strangulated.

Lumbar herniae
These may occur through Grynfeltt's space (below the 12th rib) or Petit's triangle (just above the iliac crest). They usually contain extraperitoneal fat and are often mistaken for lipomas.

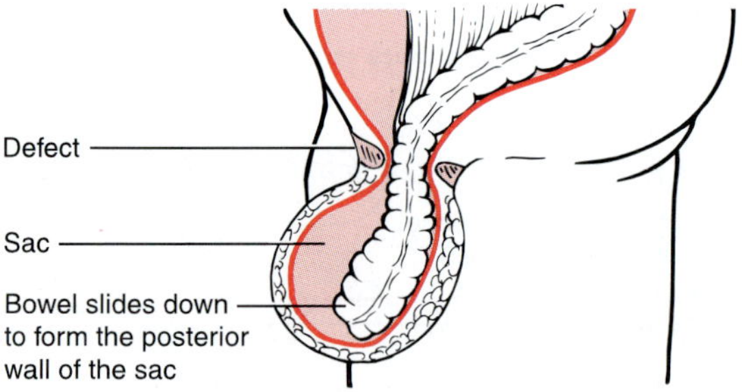

Fig. 12.3 Sliding hernia. Part of the bowel wall (sigmoid colon or caecum) forms the posterior wall of the sac.

Internal herniae

Usually they present with intestinal obstruction. They are often the result of iatrogenic causes such as defects left in the mesentery or following adhesions. Rarely, they may occur through the epiploic foramen of Winslow or into paracaecal or paraduodenal fossae.

OTHER CONDITIONS OF THE ABDOMINAL WALL

UMBILICUS

Discharge

Patent vitellointestinal duct This may result in discharge of mucus or small bowel contents. It is usually associated with a Meckel's diverticulum and usually occurs in infancy.

Patent urachus This may not present until early adult life or even old age and results from distension of the bladder usually because of outflow obstruction. Urine discharges through the umbilicus.

Abscess in a urachal cyst This may discharge through the umbilicus.

Infection This may occur deep in the umbilicus and cause discharge. It may be fungal. Inflammation of the umbilicus is called omphalitis.

Umbilical calculus This is usually black in colour and composed of inspissated desquamated epithelium and may be associated with infection and discharge. This condition is not infrequently seen in the elderly and associated with poor hygiene.

Endometriosis The umbilicus is usually painful and bleeds at the time of menstruation.

Mass

Umbilical hernia (see above)

Secondary carcinoma This is rare and presents as an umbilical nodule (Sister Joseph's nodule). It may be associated with carcinoma of the stomach, colon, ovary or breast.

RECTUS SHEATH HAEMATOMA

This is due to tearing of the inferior epigastric vessels with haematoma in the posterior rectus sheath. It may occur in athletic, muscular young men during exercise or in thin elderly females. Occasionally it occurs during pregnancy. It may be also associated with disorders of coagulation or blood dyscrasias.

Symptoms and signs Sudden onset of severe lower abdominal pain in the left or right lower abdomen. Occasionally its onset is slow and progressive. Examination in the early stages reveals a tender mass in the abdominal wall. Later bruising may be detectable in the suprapubic area.

Treatment This is usually conservative. The acute pain and discomfort should disappear within a few days. In young patients with a rectus sheath haematoma on the right side, the symptoms and signs are often mistaken for acute appendicitis.

TUMOURS OF THE ABDOMINAL WALL

Most of these are benign lipomas. Most malignant tumours of the abdominal wall are metastatic. Musculoaponeurotic fibromatoses (desmoid tumours) may occur and are part of Gardner's syndrome (familial polyposis coli, osteomas, sebaceous cysts and desmoid tumours).

SWELLINGS IN THE GROIN AND SCROTUM

These are a common clinical problem. A list of conditions is shown in Table 12.1. They are discussed further in the relevant chapters.

Table 12.1
Lumps in the groin and scrotum

Groin	**Above the inguinal ligament** Sebaceous cyst Lipoma Direct inguinal hernia Indirect inguinal hernia Imperfectly descended testis Lipoma of the cord Hydrocele of the cord (rare) Hydrocele of the canal of Nuck (rare)
	Below the inguinal ligament Sebaceous cyst Lipoma Femoral hernia Lymph nodes Saphena varix Femoral artery aneurysm (true or false) Imperfectly descended testis Neuroma of femoral nerve (rare) Synovioma of hip joint (rare) Obturator hernia (rare) Psoas abscess (rare)
Scrotum	Sebaceous cyst Indirect inguinal hernia Hydrocele Epididymal cyst (spermatocele) Epididymo-orchitis Testicular tumour Torsion of testes Varicocele Haematocele Sperm granuloma Torsion of testicular appendage

13 Acute abdomen

BASIC PRINCIPLES

Acute abdomen is the most common cause of emergency admission to a surgical unit. The term 'acute abdomen' is difficult to define but it indicates any non-traumatic disorder of acute onset in which the symptoms are predominantly abdominal and for which in some cases urgent surgery may be indicated. In practice it represents a spectrum of problems ranging from sudden onset of severe abdominal pain with a life-threatening underlying cause to minor abdominal symptoms of lengthy duration. The most important feature of the acute abdomen is to sort out the severe causes which need urgent surgery (e.g. ruptured aortic aneurysm, perforated diverticulitis) from severe abdominal pain that does not require surgery (biliary colic, ureteric colic, pancreatitis); and also from those conditions which do not need urgent investigation and treatment (e.g. mild gastroenteritis, constipation). Prompt diagnosis is essential. A careful history and examination will indicate the cause of most acute abdomens.

History

Age Certain conditions are more likely to occur in certain age groups, e.g. mesenteric adenitis in children, diverticulitis in the older patient.

Pain
- Time and mode of onset, e.g. sudden, gradual.
- Character, e.g. dull, vague, cramping, sharp, burning.
- Severity.
- Constancy, e.g. continuous pain of peritonitis; intermittent pain of intestinal colic.
- Location: where did it start, has it moved?
- Radiation, e.g. loin to groin in ureteric colic.
- Effect of respiration, movement, food, defaecation, micturition, menstruation.

Vomiting
- Did vomiting precede the pain?
- Frequency.
- Character, e.g. bile, faeculent, blood, coffee grounds.

Defaecation
- Constipation: absolute constipation with colicky abdominal pain, distension, and vomiting suggests intestinal obstruction.
- Diarrhoea: frequency, consistency of stools, blood, mucus, pus.

Fever Any rigors.

Past history
- Previous surgery, e.g. adhesions may cause intestinal obstruction.
- Recent trauma, e.g. delayed rupture of spleen.
- Menstrual history, e.g. ectopic pregnancy.

Examination

General Is the patient lying comfortably? Is the patient lying still but in pain, e.g. peritonitis? Is the patient writhing in agony, e.g. ureteric or biliary colic? Is the patient flushed suggesting pyrexia?

Pulse, temperature, respiration

Cervical lymphadenopathy (e.g. mesenteric adenitis).

Chest (e.g. referred pain from lobar pneumonia).

Abdomen
- *Inspection* Moves on respiration. Scars, distended, visible peristalsis (usually chronic obstruction in patient with very thin abdominal wall). Pain on coughing. Hernial orifices. Any obvious masses, e.g. pulsatile mass to suggest aortic aneurysm.
- *Palpation* Patient relaxed, lying flat, with arms by side. Be gentle and start as far from the painful site as possible. Check for guarding and rigidity. Rebound tenderness is unpleasant for patient and is rarely helpful. Check for masses, e.g. appendix mass, pulsatile expansile mass of aortic aneurysm. Check the hernial orifices.
- *Percussion* (e.g. tympanitic note with distension due to intestinal obstruction; dullness over bladder due to acute retention).
- *Auscultation* Take your time (30–60 s), e.g. silent abdomen of peritonitis, high-pitched tinkling bowel sounds of intestinal obstruction.

Rectal examination This is just as important as the abdominal examination. It should be carried out in the left lateral position. Insert the well-lubricated gloved finger posteriorly into the sacral hollow. Move the finger around in the arc of a circle until it impinges on the peritoneum of the rectovesical or rectouterine pouch. If the patient winces with pain when the finger impinges on the peritoneum, this is a sign of peritonitis in the most dependent part of the pelvis. The pain disappears when the finger comes off the peritoneum as it completes the circle and returns to the sacral hollow. The correct annotation of a positive rectal examination should be 'tender anteriorly'. 'Tender high up in the right' is inappropriate. There seems to be a misconception among medical students that you are feeling the area of the appendix. You are feeling for tenderness due to inflammation of the pelvic peritoneum caused by infected exudates draining to the most dependent part of the pelvis, i.e. the rectovesical or rectouterine pouch.

Vaginal examination Discharge, tenderness associated with pelvic inflammatory disease, examine the uterus and adnexa, e.g. pregnancy, fibroids, ectopic pregnancy.

Investigations • WCC: raised with a neutrophil leukocytosis • U&Es • LFTs • Amylase: a high amylase confirms the diagnosis of acute pancreatitis. A mildly raised amylase may occur with a perforated viscus, intestinal obstruction, intestinal ischaemia • CXR: exclude referred lesion, gas under diaphragm (→ Fig. 13.1) • AXR: distended bowel with air/fluid levels, gallstones (10% are radio-opaque); calcified aorta, e.g. aneurysm; air in biliary tree (cholecystoduodenal fistula with gallstone ileus) • USS: e.g. ovarian cyst, ectopic pregnancy, gallstones • KUB • IVU for stones • Angiography: e.g. acute GI haemorrhage of obscure cause, superior mesenteric embolus or thrombosis (duplex scanning may also be appropriate).

Causes

Some causes of the acute abdomen are shown in Table 13.1. With the exception of the gynaecological conditions, these conditions are covered in the relevant chapters. (For information on the site of abdominal pain in relation to suspected pathology → Table 13.2.)

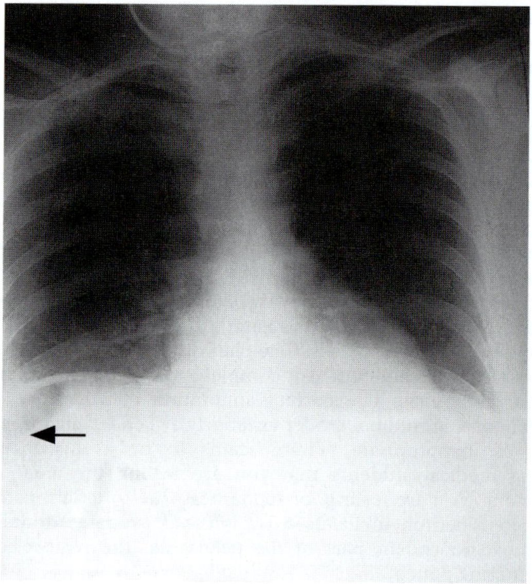

Fig. 13.1 Gas (arrow) is seen under the right hemidiaphragm following perforation of a duodenal ulcer.

Table 13.1
Causes of acute abdomen

Gastrointestinal		
	Gut	Acute appendicitis Intestinal obstruction Perforated peptic ulcer Diverticulitis Inflammatory bowel disease Acute exacerbation of peptic ulcer Gastroenteritis Mesenteric adenitis Meckel's diverticulitis
	Liver and biliary tract	Cholecystitis Cholangitis Hepatitis Biliary colic
	Pancreas	Acute pancreatitis
	Spleen	Splenic infarct and spontaneous rupture
Urinary tract		Cystitis Acute pyelonephritis Ureteric colic Acute retention
Gynaecological		Ruptured ectopic pregnancy Torsion of ovarian cyst Ruptured ovarian cyst Salpingitis Severe dysmenorrhoea Mittelschmertz Endometriosis
Vascular		Ruptured aortic aneurysm Mesenteric embolus Mesenteric venous thrombosis Ischaemic colitis Acute aortic dissection
Peritoneum		Primary peritonitis Secondary peritonitis
Abdominal wall		Rectus sheath haematoma
Retroperitoneal		Haemorrhage, e.g. anticoagulants

Table 13.2
Site of abdominal pain in relation to suspected pathology

Whole abdomen	Generalized peritonitis and mesenteric infarction
Right upper quadrant	Acute cholecystitis Cholangitis Hepatitis Peptic ulceration
Left upper quadrant	Peptic ulceration Pancreatitis Splenic infarct
Right lower quadrant	Appendicitis Ovarian cyst Ectopic pregnancy Pelvic inflammatory disease Meckel's diverticulum Mesenteric adenitis Ureteric colic Rectus sheath haematoma Right-sided lobar pneumonia
Left lower quadrant	Sigmoid diverticular disease Ovarian cyst Ectopic pregnancy Pelvic inflammatory disease Ureteric colic Rectus sheath haematoma Left-sided lobar pneumonia
Radiating pain	
Back	Peptic ulcer Pancreatitis Aortic aneurysm Acute aortic dissection
Groin	Ureteric colic Testicular torsion

Treatment
1. Relieve pain.
2. Intravenous fluids and nasogastric suction.
3. Broad-spectrum antibiotics if peritonitis or sepsis.
4. Surgery if indicated.

Indications for surgery in the acute abdomen There are no hard and fast rules but patients with the following symptoms will almost certainly require surgery:

- localized peritoneal irritation with guarding or rigidity
- spreading tenderness
- tense or progressive distension
- generalized peritonitis
- shock with bleeding or sepsis
- free gas on radiograph
- mesenteric occlusion on angiography
- blood, bile, pus or bowel contents on paracentesis.

MEDICAL CAUSES OF ACUTE ABDOMINAL PAIN

Occasionally, certain medical conditions may cause acute abdominal pain.

Referred pain It may be caused by degenerative disease of thoracic spine, herpes zoster, lobar pneumonia, pleurisy, MI.

Haematological This may be due to sickle cell crisis.

Infective and inflammatory These medical conditions are possible: tabes dorsalis, Henoch–Schönlein purpura.

Endocrine and metabolic These conditions include uraemia, hypercalcaemia, diabetic ketoacidosis, Addison's disease, acute intermittent porphyria.

PERITONITIS

Peritonitis is an inflammatory or suppurative response of the peritoneal lining to direct irritation. It may be localized or generalized, bacterial or chemical. Localized peritonitis is due to transmural inflammation of a viscus, e.g. appendicitis, cholecystitis, diverticulitis. It may remain localized through being contained by omental wrapping or adhesion of adjacent structures. In many cases, however, it becomes generalized, spreading to involve the whole peritoneum. Sudden perforation of a viscus usually results in generalized peritonitis. With the →

latter the patient is seriously ill. Hypovolaemia results from massive exudation into the peritoneal cavity, and septicaemia may result if the cause is infective, e.g. faecal peritonitis from perforated diverticulitis. Chemical peritonitis results from gastric or pancreatic juice, bile, urine or blood in the peritoneal cavity. Bile causes little reaction if sterile but causes severe peritonitis if infected or mixed with pancreatic juice. Blood and urine cause little reaction if sterile but a severe reaction occurs if they are infective. (For a classification of peritonitis → Table 13.3.)

Table 13.3
Causes of peritonitis

Acute		
	Bacterial	Primary (rare): • streptococci, pneumococci • haematogenous spread • occurs in young girls, ascites, nephrotic syndrome and postsplenectomy Secondary (common): • related to perforation, infection, inflammation or ischaemia of GI or GU tract
	Chemical	Gastric juice (e.g. perforated gastric ulcer) Pancreatic juice (e.g. acute pancreatitis) Bile (e.g. perforation of the gall bladder) Blood (e.g. ruptured spleen) Urine (e.g. intraperitoneal rupture of the bladder)
Chronic		Tuberculosis Starch (immunological reaction)

Symptoms and signs These depend on the degree of peritonitis and the precipitating cause. They also relate to the abdominal signs from the original pathology and manifestations of systemic infection. Usually there is sudden onset of abdominal pain made worse by coughing and movement. Initially it may be localized (it may remain so in some cases) but often gradually spreads to involve the whole abdomen. Nausea, vomiting, fever, abdominal tenderness (localized or generalized), guarding, rigidity, distension, absent bowel sounds when ileus supervenes. Manifestations of systemic infection include tachycardia, sweating, rigors, tachypnoea, oliguria, disorientation and shock and Gram-negative septicaemia. In advanced cases, and with delay in presentation, renal, respiratory, and cardiac failure may result.

Investigations • Hb • PCV • WCC • U&Es: dehydration, ARF • LFTs • Amylase • CXR: gas under diaphragm, small pleural effusion • AXR: distended bowel (ileus), local ileus ('sentinel' loop – appendicitis, pancreatitis) • USS: free fluid, localized collections • CT – pancreatitis.

Complications

Systemic Hypovolaemic shock, septic shock, ARDS, DIC, multiorgan failure, immunological failure.

Local Intraperitoneal sepsis: residual abscesses, e.g. subphrenic or pelvic, wound infection, anastomotic breakdown, fistula formation, adhesions.

Prognosis Overall mortality in generalized peritonitis is around 40%. Factors affecting mortality include age (elderly patients with faecal peritonitis have a high mortality), causation, duration of symptoms, degree of bacterial contamination, concomitant disease processes and organ failure.

Treatment Principles of treatment involve the following:

Resuscitation This requires pain relief with narcotic analgesics, i.v. fluids, NG aspiration, correction of electrolyte imbalance, catheterization. UO should be monitored and CVP (especially in elderly). Oxygen and antibiotics.

Treatment of causative lesion In generalized peritonitis this almost invariably requires surgery. Acute pancreatitis is the exception. Principles of operative treatment involve removal of all infected material from the peritoneal cavity, correction of the underlying cause, and attempts to prevent complications. Swab for C&S. Thorough examination of the peritoneal cavity, debridement of serosal surfaces, removal of affected organ, e.g. appendicectomy, colectomy. Formation of stomas rather than anastomosis which may leak in the presence of infection and unprepared bowel. Peritoneal lavage. Peritoneal drains. Occasionally the abdomen should be left open and the exposed bowel covered with moist swabs (laparostomy).

Postoperative care Attention should be paid to fluid and electrolyte balance. UO should be monitored. Antibiotic therapy, nutritional support and surveillance for sepsis. Ventilation may be necessary. CVVH or dialysis may be required for ARF.

INTRAPERITONEAL ABSCESSES

Following peritonitis pus may collect in either the subphrenic spaces, the pelvis or in locules between loops of bowel.

Symptoms and signs Generally unwell, swinging pyrexia, tachycardia, localized pain and tenderness, prolonged ileus, shoulder tip pain (referred from diaphragmatic irritation), hiccups, diarrhoea, chest symptoms with subphrenic abscess, boggy pelvic abscess on PR or PV examination.

Investigations • Hb • WCC • ESR • LFTs: occasionally raised • Blood culture may be positive • CXR: pleural effusion, raised hemidiaphragm, atelectasis • AXR: ileus, air/fluid levels in abscess cavities (rare) • USS • CT • Indium-labelled white cell scan.

Treatment For well-localized, non-loculated abscesses, percutaneous drainage under US or CT control. If there are multiple abscesses or they are multiloculated, open drainage at laparotomy will be required.

14

Alimentary tract

OESOPHAGUS

Most conditions of the oesophagus have dysphagia as a symptom. Dysphagia is difficulty in swallowing. It may result from local or general causes (→ Table 14.1).

Table 14.1
Causes of dysphagia

Local		
	In the lumen	Foreign body
	In the wall	Congenital atresia
		Inflammatory stricture–reflux oesophagitis
		Caustic stricture
		Achalasia
		Carcinoma
		Plummer–Vinson syndrome (oesophageal web)
		Scleroderma
		Following irradiation
	Outside the wall	Mediastinal lymphadenopathy
		Bronchial carcinoma
		Retrosternal goitre
		Pharyngeal pouch
		Para-oesophageal (rolling) hiatus hernia
		Thoracic aortic aneurysm
		Dysphagia lusoria (vascular ring)
General		Myasthenia gravis
		Bulbar palsy
		Bulbar poliomyelitis
		Hysteria

Investigation of dysphagia

History

- May be obvious cause, e.g. foreign body, ingestion of caustic substance.
- May be a previous history of oesophagitis suggesting an inflammatory stricture.
- Younger patients with history of dysphagia, worse for fluids than solids and no weight loss suggests achalasia.
- Rapid onset of dysphagia in the elderly with weight loss suggesting malignancy.

- The patient may be able to accurately locate the site and point at which the foods sticks, e.g. sternal notch with Plummer–Vinson syndrome, lower sternum with carcinoma at the cardia.

Examination There may be little to find. There may be evidence of weight loss and anaemia with malignant strictures. Koilonychia is associated with Plummer–Vinson syndrome. Glands may be palpable in the neck with carcinoma. The abdomen should be palpated to exclude liver secondaries. A lump may be palpable in the posterior triangle of the neck with pharyngeal pouch. This may gurgle when full of food.

Investigations • Hb • FBC • ESR • U&Es • LFTs • CXR: mediastinal mass, bronchial carcinoma, thoracic aortic aneurysm, gas shadow behind heart with hiatus hernia • Barium swallow and meal • Fibreoptic oesophagoscopy (should not be used if pharyngeal pouch is suspected) • Biopsy • CT scan.

Treatment It is that of the underlying cause.

FOREIGN BODY

This is usually accidental in children (small toys and coins), housewives (safety pins) and the elderly (false teeth). Deliberate swallowing occurs in the psychiatrically disturbed. Foreign bodies often impact at the narrowest parts of the oesophagus, i.e. at its commencement, where it is crossed by the left bronchus, and where it passes through the diaphragm. Smooth objects will usually pass into the stomach. Sharp and irregular objects impact.

Symptoms and signs Usually painful dysphagia. Often no signs. Mediastinitis if perforation occurs.

Investigations • CXR will show radio-opaque foreign body (→ Fig. 14.1) • Air in mediastinum if perforation has occurred • Barium swallow (Gastrograffin if suspected perforation) • Oesophagoscopy.

Treatment Oesophagoscopy and removal. A flexible endoscope may be used in association with specially designed forceps for grasping foreign bodies. Thoracotomy with oesophagotomy may be necessary. Foreign bodies that pass through the oesophagus will normally be passed per rectum. Occasionally sharp objects may perforate the bowel wall. →

Initial treatment is by observation and serial radiograph to assess the passage of the foreign body. Failure to progress and development of tenderness are indications for surgery.

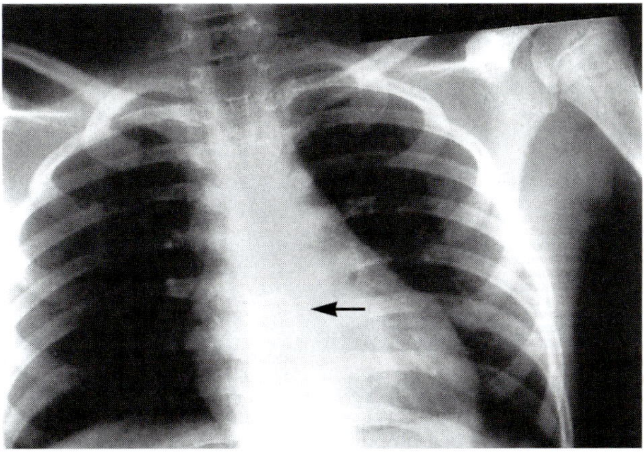

Fig. 14.1 A foreign body (wristwatch – arrow) is seen in the oesophagus.

OESOPHAGEAL PERFORATION

This may be caused by swallowed foreign bodies or corrosives; rupture at oesophagoscopy, dilatation or biopsy; penetrating wound, or following a violent vomit after a large meal (Boerhaave's syndrome).

Symptoms and signs History of foreign body, corrosive ingestion, endoscopy, violent vomit. Sudden or gradual onset of pain in chest, neck and upper abdomen. Other symptoms are dysphagia, pyrexia, shock, cyanosis, surgical emphysema in suprasternal notch.

Investigations • CXR: air in neck and mediastinum, pleural effusion • Gastrograffin swallow (*not* barium) will confirm the diagnosis and demonstrate the site.

Complication Mediastinitis.

Treatment Broad-spectrum antibiotics. Small perforations may be treated expectantly with i.v. fluids. Nil orally. Large perforations require surgical repair and drainage of the area.

INFLAMMATORY STRICTURE

This may result from prolonged acid reflux with oesophagitis. Reflux occurs through an incompetent lower oesophageal sphincter. It is often associated with a sliding hiatus hernia. Other causes of reflux oesophagitis include: prolonged vomiting, prolonged nasogastric intubation, operations which destroy the cardio-oesophageal area, e.g. resection with gastro-oesophageal anastomosis, cardiomyotomy for achalasia. As a result of long-standing reflux, the lower oesophagus may come to be lined by columnar mucosa, an appearance known as Barrett's oesophagus.

GASTRO-OESOPHAGEAL REFLUX

Many patients with reflux do not have hiatus hernia. Some patients with a hiatus hernia do not reflux. Patients with reflux should have a 24-hour ambulatory oesophageal pH study prior to surgery. The test is positive if the pH is <4 for $>4\%$ of the 24-hour period.

HIATUS HERNIA

There are two types: sliding (90%) and rolling or paraoesophageal (10%). In the rolling type the cardio-oesophageal mechanism is intact and therefore reflux does not occur. The stomach rolls up alongside the lower oesophagus pressing on it and causing dysphagia (→ Fig. 14.2).

Sliding hiatus hernia

The stomach slides through the hiatus and therefore the position of the cardio-oesophageal junction changes and reflux occurs (→ Fig. 14.2).

Symptoms and signs Retrosternal burning pain worse on bending, stooping, or lying down. Heartburn. Acid regurgitation into mouth. Pain relieved by antacids. May radiate into jaw or left arm and simulate angina. Large herniae may cause cough, palpitations, or hiccups by mechanical effect. Oesophagitis may lead to ulceration and bleeding, the latter causing symptoms of anaemia. Stricture leads to dysphagia.

Investigations • Hb • FBC • ESR • U&Es • LFTs • Barium swallow: confirms hiatus hernia and also indicates reflux when

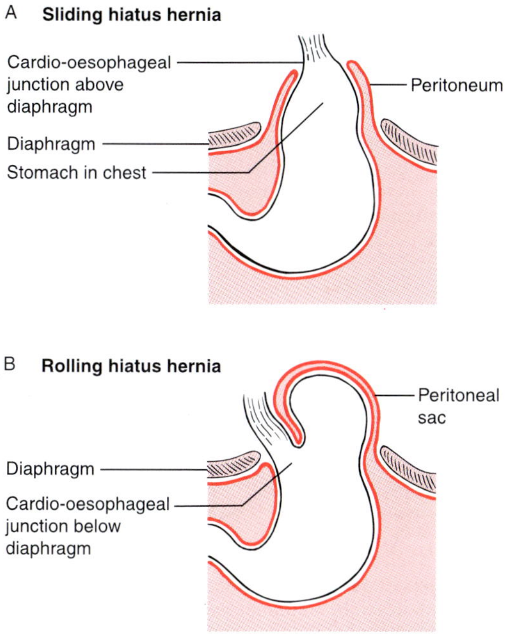

Fig. 14.2 **A.** Sliding hiatus hernia. The stomach slides up into the chest. Reflux occurs. **B.** Rolling (para-oesophageal) hernia. The stomach rolls up alongside the oesophagus and dysphagia occurs. The cardio-oesophageal mechanism is intact and therefore reflux does not occur.

patient is examined in the head-down position – stricture may be present (→ Fig. 14.3) • Upper GI endoscopy is the investigation of choice before barium studies which now rarely require to be done. Biopsy if stricture seen or diagnosis of oesophagitis is in doubt.

Treatment

Medical Lose weight, loosen corset. Sleep propped up. Antacids. Proton pump inhibitors: omeprazole or lansoprazole are now the most effective treatment. Many patients obtain relief with this regimen.

→

Surgical Indicated for failed medical treatment or complications, e.g. anaemia or severe dysphagia due to stricture. Surgery may also be indicated for young patients who do not want to take long-term acid-suppressant agents. There are several operations but a Nissen fundoplication (→ Fig. 14.4) is the most commonly performed. The hernial defect is repaired and the mobilized fundus of the stomach is wrapped around the lower end of the oesophagus to provide an antireflux mechanism. This may be done by the 'open' or laparoscopic method.

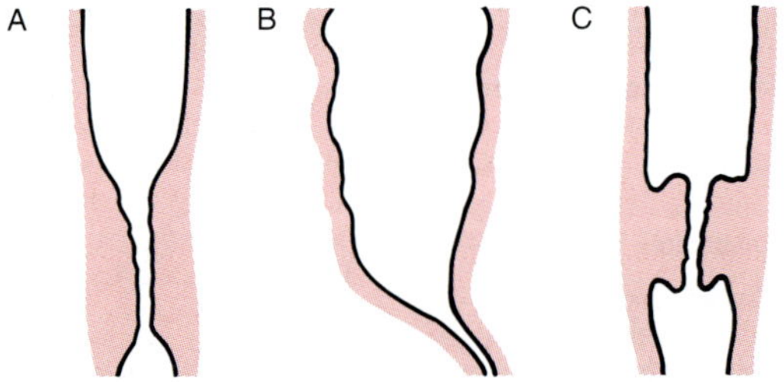

Fig. 14.3 Types of oesophageal stricture. **A.** Peptic stricture associated with reflux. **B.** Tortuous dilated oesophagus with 'rat's tail' stricture of achalasia. **C.** The irregular 'shouldered' stricture of carcinoma.

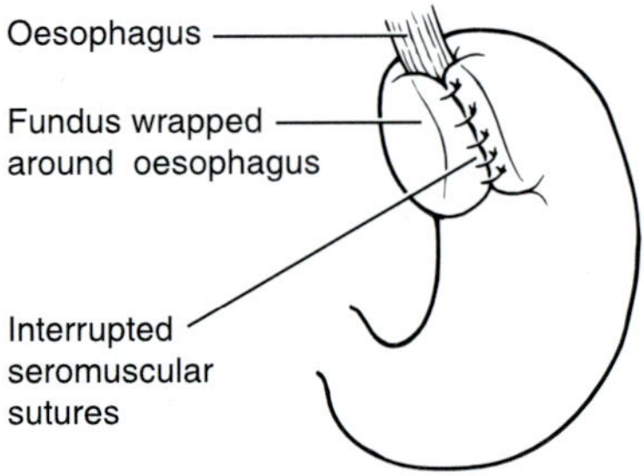

Fig. 14.4 Nissen fundoplication. The fundus of the stomach is mobilized, wrapped around the lower oesophagus, and held with seromuscular sutures.

Rolling or para-oesophageal hiatus hernia

The cardia remains in its normal position and the stomach rolls up into the chest alongside the oesophagus. The cardio-oesophageal mechanism is intact and regurgitation does not occur (→ Fig. 14.2).

Symptoms and signs Intermittent dysphagia due to a full stomach pressing on the adjacent oesophagus. Pain due to distension. Palpitations due to pressure on heart. Hiccups due to irritation of diaphragm. Respiratory embarrassment.

Investigations • CXR: air/fluid level in mediastinum • Barium meal • CT scan.

Complications Incarceration, gangrene, gastric volvulus.

Treatment Unlike sliding herniae, rolling herniae should almost always be repaired. Nissen fundoplication with repair of the diaphragmatic defect is an appropriate procedure.

ACHALASIA

This is due to failure of relaxation of the lower oesophageal 'sphincter'. It presents between 30 and 50 years and affects sexes equally. The cause is unknown but degeneration of Auerbach's plexus occurs.

Symptoms and signs Intermittent dysphagia. Gets progressively worse. May be worse for liquids than for solids. Fluid regurgitation especially at night with aspiration pneumonitis. Retrosternal pain.

Investigations • Barium swallow: dilated tortuous oesophagus above smooth tapering stricture ('rat's tail' appearance → Fig. 14.3) • Oesophagoscopy: needs aspiration of stagnant food initially, exclude benign stricture or carcinoma.

Complications Aspiration pneumonitis, oesophageal erosions. Carcinoma may develop even after treatment.

Treatment

Oesophageal dilatation This is achieved using a pneumatic dilator introduced over a guide wire under radiological control. The success rate is over 50% but repeated dilatations are necessary.

Heller's operation (i.e. cardiomyotomy) The muscle layer is divided down to the mucosa over the lower end of the oesophagus and extended for about 1 cm on to the stomach. It is a similar principle to Ramstedt's operation for pyloric stenosis in infancy.

CARCINOMA OF THE OESOPHAGUS

This occurs most commonly in males. The commonest site is the lower third of the oesophagus followed by the middle third and upper third. Postcricoid carcinoma usually occurs in females and is part of the Plummer–Vinson syndrome. Achalasia of the cardia is also a predisposing cause. Squamous cell carcinoma occurs in the upper and middle thirds but adenocarcinoma may occur in the lower third associated with areas of gastric mucosa (Barrett's oesophagus) or by growth of a carcinoma of the cardiac area of the stomach into the oesophagus. Spread occurs by the following:

- local invasion into surrounding structures, trachea, lung and aorta (massive haemorrhage may be terminal event)
- lymphatic to paraoesophageal nodes, supraclavicular and abdominal nodes
- the blood stream to liver and lung.

Symptoms and signs Dysphagia, usually rapid onset. Initially for solids then fluids. Weight loss, anorexia, anaemia. Palpable supraclavicular nodes, palpable irregular liver (secondaries).

Investigations • Hb • FBC • ESR • U&Es • LFTs • Barium swallow: 'shouldered' stricture (→ Fig. 14.3) • Upper GI endoscopy and biopsy • CXR: mediastinal widening, secondaries in lung • Bronchoscopy: to exclude invasion of oesophagus by primary lung tumour or vice versa, i.e. oesophageal tumour invading the bronchus with upper and middle third lesions • USS of liver to exclude secondaries. • CT scan to define invasion and indicate operability. • Endoluminal ultrasound to determine staging.

Treatment Resection. The stomach is mobilized and brought up into the chest and anastomosed to the remaining oesophagus in either the chest or neck. If the tumour is inoperable an expandable metal stent may be placed through the tumour using a fibreoptic endoscope. Other methods of relieving dysphagia include laser therapy. Radiotherapy may be used for primary or palliative treatment of both squamous cell carcinomas and adenocarcinomas, the latter responding nearly as well as the squamous cell carcinomas. The best response is now with a combination of chemotherapy (cisplatin and 5-FU) and radiotherapy.

Prognosis Prognosis is poor. Most patients survive less than 6 months if the primary is non-resectable. The 5-year survival following resection is less than 20%.

CORROSIVE OESOPHAGITIS

The accidental or deliberate ingestion of corrosives causes severe oesophagitis. Common substances include caustic soda, bleach and sulphuric acid. Extensive damage occurs to the mouth, pharynx, larynx and stomach as well as to the oesophagus.

Symptoms and signs History of ingestion. Burning pain from mouth to stomach. Fever. Shock. Respiratory distress if aspiration. Oedema of lips, lung, pharynx.

Investigations Early endoscopy with fine fibreoptic endoscope to assess degree of damage.

Complications Bleeding. Perforation. Stricture is a late complication.

Treatment

Emergency

Dilute acid (vinegar) or alkali (sodium bicarbonate) may be used to neutralize the ingested substance. *Never* induce vomiting. It may rupture the already damaged oesophagus.

Medical Broad-spectrum antibiotics. Steroids. TPN.

→

Endoscopic dilatation of strictures Gentle dilatation may be undertaken at 3–4 weeks.

Surgery If a severe stricture develops, oesophageal replacement by interposition of a segment of colon is required. Stomach may also be used if that has been spared from the effects of the caustic injury. Surgery is also required if perforation occurs.

Prognosis Appropriate early treatment of caustic burns usually gives good results. Extensive burns with strong acid or strong alkali progress to stricture formation and require surgery.

PLUMMER–VINSON SYNDROME (SYN. PATERSON–BROWN KELLY SYNDROME, SIDEROPENIC DYSPHAGIA)

This occurs in middle-aged females. It is an iron deficiency anaemia associated with a smooth tongue, koilonychia (spoon-shaped nails) and dysphagia. The dysphagia is due to the formation of a web in the upper oesophagus (postcricoid web). The condition is premalignant and carcinoma may develop in the upper oesophagus.

Treatment Oesophageal dilatation if symptoms from web. Follow-up to check for developing carcinoma.

STOMACH AND DUODENUM

PEPTIC ULCERATION

This occurs anywhere where pepsin and acid occur together. It is caused by an imbalance between secretion of acid and pepsin, and mucosal defence mechanisms. An acid environment and reduced mucosal defences provide ideal circumstances for pepsin to cause mucosal ulceration. If there is no acid, peptic ulceration cannot occur. Oversecretion of acid is associated with duodenal ulceration. Breakdown of the mucosal defences occurs in gastric ulceration. Exacerbating factors in peptic ulceration include stress, smoking, alcohol, NSAIDs, steroids, hyperparathyroidism, Zollinger–Ellison syndrome. →

Infection with *Helicobacter pylori* may impair mucosal defences and has recently been associated with duodenal ulcer and gastritis and to a lesser extent gastric ulcers. Common sites for peptic ulcer are the stomach and duodenum, the anterior and posterior walls of the first part of the duodenum and the lesser curve of the stomach being the most common sites. Less common sites include the oesophagus (Barrett's oesophagus), Meckel's diverticulum containing ectopic gastric mucosa and gastrojejunal anastomosis (after ulcer surgery).

Symptoms and signs

Duodenal ulcer (DU) Epigastric pain. May radiate through to back. Relieved by eating. Worse at night. Symptoms are periodic and last about 14 days and recur at 3- to 4-monthly intervals. They are often worse in spring and autumn. Vomiting is rare. If it occurs, pyloric stenosis should be suspected. Examination may reveal tenderness in epigastrium.

Gastric ulcer (GU) Epigastric pain. Not periodic. Food may precipitate pain. Pain may be relieved by vomiting. Patient may be afraid to eat and weight loss results. Examination reveals tenderness in epigastrium.

Investigations • OGD and biopsy: risk of malignancy with GU; antral biopsy for mucosal urease test (CLO test) • Serology for *H. pylori* • Breath test • Barium meal is rarely used nowadays but if a GU is diagnosed on a barium study, OGD and biopsy should be carried out • Other routine investigations include Hb, FBC, U&Es, Ca, PO_4 and occasionally serum gastrin if Zollinger–Ellison syndrome is suspected.

Treatment

Medical

- Antacids, e.g. Mist. Mag. Trisil., relieve pain but are of limited value.
- Proton pump inhibitors reduce acid secretion by inhibiting the proton pump in parietal cells. Results in greater inhibition of acid than H_2 receptor antagonists. Omeprazole and lansoprazole may be used. First-line treatment is acid suppression with proton pump inhibitor plus eradication therapy for *H. pylori*, i.e. triple therapy with omeprazole 20 mg b.d. plus two of the following three antibiotics: amoxycillin, clarithromycin, metronidazole. Check for eradication 6 weeks later by re-endoscopy and biopsy or breath test.

→

In addition to the above specific therapies, advice should be given regarding stopping smoking, stopping NSAIDs, and dealing with a stressful lifestyle.

Surgical Indications are the following:

- Failed medical treatment (unusual nowadays).
- Complications, haemorrhage, perforation, pyloric obstruction. Operations include vagotomy (→ Fig. 14.5) and drainage (→ Fig. 14.6), highly selective vagotomy (→ Fig. 14.5) and partial gastrectomy (→ Fig. 14.7).

Complications of peptic ulceration

Haemorrhage Posterior duodenal ulcers erode the gastroduodenal artery. Lesser curve gastric ulcers erode the left gastric artery. OGD to locate the site of the ulcer. A bleeding ulcer can be treated by injection, diathermy or laser coagulation at OGD. If the ulcer is not actively bleeding, a course of medical treatment may be given. The majority of patients stop bleeding spontaneously. If bleeding is massive or recurrent, surgery is required. The bleeding vessel in the base of the ulcer is oversewn to stop the bleeding. A GU is best excised or at least a biopsy should be taken to exclude malignancy. As the pylorus is opened for treating a bleeding DU, it is closed as a pyloroplasty and vagotomy added.

Perforation Anterior DUs and GUs may perforate causing generalized chemical peritonitis. Surgery involves simple suture of the ulcer with reinforcement with an omental patch. A biopsy should be taken from the edge of a GU as there is a risk of malignancy. Check *H. pylori* status and eradicate if necessary. If there is a long history of recurrent ulceration, a vagotomy and pyloroplasty may be added.

Pyloric obstruction Late complication. Vomiting of large amounts of foul-smelling vomit often containing food eaten several days previously. Eructations of foul gas. Gastric succussion splash on examination. Empty stomach with wide-bore nasogastric tube. Confirm by OGD or barium study. If surgery is required, usually vagotomy and gastrojejunostomy. Hypokalaemia and metabolic alkalosis may be present and require correction prior to surgery.

Obstruction of the midstomach may occur because of fibrosis of a large saddle-shaped ulcer astride the lesser curve of the stomach. This gives rise to the 'hourglass' appearance on a barium study. It is largely of historical interest from the days when patients kept their ulcers a long time prior to consideration of surgery.

Zollinger–Ellison syndrome

Peptic ulcer disease caused by excessive production of gastrin. Peptic ulcers may occur in unusual sites, e.g. the third part of the duodenum. There is usually a gastrin-secreting pancreatic tumour (gastrinoma). 60% are malignant; 30% associated with MEN (Type I).

Symptoms and signs Typical signs and symptoms of peptic ulcer. Diarrhoea may occur from overproduction of acid. Bleeding. Perforation. Recurrent ulcers after surgery for peptic ulcer. Ulcers resistant to medical treatment. May be family history of peptic ulcer.

Investigations • Fasting serum gastrin: raised • CT scan • Angiography.

Treatment Excision of tumour if spread to liver has not occurred. If tumour cannot be localized or has spread, acid secretion should be controlled by omeprazole. Rarely total gastrectomy may be needed to stop bleeding.

CARCINOMA OF THE STOMACH

The incidence is declining but it remains a common tumour with a poor prognosis. Widespread geographical variations occur, the incidence being high in Japan and certain coastal countries where the intake of dietary nitrate is high. Eating smoked fish and highly spiced foods has been implicated. Other associations include blood group A (suggesting a genetic factor), pernicious anaemia, atrophic gastritis, previous gastric surgery and benign gastric ulcer.

Symptoms and signs Onset silent and insidious. Vague dyspepsia, epigastric pain, weight loss, dysphagia (cardiac area), vomiting (pyloric area), anaemia, lassitude. Epigastric mass, hepatomegaly, ascites, left supraclavicular gland palpable (Virchow's node, Troisier's sign), gastric succussion splash, acanthosis nigricans.

Investigations • Hb • FBC • ESR • LFTs: alkaline phosphatase raised with liver secondaries • OGD with biopsy • USS: secondaries • CT scan for staging – may suggest linitis plastica which indicates generalized invasion of the whole wall of the stomach with cancer. • Laparoscopy to exclude peritoneal metastases.

Treatment This is surgical.

Attempt at cure Wide excision of tumour usually with 5-cm margin and clearance of nodes. For distal tumours partial gastrectomy (7/8) may suffice. For more proximal tumours, total gastrectomy. Over 60% are found to be incurable at laparotomy.

Palliative Bypass gastrojejunostomy for antral tumours. Intubation via upper GI endoscopy with an expandable mesh stent.

Prognosis In Japan where screening programmes are undertaken because of the high incidence, the 5-year survival for *early* gastric cancer is around 90%. In the UK at least 60% of cases present too late for curative surgery. Overall about 20% survive 5 years. Radiotherapy is of no value.

GASTRIC SURGERY AND ITS COMPLICATIONS

Peptic ulcer and carcinoma are the commonest indications for gastric surgery.

Operations

Vagotomy (→ Fig. 14.5) This reduces acid secretion from the stomach. It reduces gastric motility and therefore interferes with gastric emptying. A drainage procedure is therefore required:

Pyloroplasty (→ Fig. 14.6) The pylorus is cut longitudinally and sewn up transversely. In this operation, vagotomy is designed to reduce acid secretion and thus allow the ulcer to heal. The pyloroplasty is performed to allow gastric drainage.

Gastroenterostomy (→ Fig. 14.7) The most dependent part of the stomach is anastomosed to a loop of jejunum. This diverts acid away from the duodenum and allows the ulcer to heal. Vagotomy is carried out to reduce acid secretion and thus prevent stomal ulceration.

Highly selective vagotomy (→ Fig. 14.5) The vagus is sectioned such that only the body of the stomach is denervated. The nerve of Latarjet to the pylorus is left intact thus preserving motility of this region and allowing the stomach to empty without need for a pyloroplasty.

Gastrectomy This may be partial or total. Partial gastrectomy usually involves removal of about 7/8 of the stomach. The gastric

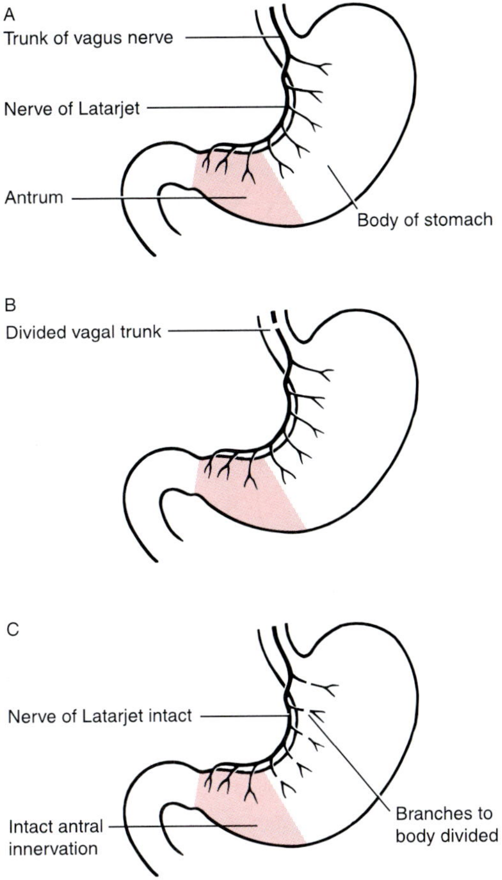

Fig. 14.5 **A.** Normal gastric vagal innervation. **B.** Truncal vagotomy. The anterior and posterior nerves are completely divided at the level of the lower oesophagus as shown in the diagram. **C.** Highly selective vagotomy. Only the vagal branches to the body of the stomach are divided. The vagal innervation of the antrum (nerve of Latarjet) is left intact.

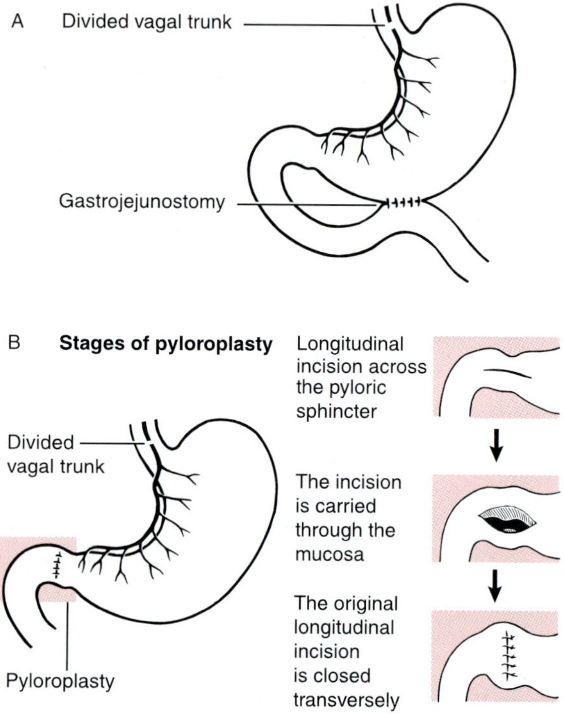

Fig. 14.6 **A.** Truncal vagotomy and gastrojejunostomy. **B.** Truncal vagotomy and pyloroplasty. The pylorus is opened longitudinally and sutured transversely thus destroying the pyloric sphincter.

remnant may be reanastomosed directly to the first part of the duodenum (Billroth I) or the duodenal stump oversewn and the continuity re-established by a gastrojejunostomy (Billroth II or Polya gastrectomy; → Fig. 14.7). If partial gastrectomy is used for GU, the ulcer is removed together with the segment of stomach. For DU, removal of the bulk of the acid-secreting area of the stomach allows the ulcer to heal. The ulcer is not usually removed. These operations are rarely used nowadays for duodenal ulceration but patients are still seen who have had the operations in the past.

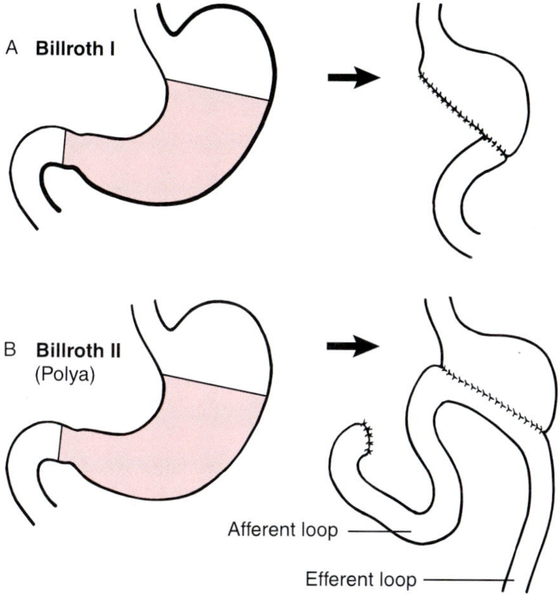

Fig. 14.7 Types of partial gastrectomy. **A.** Billroth I. The gastric remnant is anastomosed directly to the first part of the duodenum. **B.** Billroth II (Polyia). The duodenal stump is oversewn and continuity re-established by gastrojejunostomy.

Complications

Recurrent ulceration Symptoms are similar to those experienced preoperatively. Treatment is difficult. Zollinger–Ellison syndrome and hypercalcaemia should be excluded.

Epigastric fullness Particularly after partial gastrectomy. Treatment is to take small meals frequently. The symptom tends to improve with time.

Bilious vomiting Sudden emptying of the afferent loop with Billroth II. Associated biliary gastritis. May respond to metoclopramide. Severe cases need revisional surgery, e.g. Roux-en-Y anastomosis so that bile enters the GI tract lower down in the jejunum (→ Fig. 14.8).

Dumping

Early Fainting, sweating and dizziness shortly after eating. May

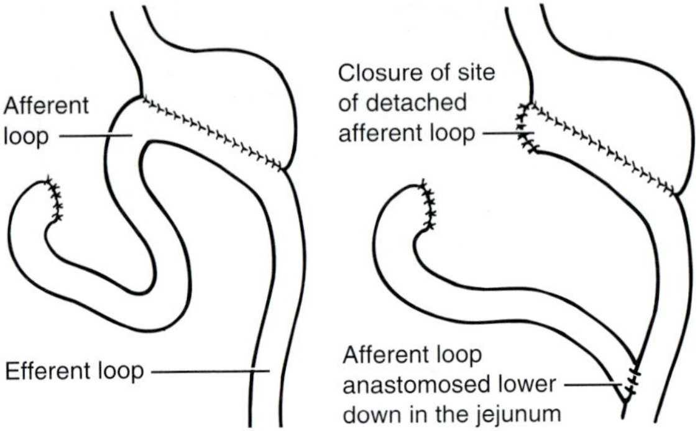

Fig. 14.8 Roux-en-Y conversion for bilious vomiting. The afferent loop is detached and reanastomosed lower down the jejunum.

be a reflex caused by osmotic effect of large volumes of food 'dumped' into the jejunum. Less common after highly selective vagotomy. Patient may need to lie down and rest for half an hour. Symptoms may be improved by eating small dry meals frequently and avoiding heavy carbohydrate meals. Early dumping may subside spontaneously with time.

Late Due to hypoglycaemia and occurs $1\frac{1}{2}$–3 hours after a meal. Responds to glucose (sucking barley sugars).

Diarrhoea This may be disabling after vagotomy. Codeine phosphate and small dry meals may help. The incidence is less after highly selective vagotomy.

Nutritional disturbances

Weight loss May be due to reduced caloric intake or poor absorption.

Steatorrhoea Due to poor mixing of food and enzymes, e.g. long afferent loop where food passes into the jejunum before it is adequately mixed with digestive enzymes coming from the afferent loop. Blind loop syndrome may be responsible, i.e. stasis in the long afferent loop with colonization with abnormal bacteria, which restricts digestion and absorption of food. Surgical correction of the afferent loop may be necessary.

Anaemia Iron deficiency anaemia due to reduced hydrochloric acid which is required for iron absorption. With total gastrectomy, megaloblastic anaemia may occur, owing to loss of intrinsic factor and subsequent B_{12} deficiency. Vitamin B_{12} injections are required.

Bolus obstruction Destruction of the pylorus allows unmasticated food to pass into the small intestine. This may swell and lodge in the terminal ileum. This occurs particularly with orange pith and dried fruits. Patients should be warned not to eat these foods if the pylorus is not intact.

Carcinoma It may occur in the gastric remnant. This is rare.

UPPER GASTROINTESTINAL TRACT BLEEDING

This causes either haematemesis (vomiting of blood) melaena (passage of altered blood PR – usually black and tarry with a characteristic smell), or both. Causes include peptic ulceration, acute gastric erosions, oesophageal varices, oesophagitis, Mallory–Weiss syndrome, and carcinoma. Rarer causes include leiomyoma, angiomatous malformations, haemobilia and bleeding disorders. Drugs which may precipitate bleeding include steroids, NSAIDs, and anticoagulants. Principles of treatment include replacement of blood loss, diagnosis of the cause and treatment of the condition.

Symptoms and signs Clinically anaemic. With severe bleed, shock will occur. History of aspirin, NSAIDs, steroid or anticoagulant. Stigmata of liver failure. Abdominal mass.

Investigations • Hb • FBC • U&Es • LFTs • Clotting screen • Cross-match blood • OGD • Angiography if source of bleeding is obscure.

Treatment

- Bed rest, pulse, BP, CVP line. Infusion of crystalloid, colloid, blood.
- Treat shock.
- Catheterize.
- Establish diagnosis by endoscopy.
- Control varices with Sengstaken tube or injection.
- Give intravenous H_2 receptor antagonist.

Indications for intervention are the following:

- massive uncontrolled bleeding
- rebleeding especially if bleeding vessel or clot on ulcer has been seen at endoscopy
- more than 4 unit bleed in 24 hours unless the cause is varices.

→

Interventional options are non-operative or operative.

Non-operative Laser coagulation. Local cautery. Injection of adrenaline. Varices may be treated by sclerotherapy. Octreotide infusion for varices. Angiomatous malformations may be treated by embolization.

Operative • Peptic ulcer: oversewing of the ulcer + vagotomy and drainage. Partial gastrectomy may be necessary • Acute erosions: vagotomy and drainage or partial gastrectomy • Oesophageal varices: oesophageal transection. Portocaval or distal splenorenal shunting • Carcinoma: partial or total gastrectomy.

Prognosis The overall mortality for an upper GI bleed is 10%. Adverse prognostic factors include old age, shock at presentation, rebleeding and oesophageal varices.

OTHER CONDITIONS OF THE STOMACH AND DUODENUM

Stomach

Leiomyoma Commonest benign tumour of stomach. Epigastric discomfort, indigestion, haematemesis or melaena due to ulceration of mucosa overlying tumour. Barium meal shows space-occupying lesion. Surgical excision is required.

Lymphoma Symptoms are those of peptic ulcer or gastric carcinoma. OGD and biopsy to confirm diagnosis. Treatment is by surgical resection followed by radiotherapy or chemotherapy. 50% of patients survive 5 years or more.

Duodenum

Other than peptic ulcer, conditions of the duodenum are rare. A duodenal diverticulum may occur on the medial wall near the ampulla of Vater. Most are asymptomatic. Rarely bleeding and perforation may occur. Symptomatic diverticulae should be excised. Tumours of the duodenum are rare. Adenocarcinoma does *not* occur in duodenal ulcers. Rarely it may occur in other parts of the duodenum and if it arises near the bile ducts, may cause obstructive jaundice.

CONDITIONS OF THE SMALL BOWEL

Meckel's diverticulum

A remnant of the vitellointestinal duct of the embryo. Classically it occurs in 2% of patients, is 2 inches long, and 2 feet from the ileocaecal junction ('rule of 2s'). It occurs on the antimesenteric border of the terminal ileum.

Symptoms and signs Symptomless. Incidental finding at laparotomy. Symptoms typical of acute appendicitis may occur. Rectal bleeding (ectopic gastric mucosa). Rarely umbilical discharge (fistula), intestinal obstruction (due to entrapment around the band from the apex of the diverticulum to the back of the umbilicus), small bowel volvulus, or intussusception (ileo-ileal).

Investigations • Technetium scan for GI bleeding may show gastric mucosa in a Meckel's • Laparotomy is required for complications of Meckel's – the cause is not usually apparent until laparotomy is undertaken.

Treatment Excision of the diverticulum.

Crohn's disease

This is dealt with in the section on inflammatory bowel disease (p. 253).

Typhoid

It is caused by *Salmonella typhi*. About 200 cases occur in the UK annually. It may occur in the immigrant population and in those who have travelled in countries where the disease is endemic. The organism enters Peyer's patches and may result in perforation or bleeding usually involving the ileum. This usually occurs during the third week of the disease. The patient shows signs of perforation with peritonitis. Surgical closure of the perforation is required. The bowel is very friable. Chloramphenicol i.v. is given for 2 weeks postoperatively.

Tuberculosis

This may present as an acute abdomen in recent immigrants. It chiefly affects the terminal ileum and the ileocaecal region. Differentiation from Crohn's disease is essential.

Symptoms and signs Ill patient: fever, diarrhoea, colicky abdominal pain. Weight loss. May be history of pulmonary TB. Mass in RIF. Chest signs.

Investigations • CXR • Mantoux • Sputum culture • AXR: small bowel obstruction • Barium studies show thickening, ulceration and narrowing of terminal ileum • USS: may show mass • CT: may show abscess • Diagnosis may be made only at laparotomy.

Treatment Antituberculous therapy for 6 months to 2 years. Surgery is required if diagnosis is unclear, for perforation, abscess, bleeding or obstruction.

TUMOURS OF THE SMALL INTESTINE

These form less than 5% of all tumours of the GI tract. Obstruction and bleeding are the usual symptoms.

Benign

These include adenomas, leiomyomas and lipomas. Obstruction, intussusception, or bleeding may occur. Polyposis of the small bowel (mainly jejunum) may occur in association with pigmentation of the lips and mouth (Peutz–Jeghers syndrome). Bleeding or intussusception may occur.

Malignant

Adenocarcinoma is rare and usually affects the jejunum. Bleeding and obstruction may occur. Lymphoma may present as intestinal obstruction or a palpable mass. Consider lymphoma in patients with coeliac disease. Palliation of these tumours is by radiotherapy or chemotherapy.

Carcinoid tumour

These occur most commonly in the appendix but can occur anywhere in the GI tract and occasionally in the lung. Those in the small bowel grow slowly but most of those greater than 2 cm have metastasized at the time of surgery. The tumours arise from argentaffin cells.

Symptoms and signs May be none before metastases occur. Carcinoid syndrome is associated with liver metastases. Flushing (caused by alcohol, coffee), diarrhoea, bronchospasm, pulmonary stenosis. Loud borborygmi may be heard on auscultation. Hepatomegaly, palpable abdominal mass.

Investigations • Raised 24-hour excretion of 5-HIAA • USS • CT.

Treatment Resection of primary tumour. Partial hepatectomy if metastases confined to one lobe. Methysergide blocks 5-HT and may be beneficial in patients with metastases. Phenoxybenzamine may be helpful in reducing flushing. Other procedures include hepatic embolization, systemic chemotherapy and hepatic infusion chemotherapy.

Prognosis Malignant carcinoid of the small bowel has a 25% 5-year survival.

SMALL BOWEL OBSTRUCTION

Mechanical obstruction of the small bowel may be simple (one point of obstruction) or closed loop (obstruction at two points enclosing a segment of bowel). If the bowel is viable, the obstruction is termed non-strangulating. If the blood supply is compromised, strangulating obstruction occurs with subsequent infarction of bowel. Strangulation occurs when the obstructing mechanism cuts off the mesenteric arterial blood flow, e.g. the neck of the sac with a loop of bowel trapped in a hernial sac, or the twist of a volvulus. Mechanical obstruction is more common in the small bowel than in the large bowel.

Causes Causes may be found in the following:

- in the lumen: gallstone ileus, food bolus (following pylorus-destroying operations, i.e. gastrojejunostomy or pyloroplasty)
- in the wall: congenital atresia, Crohn's disease, tumours, e.g. lymphoma or carcinoma
- outside the wall: herniae, adhesions, volvulus, intussusception.

Symptoms and signs Colicky abdominal pain. The patient cannot get into a comfortable position. Vomiting. Constipation. Symptoms depend on whether the obstruction is high or low. High obstruction is characterized by early vomiting (bilious), and late constipation. Low obstruction is characterized by early constipation, and late vomiting (faeculent). Distension, marked with low obstruction, tympanitic abdomen, high-pitched tinkling bowel sounds. Hernial orifices should be carefully examined. Pyrexia, tachycardia, continuous pain and localized tenderness suggest actual or impending strangulation.

Investigations • Hb • FBC • WCC with neutrophilia may indicate strangulation • U&Es • AXR: distended loops of small bowel in central abdomen (→ Fig. 14.9). Erect films show air/fluid levels. Absent or diminished colonic gas. Dilated proximal small bowel shows lines close together (valvulae conniventes) crossing completely the lumen of the bowel. These get progressively fewer the more distal the distended loop and are absent in the terminal ileum. Look for gas in the biliary tree (gallstone ileus with cholecystoduodenal fistula).

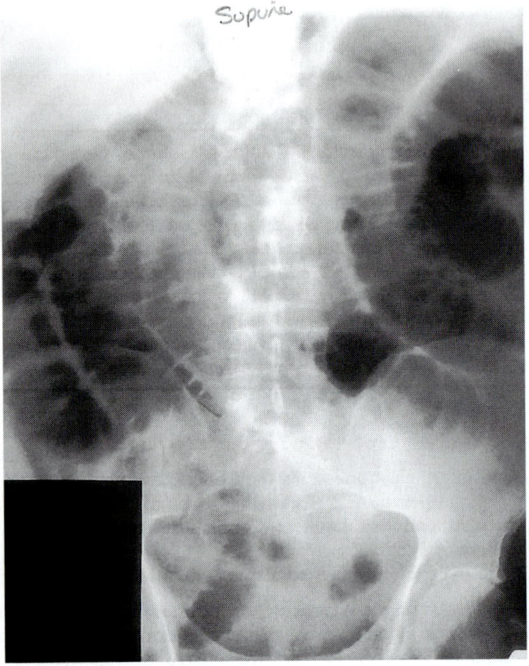

Fig. 14.9 Small bowel obstruction. Distended loops of small bowel are visible in the central abdomen.

Treatment

Conservative

- Intravenous fluids and nasogastric aspiration.
- Nil orally.
- 2-hourly temperature and pulse.
- Abdominal examination 8-hourly.

Some cases of simple mechanical obstruction, e.g. due to adhesions, will settle on this regimen.

Indications for surgery Strangulating obstruction, e.g. a tender irreducible hernia requires urgent surgery. If a conservative 'drip and suck' regimen has been undertaken for obstruction, surgery is indicated for signs of incipient strangulation (pyrexia, tachycardia, localized tenderness). Surgery is also →

required for simple obstruction which fails to settle, e.g. adhesions, gallstone ileus. At surgery the affected bowel is inspected for viability. Indications of non-viability include:

- absence of peristalsis
- loss of normal sheen
- loss of pulsation in bowel mesentery
- colour: green or black bowel is non-viable and resection is required. Plum-coloured bowel may respond to wrapping for a few minutes in warm saline-soaked packs. If colour returns and it will transmit a peristaltic wave, it is viable.

Prognosis Small bowel obstruction has a very low mortality rate if it is simple. Strangulating obstruction increases the mortality and if small bowel resection is required, especially in the elderly, the mortality rate may reach 25%.

APPENDICITIS

This is the commonest cause of the acute abdomen in the UK. It usually occurs when there is an obstruction in the lumen of the appendix either by a faecolith or foreign body or by enlargement of lymphoid follicles in its wall. It most often affects children, teenagers and young adults. It is rare at the extremes of life. In the infant, the lumen of the appendix is wide in relation to the remainder of the bowel and the diet is soft and hence obstruction within the lumen is less likely. In the elderly the lumen tends to be obliterated. Rarer causes of appendicitis include carcinoma of the caecum obstructing the appendiceal lumen, carcinoid tumour and obstructing fibrous bands. Occasionally a carcinoma obstructing the lumen of the appendix will cause it to distend and fill with mucus, i.e. a mucocele of the appendix.

Symptoms and signs Central abdominal cramping or colicky pain. Nausea. Vomiting is uncommon. Occasionally the patient may pass a loose stool. Frank diarrhoea is uncommon. Central abdominal pain lasts approximately 8 hours. It is followed by the development of a sharp, stabbing somatic type of pain in the RIF made worse by coughing or moving. Low-grade pyrexia (37.2–37.8°C). Flushed. Characteristic fetor (sweet faecal smell to breath). White furred tongue. Tachycardia (< 100 in first 24 hours). Tender with guarding in RIF over McBurney's point. Examination PR: tender anteriorly in the rectovesical or recto-uterine pouch.

> In infants diarrhoea and vomiting may be the only symptoms. This may lead to difficulty in diagnosis and confusion with gastroenteritis. In elderly patients there may be confusion and later shock may develop.

Investigations • WCC: usually $>10 \times 10^9$/l with neutrophil leukocytosis • USS: may show a mass or abscess; not useful in early appendicitis.

Differential diagnosis In the classical case of acute appendicitis there are few conditions that enter into the differential diagnosis. These include mesenteric adenitis, Meckel's diverticulitis, Crohn's disease (regional ileitis), mesenteric embolus and right-sided colonic diverticulitis. All these conditions will initially cause central abdominal cramping pain with subsequent tenderness in the RIF.

In the atypical case, other causes of intra-abdominal pathology, urinary tract disease, gynaecological problems and extra-abdominal conditions must be considered.

Abdominal disease Cholecystitis, gastroenteritis, pancreatitis, perforated DU, intestinal obstruction, diverticulitis, non-specific abdominal pain.

Urinary tract Acute pyelonephritis, renal colic, cystitis. An inflamed appendix adherent to the bladder may cause frequency and pyuria. Organisms will be absent on urinary microscopy.

Gynaecological causes Salpingitis. Ectopic pregnancy. Degeneration of a fibroid. Mittelschmerz. Pelvic inflammatory disease.

Extra-abdominal causes Referred pain from nerve roots, e.g. herpes zoster, degenerative and malignant disease affecting roots T11, T12. Referred pain from right lower lobar pneumonia. Referred pain from a right-sided testicular torsion.

> ***Treatment*** The treatment of acute appendicitis is appendicectomy. Prophylactic metronidazole by suppository should be given 1 hour preoperatively to reduce the risk of wound infection.

Complications Appendicitis may resolve spontaneously. The appendix may become surrounded by adjacent small bowel and omentum and give rise to an appendix mass. It may perforate giving rise to generalized peritonitis or it may perforate amidst local adhesions giving rise to an appendix abscess. Often it is difficult to diagnose appendicitis. If the symptoms have been present for 48 hours ('48 hour rule') and the diagnosis is truly appendicitis, then the patient should either have developed an appendix mass or generalized peritonitis. If neither of these two are present, then the diagnosis of appendicitis should be reviewed.

Appendix mass

Omentum and small bowel adhere to the inflamed appendix. This usually happens 2–5 days after onset of initial symptoms. This should be initially treated conservatively. Mark out the site of the mass on the abdominal wall. i.v. fluids, analgesia, and antibiotics (cefuroxime and metronidazole) should be administered. If the mass resolves it is usual to carry out an interval appendicectomy after 3 months. If the mass gets bigger it is likely that an abscess is forming, i.e. the appendix has perforated within the appendix mass.

Appendix abscess

If an appendix mass enlarges and the temperature fails to settle, an appendix abscess is developing. The patient may appear toxic with a tachycardia. An appendix abscess requires either surgical drainage and appendicectomy, or percutaneous insertion of a drain under ultrasound control. Interval appendicectomy is required subsequently.

Other complications include subphrenic abscess, pelvic abscess, paralytic ileus, septicaemia, portal pyaemia (rare). Long-term complications may be due to adhesions resulting in intestinal obstruction in a small proportion of patients. Tubal adhesions with infertility may occur in females.

Appendicitis in pregnancy

This is no commoner than at other times. Pain and tenderness are higher because of displacement of the appendix by the enlarging uterus. Prompt assessment and intervention are essential. There is a risk of abortion in the first trimester but if treatment is delayed until perforation occurs the risk is considerably higher (approximately 25%).

CONDITIONS OF THE COLON, RECTUM AND ANUS

COLONIC POLYPS

A polyp is a lesion that projects into the lumen.

Hamartomas

Juvenile polyps May occur in large or small bowel. Cause bleeding or obstruction. May auto-amputate in adolescence.

Peutz–Jeghers syndrome Diffuse GI polyposis with mucocutaneous pigmentation of lips and gums. The polyps have no malignant potential. Surgery is indicated only for symptoms, i.e. obstruction or bleeding.

Neoplastic polyps

Adenomatous polyps and villous adenomas These have malignant potential especially the villous adenoma.

Familial polyposis coli This is an autosomal dominant condition with multiple polyps involving colon and rectum. Duodenal adenomas may also occur and progress to malignancy. It first appears in adolescence. If untreated, malignancy will develop before the age of 40. Treatment is classically by subtotal colectomy with ileorectal anastomosis. However, now, most patients are offered restorative proctocolectomy with ileo-anal pouch. Ileorectal anastomosis is still a reasonable option. Occasionally, rectal polyps regress after this procedure. Regular (6-monthly) inspection of the rectum by sigmoidoscopy is undertaken and any polyps excised. Sulindac may reduce polyp formation. Recurrence is high with carcinoma developing in the rectum. Other operations include total colectomy with mucosal proctectomy, and ileo-anal anastomosis or in some cases panproctocolectomy with ileostomy. There is a need for upper GI surveillance as most of the mortality is from development of ampullary/duodenal carcinomas developing from duodenal adenomas.

Gardner's syndrome A variant of familial polyposis, it is associated with desmoid tumours, osteomas of the mandible and multiple sebaceous cysts.

Inflammatory pseudopolyps These may arise in ulcerative colitis. Lymphoid hyperplasia may also be apparent as a polyp.

Symptoms and signs of polyps Passage of blood and mucus PR. Rarely obstruction or intussusception.

Investigations • Sigmoidoscopy and biopsy • Barium enema (→ Fig. 14.10) • Colonoscopy.

Treatment Pedunculated polyps or small sessile polyps may be removed at sigmoidoscopy or colonoscopy. If invasive carcinoma is found, colectomy is required.

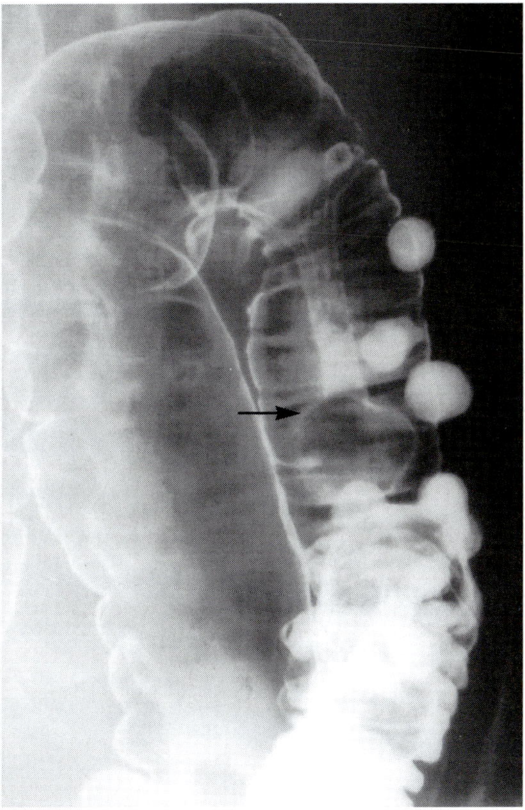

Fig. 14.10 A barium enema showing part of the sigmoid colon. A large pedunculated polyp is seen (arrow). There is also marked diverticular disease.

COLORECTAL CANCER

Commonest GI cancer. Usually presents after middle life but can occur earlier. The highest incidence of colorectal cancer is seen in Western Europe and North America; the lowest incidence occurs in Asia and South Africa. The precise cause is unknown but environmental and genetic factors are important. Lack of dietary fibre, increased fat, increased bile acids, have been →

implicated. Other predisposing factors include inflammatory bowel disease, familial polyposis coli, colorectal polyps, and previous irradiation. Apart from familial adenomatous polyposis, there are other groups of patients who have hereditary predisposition to develop large bowel cancer. There are two types of autosomal dominant hereditary non-polyposis colorectal cancer (HNPCC). These are: (i) cancer family syndrome (CFS), which occurs with early onset at around 20–30 years and is associated with other adenocarcinomas especially endometrial carcinoma and breast carcinoma; (ii) hereditary site-specific colonic cancer (HSSCC), which shows the same characteristics except for the extracolonic carcinomas. It has also been demonstrated that the frequency of colorectal cancer developing in first-degree relatives of patients with large bowel carcinoma is significantly higher than expected. The relative sites of distribution in the colon are shown in Figure 14.11.

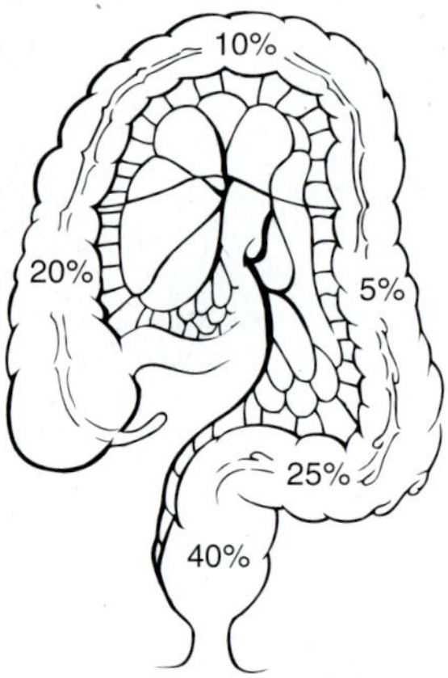

Fig. 14.11 Anatomical distribution of colorectal cancer.

Symptoms and signs Clinical features depend upon the sites. Right colon: anaemia, palpable mass, change in bowel habit. Left colon: change in bowel habit, lower abdominal colicky pain. Blood or mucus on or mixed with stool. With sigmoid cancers, spurious diarrhoea may occur. Rectal cancers present with frequency of defaecation because of tenesmus (a sense of incomplete evacuation). Blood and mucus PR. Patients may present with symptoms due to direct spread; sacral pain or sciatica due to direct invasion of the nerve. Jaundice due to liver or porta hepatis node metastases. Examination may reveal an abdominal mass or hepatomegaly. Examination PR may show blood on examining glove or mass may be palpable.

25% of large bowel cancers present as emergencies. Obstruction may occur, e.g. small bowel obstruction with caecal cancers growing over the ileocaecal valve or obstruction occurring on the left side where the bowel lumen is narrow and the faeces more formed. Perforation may occur because of either direct perforation of the cancer or perforation of the caecum with a closed-loop obstruction where the ileocaecal valve is competent. Massive haemorrhage is rare.

Investigations • Hb • FBC • U&Es (ureteric involvement) • LFTs (liver secondaries, alkaline phosphatase raised) • Sigmoidoscopy • Biopsy • Barium enema (5% of tumours are metachronous); 'Apple core' lesion may be visible (→ Fig. 14.12) • Colonoscopy • USS: liver secondaries, ureteric obstruction.

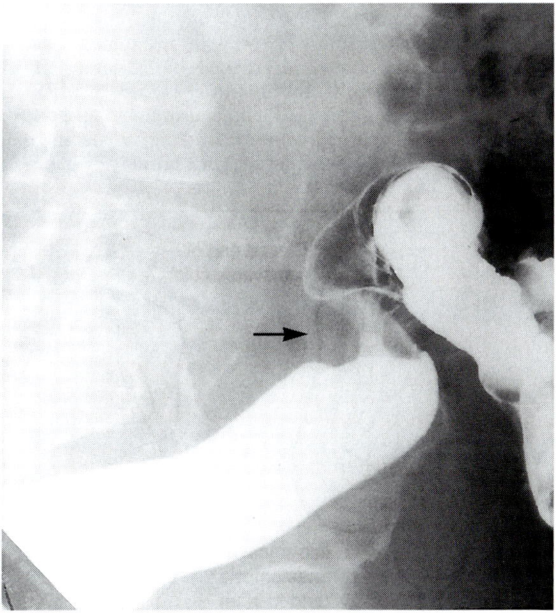

Fig. 14.12 A barium enema showing a colonic carcinoma. A typical 'apple core' lesion is visible (arrow).

Treatment (→ Fig. 14.13).

Elective

- Caecum and right colon: right hemicolectomy.
- Transverse colon: extended right hemicolectomy.
- Descending colon: left hemicolectomy.
- Sigmoid colon: sigmoid colectomy.
- Rectum and rectosigmoid: anterior resection with primary anastomosis. If low rectal tumour, abdominoperineal excision of the rectum should be carried out with a permanent colostomy. For any operation on the left side of the colon, the patient should be warned about a temporary defunctioning colostomy until the primary anastomosis has healed.

Emergency Correct fluid and electrolytes imbalance. In closed-loop obstruction a caecum of greater than 10 cm in diameter on AXR is an indication for urgent surgery especially if it is tender. Right-sided tumours may be treated with right hemicolectomy with primary anastomosis. Lower left-sided tumours should be treated by resection of the tumour and Hartmann's procedure, i.e. closure of the rectal stump and fashioning of an LIF end colostomy. Continuity of the bowel is re-established some weeks later. Some surgeons carry out an on-table colonic lavage with primary anastomosis covered by a loop ileostomy.

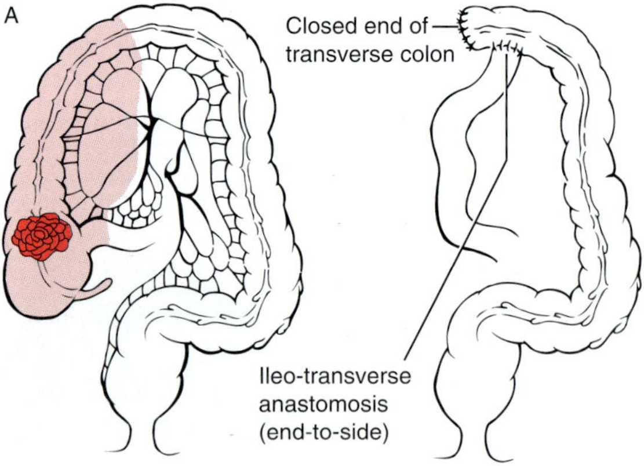

Fig. 14.13 Operations for colorectal cancer. The diagrams indicate the extent of resection and the method of re-establishing continuity. **A.** Right hemicolectomy.

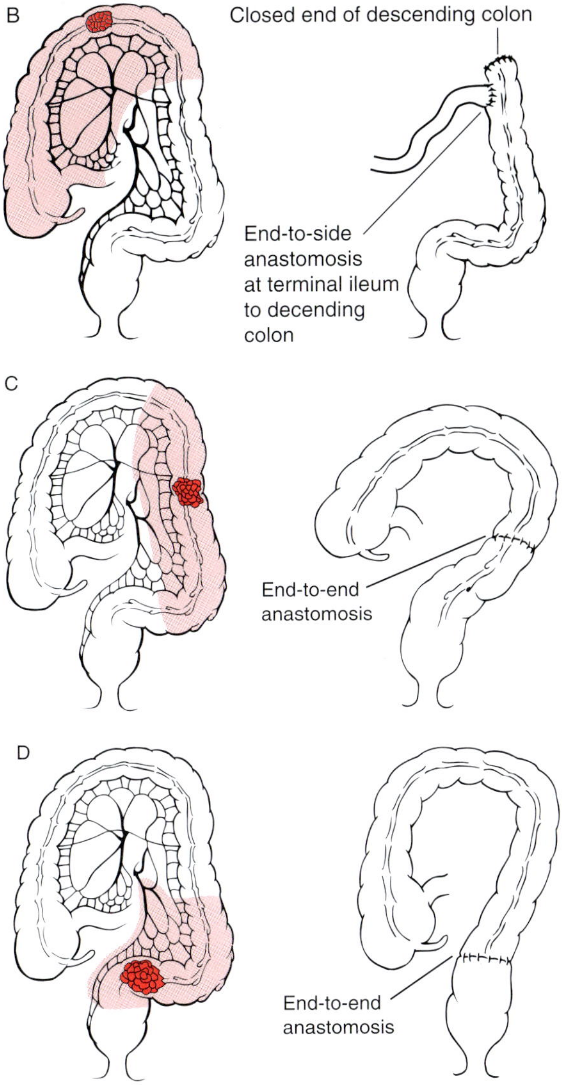

Fig. 14.13 (*Contd*) **B.** Extended right hemicolectomy. **C.** Left hemicolectomy. **D.** Sigmoid colectomy.

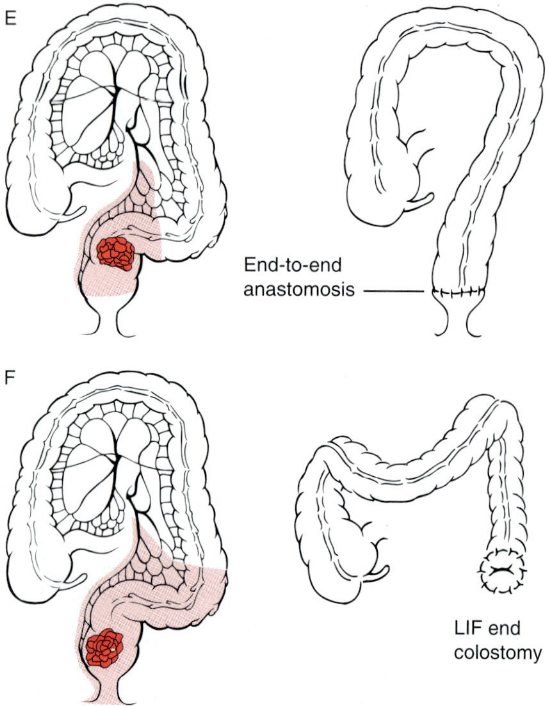

Fig. 14.13 (*Contd*) **E.** Anterior resection. **F.** Abdominoperineal resection of the rectum with permanent colostomy. The shaded area is the area resected.

Prognosis This is based on Dukes' classification, originally described for rectal cancer but now applied to all colorectal adenocarcinomas (→ Table 14.2).

Screening Populations at risk include asymptomatic relatives of patients with colorectal cancer and patients who have large bowel polyps. Screening methods include regular rigid sigmoidoscopy, flexible endoscopic screening or screening for faecal occult bloods. Serum markers such as carcinoembryonic antigen (CEA) may also be used for follow-up after resection. Ultrasound may be used for liver surveillance following successful resection. If an isolated secondary occurs, liver resection may be carried out.

Table 14.2
Dukes' classification

A	Confined to bowel wall, 80% 5-year survival
B	Through wall into surrounding tissue, 60% 5-year survival
C	Lymph node involvement, 30% 5-year survival

*If distant metastases are present, the 5-year survival is only 5%

INFLAMMATORY BOWEL DISEASE

The two main disorders are Crohn's disease and ulcerative colitis.

Crohn's disease

This is a chronic inflammatory disorder which may occur anywhere in the alimentary tract from the mouth to the anus. Common sites include the terminal ileum (regional ileitis), colon and rectum. Unlike ulcerative colitis the whole thickness of the bowel wall is involved. The aetiology is unknown. The disease occurs most commonly in the 15–35 age group. Familial clustering occurs. Malignancy may rarely occur in both small and large bowel.

Symptoms and signs Malaise, anorexia, fever, nausea, abdominal pain, weight loss, diarrhoea, rectal bleeding. Perianal inflammation with abscess, fissure, and fistulae formation may occur. Pallor, malnutrition, abdominal mass, perianal sepsis, fissures, fistulae, clubbing, erythema nodosum, pyoderma gangrenosum, uveitis.

Investigations • Hb • FBC • ESR • Folate • B_{12} • U&Es: electrolyte imbalances • LFTs: albumin reduced • CRP: elevated levels • Radiographs – AXR: obstruction, perforation, toxic dilatation • Small bowel enema and barium enema: skip lesions in small bowel, strictures (→ Fig. 14.14), 'rosethorn' ulcers, 'cobblestone' mucosa • Sigmoidoscopy and biopsy • Colonoscopy and biopsy • USS • CT: abscesses.

Complications Extra-alimentary manifestations (see above). Toxic dilatation. Stricture. Internal fistulae. Haemorrhage. Abscess formation. Perianal complications. Gallstones. Renal calculi. Psychological problems. Risk of carcinoma.

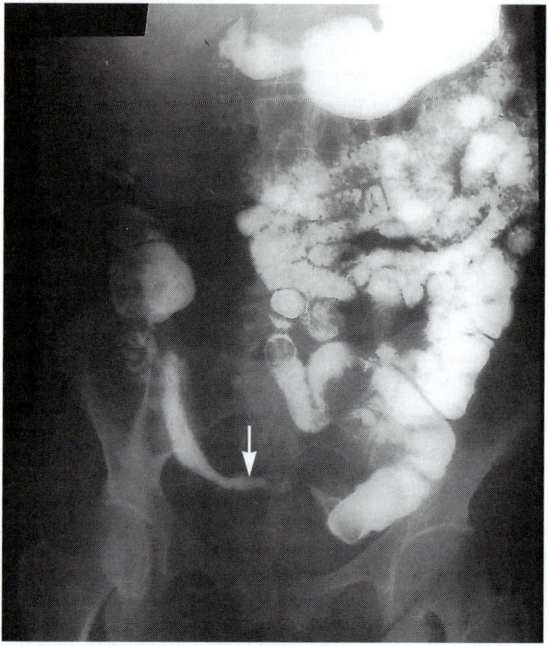

Fig. 14.14 Small bowel enema showing Crohn's disease. A stricture is seen in the terminal ileum (arrow).

Treatment

Medical Correction of fluid and electrolyte imbalance. Nutritional support. Steroids: 40 mg daily of prednisolone in acute exacerbations. Rectal disease may respond to predsol enemas. Mesalazine may help colonic disease and may reduce the frequency of relapses. Other drug therapies include azathioprine (useful as steroid-sparing drug in some cases), cyclosporin, metronidazole (especially for colonic disease with perianal sepsis). Antidiarrhoeal agents may be used for symptomatic control but should be stopped if obstructed symptoms occur.

Surgical Indicated for toxic dilatation, acute haemorrhage, perforation, obstruction, abscess formation, fistula formation, failure of medical treatment, uncertainty of diagnosis, development and prevention of carcinoma. Surgery involves segmental →

resection of bowel, sparing as much bowel as possible. For short strictures stricturoplasty may be carried out. Procto-colectomy with ileostomy may be required. Unlike ulcerative colitis, surgery in Crohn's disease cannot be guaranteed to be curative.

Prognosis Acute regional ileitis may be cured by right hemi-colectomy. Colonic Crohn's often responds well to medical treatment but at least 50% of patients will require surgery at some time. The mortality rate is about 14% over 30 years. The disease pursues a course of remissions and exacerbations.

Ulcerative colitis

This is a chronic inflammatory disease which involves the whole or part of the colon. The inflammation is confined to the mucosa and nearly always involves the rectum, extending to involve the distal or total colon. The aetiology is unknown but immuno-logical, dietary and genetic factors may be involved. The majority of cases present between 25 and 30 years. Familial clustering occurs. Malignant change occurs in the colon with time.

Symptoms and signs Diarrhoea, rectal bleeding, abdominal pain, fever, weight loss. The disease may be acute and fulminant, intermittent or chronic. Pallor, mulnutrition, abdominal tender-ness, abdominal distension, erythema nodosum, pyoderma gangrenosum, arthritis, uveitis, jaundice (sclerosing cholangitis).

Investigations • Hb • FBC • U&Es: dehydration and electro-lyte imbalance in severe cases • LFTs: hypoproteinaemia or abnormal because of complications of sclerosing cholangitis • AXR: acute toxic dilatation, perforation • Barium enema – double contrast (→ Fig. 14.15): loss of haustrations, mucosal distortion, colonic shortening, stricture due to carcinoma. Barium enema should not be performed on ill patients with toxic dilatation in case of perforation • Sigmoidoscopy: red, inflamed mucosa, contact bleeding, pseudopolyps • Biopsy • Colono-scopy: assess extent of disease, exclude carcinoma.

Complications Local complications include toxic dilatation, haemorrhage, stricture, perforation, and carcinoma. Extracolonic complications include seronegative arthritis (sacroileitis, ankylosing spondylitis), sclerosing cholangitis, chronic active hepatitis, uveitis, and amyloid.

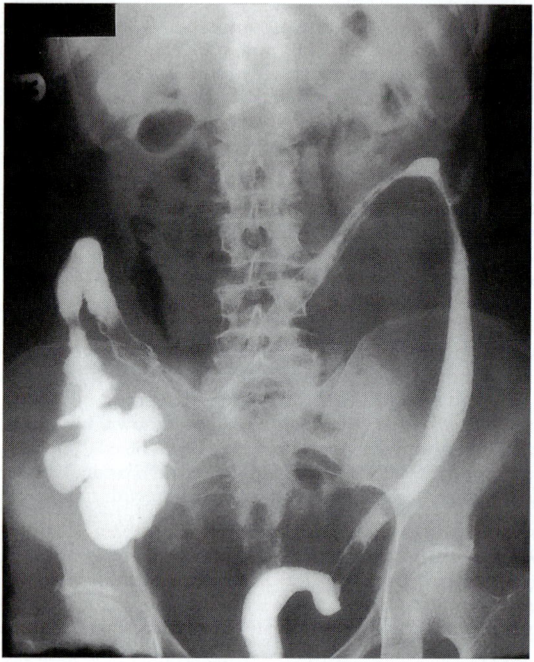

Fig. 14.15 Ulcerative colitis. There is shortening of the colon with loss of haustrations ('lead pipe' appearance).

Treatment

Medical Acute severe ulcerative colitis is treated with i.v. fluids, blood transfusion, parenteral nutrition and parenteral steroids. This regimen is instituted usually for 5 days. Regular examination of the patient is undertaken. If the patient deteriorates or toxic dilatation or perforation supervene, urgent surgery is required.

In the less ill patient oral steroids may be given until the disease is controlled. Those who respond to the above regimens may be treated with sulphasalazine or mesalazine orally to maintain the remission. Distal colitis and proctitis may be controlled by predsol retention enemas for relapses and sulphasalazine for maintenance.

→

Surgical Indications for surgery include acute toxic dilatation, perforation, failure to respond to medical treatment, chronic disease, severe arthritic symptoms, carcinoma. Surgery usually involves panproctocolectomy with ileostomy but other procedures now available include retention of the rectum with mucosal proctectomy or fashioning of an ileal pouch with maintenance of anal sphincters.

Prognosis The mortality rate with toxic dilatation or perforation is around 5%. The risk of colorectal cancer increases after 10 years' duration of disease, being about 2% at 10 years and up to 30% at 30 years. The risk is greater in those with total colitis and severe disease. Dysplasia often precedes carcinoma. Colonoscopic surveillance should be carried out at least 2-yearly.

DIVERTICULAR DISEASE

Diverticulae are outpouchings of mucosa through the bowel wall associated with increased intraluminal pressure (pulsion diverticulae). They occur between the taenia coli where vessels penetrate the bowel wall. They occur most commonly in the sigmoid colon and descending colon but may occur anywhere in the colon. They are rare before the age of 40 but thereafter there is an increase in incidence with age such that about 40% of patients over 70 have them. Diverticular disease is rare in countries where there is considerable roughage in the diet and is largely a condition occurring in western civilized societies where the diet is refined.

Symptoms and signs Diverticular disease may be asymptomatic (diverticulosis). *Acute diverticulitis* gives rise to lower abdominal colicky pain with localizing somatic pain usually in the LIF. Diarrhoea, constipation, and abdominal distension may occur. Fever. Tender in LIF. *Chronic diverticular disease* may cause lower abdominal colicky pain, alternating constipation and diarrhoea and excessive flatus together with abdominal distension. There may be little to find on abdominal examination.

Investigations • Hb • FBC (WCC raised in acute but normal in chronic) • Sigmoidoscopy to exclude carcinoma • Barium enema (→ Fig. 14.16) or colonoscopy

Differential diagnosis Carcinoma of the colon. Crohn's disease. Ischaemic colitis.

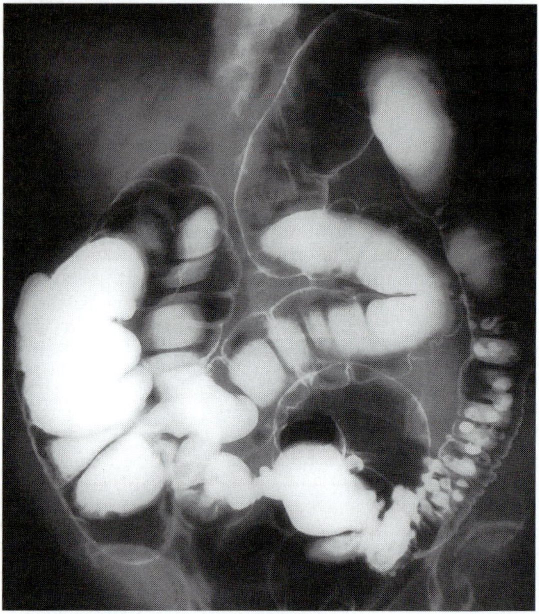

Fig. 14.16 Diverticular disease. A barium enema showing numerous diverticulae in the sigmoid colon.

Complications Acute diverticulitis. Stricture formation. Perforation with either generalized peritonitis, paracolic abscess, or fistula formation (vesicocolic, vaginocolic, ileocolic). Haemorrhage. Large bowel obstruction.

Treatment

Uncomplicated, symptomatic diverticular disease High-fibre diet. Antispasmodic, e.g. colofac. Bulking agent, e.g. fybogel.

Acute diverticulitis Bed rest. Fluids only or nil orally. Analgesic. Antibiotics: cefuroxime and metronidazole i.v. When symptoms settle, treatment is as for uncomplicated symptomatic diverticular disease.

Perforation with generalized faecal peritonitis Laparotomy. Peritoneal lavage. Resect perforated area. In case of sigmoid diverticulae treatment is by Hartmann's procedure. Drain →

peritoneal cavity. Antibiotics as for acute diverticulitis. In the elderly, perforated diverticulitis with faecal peritonitis carries a high mortality.

Perforation with paracolic abscess Percutaneous drainage followed by elective resection.

Perforation with fistula formation This involves bladder, vagina or small bowel. A vesicocolic fistula presents with dysuria and pneumaturia (passing wind in urine), a vaginocolic fistula presents with the passage of faeces PV and ileocolic fistula with diarrhoea. Vesicocolic fistulae show gas in the bladder on a plain radiograph. Barium enema may show the communication. Primary resection and anastomosis is the treatment of choice for ileocolic and vaginocolic fistulae. Vesicocolic fistulae may be treated by defunctioning colostomy followed by resection, followed by closure of colostomy. In an adequately prepared bowel, primary resection with end-to-end anastomosis of colon and closure of bladder with interposition of omentum between colonic anastomosis and bladder may be more appropriate treatment.

Haemorrhage Usually self-limiting. May be profuse and require transfusion. Exact site may be difficult to establish. Angiography may be required. If haemorrhage is life-threatening, total colectomy with ileostomy and preservation of rectal stump may be required. Continuity of the bowel is re-established subsequently.

Intestinal obstruction Progressive diverticular disease causes stricture. Treatment is by resection with either a Hartmann's procedure which is followed by subsequent restorative surgery, or a primary anastomosis protected by a temporary defunctioning colostomy.

VOLVULUS

This is a twisting of a loop of bowel around its mesenteric axis. Partial or complete obstruction may result. Occlusion of the arteries at the base of the involved mesentery leads to gangrene and perforation. The sigmoid colon and caecum may be involved, the sigmoid being the more common.

Sigmoid volvulus

Middle-aged and elderly males are more often affected. The twist is usually anticlockwise. A large redundant sigmoid colon and constipation are predisposing factors.

Symptoms and signs Sudden onset of lower abdominal colicky pain associated with gross abdominal distension. May be history of recurrent mild attacks associated with partial volvulus relieved by passage of large amounts of faeces and flatus. Distended tympanitic abdomen.

Investigations • AXR: distended loop of bowel the shape of a 'coffee bean' arising out of the pelvis on the left side • Barium enema may be helpful in doubtful cases – the barium column resembles a 'bird's beak' because of the way the lumen tapers towards the volvulus (→ Fig. 14.17).

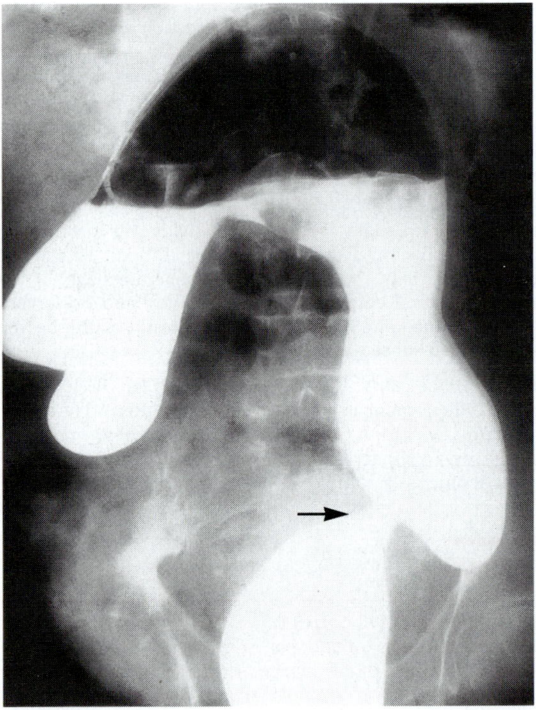

Fig. 14.17 Barium enema showing a sigmoid volvulus. A 'bird's beak' deformity is seen (arrow). In this case, barium has passed into the volvulus – often it does not.

Treatment Decompression by sigmoidoscopy. A rectal flatus tube should be left in situ for 48 hours. If the patient is fit, elective resection of the sigmoid is carried out at a later date. If decompression is unsuccessful or there are signs of gangrene or perforation, laparotomy with resection is undertaken, the two ends of the colon being brought out as a double-barrelled colostomy (Paul–Mickulicz procedure), which is later closed.

Caecal volvulus

This occurs when the caecum and ascending colon are excessively mobile, or if there has been a defect in rotation, the caecum retaining its mesentery.

Symptoms and signs Sudden onset of abdominal pain, vomiting and constipation. Tympanitic mass in LUQ. Tender mass if impending infarction.

Investigations • AXR: dilated caecum in left upper quadrant (→ Fig. 14.18).

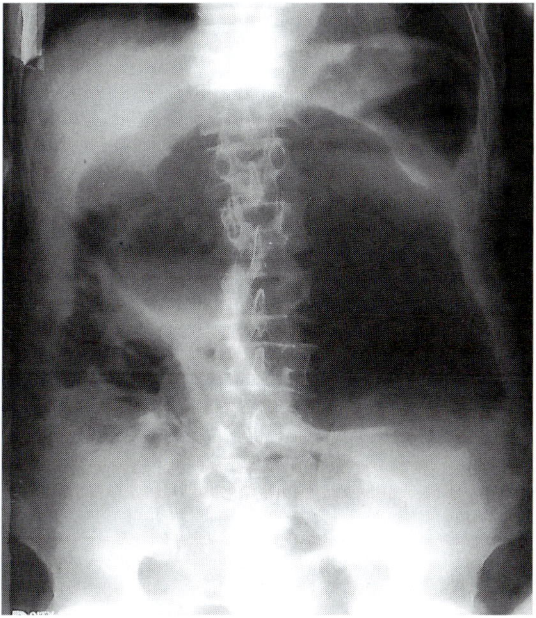

Fig. 14.18 Caecal volvulus. A hugely dilated caecum is seen in the epigastrium and left upper quadrant.

Treatment Laparotomy. If bowel is viable, untwisting with caecostomy. There is a high incidence of recurrence, however, and right hemicolectomy may be the best option. If caecostomy is carried out it may close spontaneously or may require subsequent closure. If the bowel is gangrenous at laparotomy, a right hemicolectomy is required.

Prognosis The mortality rate is high usually owing to delayed diagnosis.

Irradiation proctitis

This may complicate irradiation of pelvic lesions, e.g. cervix, uterus, bladder, prostate. Bleeding, diarrhoea and tenesmus may result. Later ulceration and stricture formation may also occur. Early symptoms appearing soon after irradiation may respond to steroid enemas. Diverting colostomy may be required for severe symptoms.

Angiodysplasia

Vascular anomalies which may be degenerative may cause bleeding from the large bowel. This is most common in the elderly. It is commonest in the right colon.

Symptoms and signs Bleeding PR which may be torrential but is often repeated small bleeds.

Investigations • Colonoscopy • Selective mesenteric angiography in the actively bleeding phase.

Treatment Coagulation under direct vision at colonoscopy. Embolization at angiography. Extensive areas require colectomy.

LARGE BOWEL OBSTRUCTION

The major causes are carcinoma, diverticular disease and volvulus. In 20% of patients the ileocaecal valve is competent and decompression into the small bowel does not occur. Closed-loop obstruction therefore occurs, the caecum progressively distending. Ischaemia and perforation of the caecum may occur.

Symptoms and signs Colicky abdominal pain, constipation, and vomiting (late). Constant severe pain suggests ischaemic bowel. Distended tympanitic abdomen. Obstructed bowel sounds. Rectum may be empty on examination PR.

Investigations • Sigmoidoscopy: rectosigmoid lesions may be seen • AXR: distended large bowel with air/fluid levels surrounding the abdomen like a picture frame (→ Fig. 14.19). • Limited barium enema may show 'apple core' lesion. • Instant enema to exclude pseudo-obstruction.

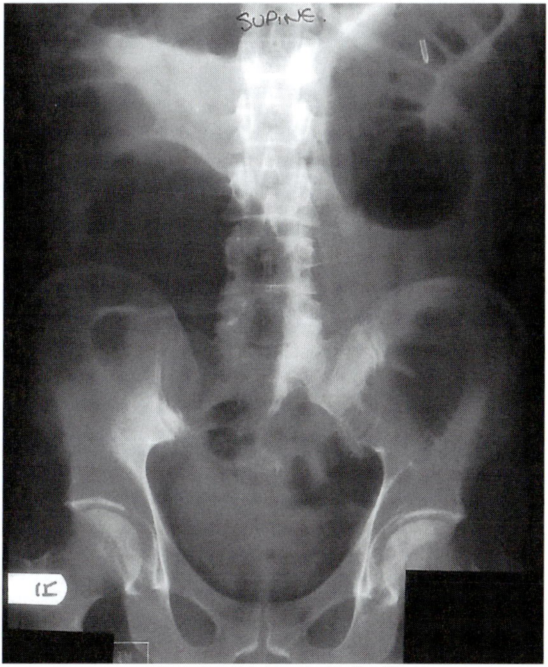

A

Fig. 14.19 A plain AXR showing large bowel obstruction.
A. Supine film. The left colon is distended down to the pelvis where there is sharp 'cut-off' of the gas shadow.

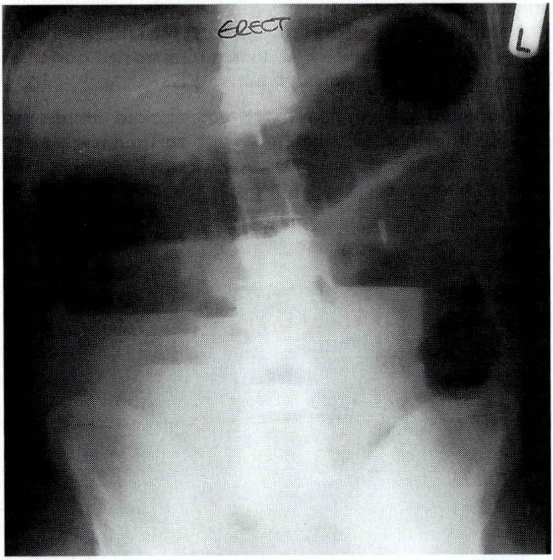

B

Fig. 14.19 (*Contd*) **B.** Erect film. This shows air/fluid levels in the large bowel. Again the sharp 'cut-off' is seen in the pelvis. This represents the point of the obstructing lesion, which in this case was in the lower sigmoid colon.

Treatment Drip and suck. Correct electrolyte imbalance. A caecum 10 cm or greater in diameter on radiograph is an urgent indication for surgery, especially if tender to palpation. Laparotomy with decompression of the obstruction. Right-sided lesions are treated by right hemicolectomy. Left-sided lesions may be treated by left hemicolectomy with covering colostomy. Low left-sided lesions are treated by resection of the tumour with Hartmann's procedure. However, on-table lavage of the colon and primary anastomosis may be carried out in experienced hands. A carcinoma on the apex of the sigmoid loop may be treated by resection and a Paul–Mickulicz double-barrel colostomy. In a poorly patient a defunctioning colostomy or caecostomy may be carried out and elective resection delayed until a later date when the patient is fitter. Sigmoid volvulus may be treated by resection and a Paul–Mickulicz procedure. Colonic stenting may be carried out in those unfit for surgery.

Prognosis The overall mortality rate approaches 15%. Perforation is the main cause of mortality.

ANAL CONDITIONS

HAEMORRHOIDS

These are enlarged vascular cushions in the lower rectum and anal canal. They are not simply varicosities. At least 10% of the population have symptomatic haemorrhoids at some time in their life. The classical position of haemorrhoids corresponds to branches of the superior haemorrhoidal artery occurring at the 3 o'clock, 7 o'clock and 11 o'clock positions with the patient in the lithotomy position.

Symptoms and signs Asymptomatic. Rectal bleeding (on toilet paper or drips into toilet on defaecation). Prolapse. Itching. Piles are not painful unless they thrombose. First-degree piles remain in the rectum and manifest only by bleeding. Second-degree piles prolapse on defaecation but reduce spontaneously. Third-degree piles prolapse and require manual reduction. Check Hb if bleeding is prolonged or heavy. Examine abdomen to exclude other lesions. Digital rectal examination.

Investigations • Sigmoidoscopy to exclude other lesions • Proctoscopy to confirm presence of piles. Remember at least 10% of population have piles. Abdominal pain is not associated with piles • If there is any doubt as to the cause of bleeding, carry out a barium enema.

- Injection treatment: inject 2–3 ml of phenol in almond oil into the submucosa above the pile. This is suitable for first-degree and small second-degree piles.
- Other non-operative approaches include rubber band ligation, cryosurgery and photocoagulation.
- Large second-degree piles and third-degree piles require haemorrhoidectomy.
- Thrombosed piles may be treated by bed rest, analgesia and ice packs. The piles may thrombose with cure or remain as skin tags which require subsequent excision. Some surgeons advocate emergency haemorrhoidectomy. Whatever treatment is used, subsequent regulation of bowel habit with high-fibre diet and bulk laxatives is required.

Treatment

Complications of haemorrhoidectomy Acute retention of urine. Haemorrhage (slipped ligature in the early postoperative period or secondary haemorrhage 8–10 days postoperatively). Stricture may occur with anal stenosis if too much skin has been excised.

Differential diagnosis Perianal haematoma, rectal prolapse, fissure-in-ano, inflammatory bowel disease, anal polyp, carcinoma, proctalgia fugax.

RECTAL PROLAPSE

This may be partial or complete. Partial prolapse involves the mucosa alone and prolapse is usually no more than a few centimetres. Complete prolapse involves all layers of the rectal wall and is most common in elderly females.

Symptoms and signs Protruding mass from anus especially during defaecation. May reduce spontaneously. May need manual reduction and eventually becomes difficult to reduce. Blood and mucus PR from ulceration of exposed mucosa. Palpate prolapse between fingers. Mucosal prolapse reveals two layers of mucosa about 2–4 cm long with radial folds. Lax sphincter on examination PR. Complete prolapse is thick, up to 12 cm long and patient may be unable to contract sphincter muscles after prolapse reduced.

Differential diagnosis Prolapsing haemorrhoids, polyps, intussusception.

Treatment Mucosal prolapse usually responds to sclerosants injected submucosally as for piles. Excision of prolapse mucosa may be necessary. Complete prolapse is treated by abdominal rectopexy. The rectum is mobilized and fixed to the sacrum usually by inserting a Teflon prosthesis to hold it in position (Ripstein's procedure). Other procedures include excision of mucosa and longitudinal plication of the rectal muscle (Delorme procedure); and circumferential narrowing of the anus by inserting a suture subcutaneously around the anal orifice (Thiersch wire – although nylon rather than wire is used nowadays).

Complications Abdominal rectopexy usually gives good results but residual incontinence due to chronic stretching of the sphincter may result. Thiersch wire procedure may result in infection and faecal impaction.

Rectal prolapse in children

Usually self-correcting. Parents require reassurance. Keep act of defaecation as short as possible and avoid straining. Repeat simple reduction is all that is required. A mild laxative may be necessary. In a few cases subcutaneous injection sclerosant may be required.

PERIANAL HAEMATOMA

Symptoms and signs Acute perianal pain. Worse on sitting, walking and defaecation. Tense, smooth, tender blue lump at anal verge.

Treatment Symptoms may subside spontaneously after 2-3 days during which time analgesia is given. If patient presents in acute phase, incision under LA should be carried out.

FISSURE-IN-ANO

This is a tear at the anal margin due to passage of a constipated stool. The fissure is usually in the midline posteriorly but may occasionally be anterior. Multiple fissures may be due to Crohn's disease.

Symptoms and sign Acute anal pain, severe on defaecation. Blood on toilet paper. Part the buttocks and the fissure may be apparent. Acute sphincter spasm. Examination PR impossible. Occasionally 'sentinel' pile. This is a skin tag at the anal verge external to the fissure.

Differential diagnosis Crohn's disease, trauma (beware abuse in children), carcinoma, herpes, TB, syphilis and psoriasis.

Treatment

Conservative If symptoms are relatively mild, LA gel or suppository may be applied. This is best applied some half hour before defaecation. Attention should be given to correcting constipation with a stool-softening laxative and high-fibre diet. An alternative treatment is to apply 0.2% →

GTN ointment locally, which relaxes the internal anal sphincter. This should be applied twice daily for 6 weeks. Many fissures heal with this regimen at the expense of headache due to absorption of GTN.

Surgical Acutely painful fissures should be treated as surgical emergencies. A lateral subcutaneous internal sphincterotomy should be carried out to relieve spasm and to allow the fissure to heal. A laxative and high-fibre diet should be taken in the postoperative period. Chronic fissures should be treated by lateral subcutaneous internal sphincterotomy. Recurrent fissures should be treated by excision of the fissure, which is sent for histological examination to exclude underlying causes.

ANORECTAL ABSCESSES (→ Fig. 14.20)

These develop in tissue spaces adjacent to the anorectal area. They may be perianal (in a hair follicle, sebaceous gland or perianal haematoma), ischiorectal (in the ischiorectal fossa), intermuscular (between internal and external sphincters), or pelvirectal (spreading from a pelvic abscess – rare). In many cases the infection may start in the anal crypt and spread along tissue planes.

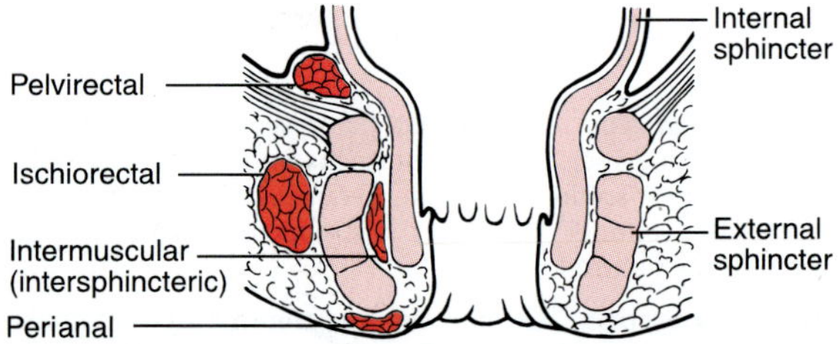

Fig. 14.20 The anatomy of anorectal abscesses.

Symptoms and signs Constant, throbbing, perianal pain worse on sitting. With pelvirectal abscesses, the pain may also be in the lower abdomen. Indurated tender mass perianally. Boggy mass on examination PR, in ischiorectal fossa or anteriorly if pelvirectal abscess. Fever.

Treatment Prompt surgical drainage to prevent fistula formation. There is no role for antibiotics except in diabetics and the immunocompromised and then only as an adjunct to surgery. Incision, curettage and packing are required.

Complications Fistula-in-ano occurs in up to 30% of patients.

FISTULA-IN-ANO

A fistula is an abnormal communication between two epithelial surfaces. In this instance there is an internal opening in the anal canal and one or more external openings on the perianal skin. The majority arise from delay in treatment, or inadequate treatment, of anorectal abscesses. Rarer causes include Crohn's disease, tuberculosis and carcinoma. It may be difficult to locate the internal opening. Application of Goodsall's rule ('if the external opening lies anterior to a line drawn transversely through the centre of the anus, the track passes radially through a straight line towards the internal opening (→ Fig. 14.21). If the external opening is behind this line the track curves in a horseshoe manner to open into the midline posteriorly'). Fistulae may be classified as subcutaneous, submucous, low anal (below puborectalis), high anal (opening in close relation to the anorectal junction) or pelvirectal (penetrating levator ani) (→ Fig. 14.22).

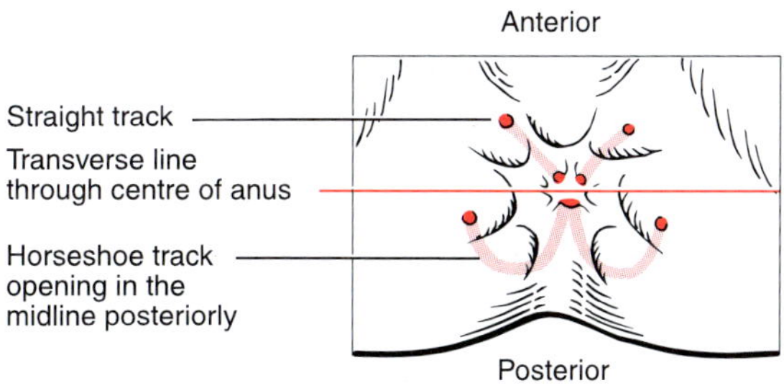

Fig. 14.21 Goodsall's rule.

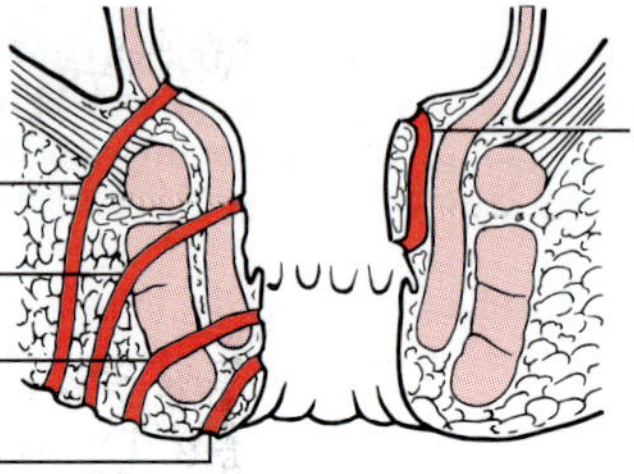

Fig. 14.22 The anatomy of fistula-in-ano.

Symptoms and signs History of abscess which drains spontaneously or was surgically drained. Persistent drainage of pus, mucus, blood or faecal matter associated with perianal irritation and discomfort. Drainage may be intermittent if the fistula heals and opens recurrently. Single opening near anus. Examination PR reveals indurated track, pressure on which may cause discharge. Proctoscopy or sigmoidoscopy to define internal opening.

Differential diagnosis Pilonidal sinus, hidradenitis suppurativa, incontinence, Crohn's disease, trauma.

Treatment The track is identified by probing and laid open under GA, so that it heals by granulation tissue from the base. With high fistulae or pelvirectal fistulae there is a danger to puborectalis when opening the track. Incontinence may result. Fortunately the latter types are rare but require specialist treatment often by a two-stage operation.

PRURITUS ANI

This is itching in the perianal area. It is a symptom of various conditions. Local causes include poor hygiene, sweating, fistula, haemorrhoids, neoplasia, warts, fungal infections, contact dermatitis (deodorants), worms, antibiotics (possibly via the complication of diarrhoea or fungal infection). General causes include diabetes mellitus, obstructive jaundice, Hodgkin's disease. Dermatological diseases include scabies, pediculosis, psoriasis and atopic eczema. The majority of causes are probably idiopathic or psychogenic. Often an 'itch/scratch' vicious circle is created and symptoms persist even after the initial cause has been eradicated.

Symptoms and signs Worse at night whatever the cause. History of precipitating cause, e.g. antibiotics, diabetes, pruritus elsewhere. Perianal skin may be normal, or inflamed, moist or macerated. Examination PR and proctoscopy to exclude anal conditions, e.g. fistulae.

Investigations • Hb • WCC • Blood sugar • Perianal scrapings and microscopy for fungus.

Treatment Specific for the underlying disease. Non-specific treatment includes advice on hygiene, diet, wearing loose underclothes, cleansing after defaecation with simple soap and application of glycerine and witch hazel. Application of hydrocortisone and LA cream may help. Occasionally the condition is difficult to treat.

VENEREAL DISEASES

Condylomata acuminata (anal warts) Caused by human papilloma virus. Usually venereal. Over 50% of patients admit to anal intercourse. May be few or a continuous carpet of warts extending into the anal canal. Symptoms include bleeding and pruritus. Small groups may be treated with topical podophyllin. Widespread lesions require surgical excision or diathermy. Recurrence is common.

Gonorrhoea Gonococcal proctitis presents with pain, bleeding and purulent rectal discharge. Proctoscopy reveals ulcerated friable mucosa and pus in the rectal lumen. Culture confirms diagnosis. Treatment is usually by i.m. procaine penicillin and probenecid.

Herpes Severe perianal pain, constipation, discharge and ulceration. Examination reveals vesicles and ulcers. Treatment is by topical or oral acyclovir.

Syphilis Perianal or anal ulcers. May resemble anal fissure. Often painless. Diagnosis is confirmed by dark field examination of discharge and serology. Penicillin is treatment of choice. Contact follow-up is important.

AIDS Anorectal manifestations include fissure, perianal sepsis, ulceration, fungal or viral infections, rectal lymphoma and Kaposi's sarcoma.

ANAL MALIGNANCIES

Anal tumours are rare and include epidermoid tumours, malignant melanoma, lymphoma (often in association with AIDS), and Kaposi's sarcoma (associated with AIDS). Adenocarcinoma occurs in the upper part of the anal canal but may spread across the dentate line and appear at the anal margin. The most common of the tumours is the epidermoid carcinoma (squamous cell carcinoma). Patients should be checked for a history of homosexuality with penetrative anal sex.

Symptoms and signs Bleeding, pruritus, pain, discharge, palpable mass in anal canal. Patients may think they have haemorrhoids. Rectal examination may reveal visible tumour growing out of the anus. Hard, irregular, ulcerated mass. Palpable inguinal nodes. Hepatomegaly if secondaries.

Investigations • Biopsy • USS liver.

Treatment Small, non-invasive lesions may be locally excised and treated with radiotherapy. Larger lesions invading the sphincters will require abdominoperineal resection, although recent evidence suggests survival rates may be as good with radiotherapy combined with chemotherapy.

Prognosis 50% of patients survive 5 years.

RECTAL BLEEDING

Bleeding PR is a common clinical problem. The commonest causes are haemorrhoids, fissure-in-ano and colorectal cancer. Massive rectal bleeding may be due to diverticular disease, angiodysplasia, or a cause in the upper GI tract, e.g. peptic ulcer or an aorto-enteric fistula. If bright red rectal haemorrhage is coming from the upper GI tract, the bleeding is massive with rapid gut transit time and the patient will always be shocked. (For causes of rectal bleeding → Table 14.3.)

Symptoms and signs Check colour and amount of blood. Bright red bleeding in small amounts usually indicates that the source is in the anal canal or rectum. Large amounts suggest diverticular disease or angiodysplasia. Bleeding for haemorrhoids may occasionally be considerable. Blood on toilet paper suggests haemorrhoids or fissure-in-ano. Dripping into the toilet at defaecation suggests haemorrhoids. Blood streaked on stools suggests rectosigmoid or rectal carcinoma. Blood and mucus on defaecation suggest rectal carcinoma. Blood, mucus and pus associated with abdominal pain, diarrhoea and fever, suggest colitis. Bleeding associated with change in bowel habit and abdominal pain suggests colonic cancer. Bleeding associated with pain on

Table 14.3
Causes of rectal bleeding

Haemorrhoids Fissure-in-ano Carcinoma of anus

Colorectal carcinoma
Colorectal polyps
Diverticular disease
Inflammatory bowel disease:
  Crohn's disease
  Ulcerative colitis
Ischaemic colitis
Angiodysplasia
Irradiation colitis or proctitis
Rectal prolapse

Meckel's diverticulum Intussusception Mesenteric infarction Aortoenteric fistula
Massive upper GI haemorrhage
Trauma
Bleeding diathesis

defaecation suggests fissure-in-ano or carcinoma of the anal canal. Check for abdominal pain, anal pain, change in bowel habit, abdominal distension. Symptoms of anaemia, weight loss, jaundice. Abdominal mass, e.g. colonic tumour, hepatomegaly (metastases). Abdominal tenderness, distended abdomen – shifting dullness (ascites) – obstructed bowel sounds. Inspection PR for piles, warts, fissure, tumour. Rectal mass (90% of rectal cancers can be felt on examination PR).

Investigations • Hb • FBC • ESR • U&Es (ureteric involvement with colorectal tumours) • LFTs (liver metastases) • Clotting screen • Proctoscopy: haemorrhoids • Sigmoidoscopy and biopsy • Barium enema • Colonoscopy • Selective mesenteric angiography, preferably in bleeding phase • Radiolabelled autologous red cells • Technetium scanning (taken up by ectopic gastric mucosa in Meckel's) • Gastroscopy if upper GI haemorrhage suspected.

Treatment Principles of treatment include:

- resuscitation if massive bleeding
- diagnosis of the cause
- definitive treatment of the cause.

The treatment of the various conditions is covered elsewhere in this book.

LIVER

Diseases of the liver usually present to the surgeon as jaundice, hepatomegaly, or ascites. This section will deal only with liver disease as far as it concerns the surgeon. (For causes of hepatomegaly → Table 14.4.)

Table 14.4
Causes of hepatomegaly

Regular generalized enlargement without jaundice	Cirrhosis Congestive cardiac failure Reticuloses Budd–Chiari syndrome (hepatic vein obstruction) Amyloid
Regular generalized enlargement with jaundice	Viral hepatitis Biliary tract obstruction Cholangitis
Irregular generalized enlargement without jaundice	Secondary tumours Macronodular cirrhosis Polycystic disease Primary tumours
Irregular generalized enlargement with jaundice	Cirrhosis Widespread liver secondaries
Localized swellings	Riedel's lobe Hydatid cyst Amoebic abscess Primary carcinoma

INFECTIONS IN THE LIVER

Abscess

This is rare and usually caused by pyogenic bacteria. Causes are due to the following:

- portal pyelophlebitis secondary to acute abdominal infection, e.g. appendicitis, diverticulitis, peritonitis
- biliary disease, e.g. cholecystitis, ascending cholangitis
- trauma
- direct extension from subphrenic abscess, empyema of gall bladder
- septicaemia
- infection of a liver cyst
- rarely there is no cause, i.e. cryptogenic.

Symptoms and signs Those of underlying disease. Fever, toxic, rigors, jaundice, upper abdominal pain, may be of acute onset with no apparent underlying cause. Tender hepatomegaly.

Investigations • WCC • LFTs: abnormal • Blood cultures positive • USS • CT • Indium-labelled WC scan.

Differential diagnosis Tumour, amoebic abscess.

Treatment Multiple small abscesses require antibiotics, e.g. gentamicin and metronidazole. Prognosis is poor. These often complicate septicaemia in an immunocompromised patient. Solitary or multiple large abscesses may be treated by percutaneous drainage under US control. Occasionally open surgical drainage is required.

Amoebic abscess

Due to infection with protozoan parasite *Entamoeba histolytica.* More than 50% occur in the absence of amoebic dysentery. Abscesses may be single (common) or multiple. They may be small or very large containing up to 3 litres of pus. More common in the right lobe of the liver. Cases in Europe occur in immigrants or those who have returned from areas where the disease is endemic.

Symptoms and signs Insidious onset. Right hypochondrial pain. Malaise. Pyrexia. Weight loss. Occasionally rigors and diarrhoea. Jaundice uncommon.

Investigations • USS • CT.

Treatment Metronidazole. Large cysts require percutaneous drainage and US control. Surgery is rarely required and usually only if cyst rupture has occurred.

Hydatid disease

Due to infection with an *Echinococcus granulosus* (tapeworm). The tapeworm develops in the dog intestine and ova are shed in the faeces. These contaminate grass or vegetables and are ingested by sheep, cattle or humans. The ova then pass to the liver via the portal circulation where they develop into hydatid cysts. These may also enter the kidneys and lungs. The disease occurs in sheep- and cattle-rearing countries of the world, e.g. Australia, Africa and Wales.

Symptoms and signs Symptomless mass. Abdominal pain. Jaundice (due to pressure on ducts). Rupture into the peritoneal cavity results in peritonitis and shock.

Investigations • AXR: calcified outline of cyst • Hydatid serology • USS • CT.

Treatment Medical treatment is by albendazole. This may result in shrinkage in some cases but usually surgery is indicated. Care must be taken to avoid spilling cyst contents into the peritoneal cavity as anaphylactic shock may occur. The cyst is usually aspirated under direct vision and a scolicidal agent injected into the cyst, e.g. hypertonic saline. The cyst is then carefully excised and the cavity closed. Albendazole is given pre- and postoperatively.

LIVER TUMOURS

Secondary tumours are common arising from the GI tract, lung and breast. More than 25% of patients who die of malignant disease have liver secondaries. Primary tumours are rare. The commonest malignant primary tumours are hepatocellular carcinoma and cholangiocarcinoma. Benign tumours are rare and include adenoma and cavernous haemangioma.

PRIMARY MALIGNANT TUMOURS

Hepatocellular carcinoma

About 50% of these carcinomas occur in patients with cirrhosis. It is common in Africa and the Far East, and more common than cholangiocarcinoma. It is associated with hepatitis B, the contraceptive pill, aflatoxin, anabolic steroids.

Symptoms and signs Pre-existing cirrhosis. Abdominal pain. Weight loss. Fever. Ascites. Jaundice. Hepatomegaly.

Investigations • Hb • ESR • LFTs abnormal • α-fetoprotein raised (mainly in cirrhotics) • CXR: raised diaphragm, lung secondary • USS • CT • Liver biopsy under US control • Arteriography prior to resection to assess resectability and blood supply.

Treatment Surgical resection if confined to one lobe. Liver transplantation. Chemotherapy directly into hepatic artery.

Prognosis Small tumours confined to one lobe treated by hepatic lobectomy have a good prognosis. Otherwise the prognosis is poor, death usually occurring within 1 year.

Cholangiocarcinoma

The tumour arises from the cells of the intrahepatic bile duct system. It is less common than hepatocellular carcinoma. There is an association with primary sclerosing cholangitis, liver fluke infestation and anabolic steroids.

Symptoms and signs Usually presents with jaundice.

Investigations • Hb • LFTs: bilirubin↑, alkaline phosphatase↑ • USS • CT • Liver biopsy under US control • ERCP.

Treatment Rapid, direct, and lymphatic spread makes surgical cure rare. Surgical resection with hemihepatectomy is sometimes possible. Palliation of jaundice via surgical bypass or endoscopic stenting. Rarely liver transplantation may be feasible.

Prognosis Bad. Most patients are dead within 6 months.

Hepatic metastases

Common. More than 90% of patients with hepatic metastases have metastatic disease elsewhere.

Symptoms and signs Those of the primary tumour. Previous surgery for primary. Anorexia, vomiting, weight loss, cachexia. Upper abdominal pain or discomfort. Jaundice. Ascites. Hard, irregular, palpable liver.

Investigations • Hb • LFTs: alkaline phosphatase↑, bilirubin↑, albumin↓ • CEA for colorectal secondaries • USS • CT (→ Fig. 14.23) • Biopsy under US control.

Treatment Younger patients with metastases from colorectal cancer, confined to one lobe of the liver and up to four in number, should be treated by partial hepatectomy. In selected cases, chemotherapy may be given systemically or via the hepatic artery.

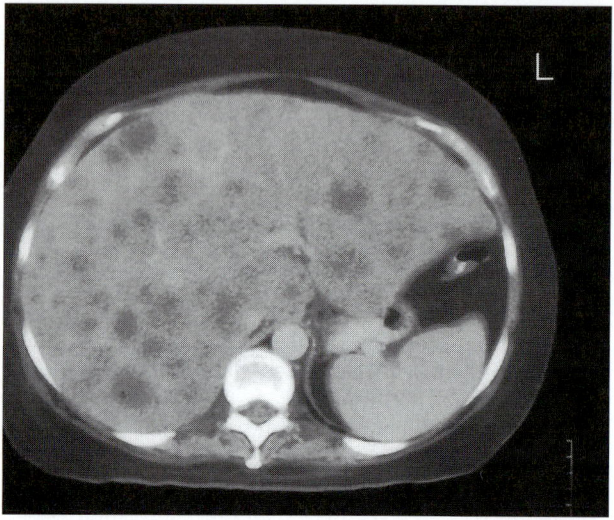

Fig. 14.23 CT scan of abdomen. Numerous liver metastases are seen in both the right and left lobes of the liver.

Prognosis Depends upon the type of metastatic tumour. Most patients survive less than 2 years but there is a 35–40% 5-year survival rate for patients with colorectal secondaries that are completely resected.

PORTAL HYPERTENSION

Portal hypertension occurs when portal venous pressure equals or exceeds 15 mmHg (20 cm water). Collateral channels open up between the portal and systemic circulations, the clinically most important of these being at the gastro-oesophageal junction, leading to the development of the oesophageal varices which may be responsible for torrential bleeding. Other consequences of portal hypertension include splenomegaly, ascites (in hepatic and posthepatic forms) and the manifestations of hepatic failure (encephalopathy).

Causes

Prehepatic Congenital malformations, neonatal umbilical sepsis. Exchange transfusion via umbilical catheter. Tumour.

Hepatic Cirrhosis, schistosomiasis.

Posthepatic Budd–Chiari syndrome (obstruction of the hepatic veins which may be due to idiopathic hepatic vein thrombosis, congenital obliteration, or blockage of the hepatic vein by tumour), constrictive pericarditis.

Symptoms and signs Jaundice. Mental changes. Flapping tremor. Coma. Haematemesis and melaena. Ascites. Spider naevi, liver palms, clubbing, gynaecomastia, testicular atrophy, caput medusae. Peripheral oedema. Leukonychia. Dupuytren's contracture. Xanthoma. Keyser–Fleischer rings. Bruising.

Investigations • Hb • FBC • LFTs • Coagulation screen • OGD.

Treatment of bleeding oesophageal varices

Acute bleed Resuscitate. CVP monitoring. Blood transfusion. FFP. Platelets. Urgent endoscopy to confirm diagnosis. Inject the varices with sclerosant at the time of endoscopy. If a good view cannot be obtained because of gross bleeding, the following measures should be undertaken:

- tamponade with a Sengstaken–Blakemore tube
- administer vasopressin i.v. to lower portal venous pressure
- administer i.v. metoclopramide which constricts lower oesophageal sphincter and empties stomach of blood
- somatostatin may be beneficial by reducing portal venous pressure.

The control of bleeding by tamponade is temporary while the next stage of treatment is planned. Usually this is sclerotherapy which is effective in 90% of patients. Patients who fail to respond should be considered for oesophageal transection or shunting.

Definitive treatment after bleeding

- Chronic injection sclerotherapy. The varices are injected at monthly intervals until they are obliterated. Endoscopic follow-up is carried out on a regular basis. Complications of this technique include ulceration, stricture, and dysphagia.
- Portosystemic shunting. Splenoportogram and CT are carried out to assess the patency of the portal vein. Shunts may be portocaval, mesocaval, or splenorenal. They may be carried out as an emergency to lower portal pressure but it is rare to do so since the advent of injection sclerotherapy. Shunting is usually carried out in the elective stage when there have been previous bleeding episodes.

→

For a successful shunt operation, hepatic function needs to be reasonably good. Jaundice, hypoalbuminaemia, ascites, and encephalopathy indicate a bad prognosis with shunt operations. Liver transplantation is preferable except when the obstruction is prehepatic with good liver function.

Prophylaxis Many patients with varices never bleed. If varices are known to be present, oral β-blockade with propranolol significantly decreases the incidence of bleeding and rebleeding.

Prognosis Up to 40% of patients having their first variceal bleed will die. Long-term survival after portocaval shunt operations is poor. The 5-year survival after portocaval shunting for alcoholic liver disease is about 45%. Some degree of encephalopathy develops in 14–30% of patients.

EXTRAHEPATIC BILIARY SYSTEM

CHOLELITHIASIS (GALLSTONES)

This is common and present in 10% of the population over 50. It is more common in females especially in multiparous women. Obesity, drugs, contraceptive pill, clofibrate, haemolytic disorders, ileal disease (resection, Crohn's disease) are aetiological factors. Factors which may produce lithogenic bile include increased cholesterol content, reduced bile acids, biliary stasis. Classically three types of stone are described:

- cholesterol stones (may be solitary), cholesterol 'solitaire' – radiolucent
- pigment – occur with haemolysis – small, black, irregular and friable – radiolucent
- mixed – often faceted – contain calcium, pigment, and cholesterol – 10% are radio-opaque (→ Fig. 14.24).

About 80% of stones are asymptomatic. Symptoms are related to the complications they cause.

Complications

Gall bladder Acute cholecystitis, chronic cholecystitis, acute-on-chronic cholecystitis. Empyema (pus in the gall bladder). Mucocele (mucus in the gall bladder). Carcinoma. Perforation of gall bladder.

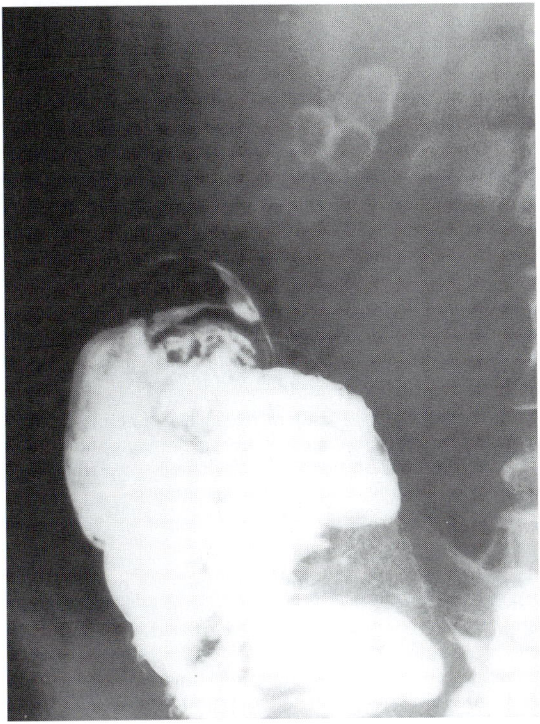

Fig. 14.24 Gallstones. An incidental finding on barium enema. There are several radio-opaque gallstones in the right hypochondrium.

In the ducts Obstructive jaundice, cholangitis, pancreatitis.

In the gut Gallstone ileus (associated with cholecystoduodenal fistula).

Acute cholecystitis

Gallstones are the most common cause. Rarely acalculous cholecystitis may occur. Sometimes it is associated with typhoid fever. Most cases are in fact acute-on-chronic, many patients having demonstrated symptoms of chronic cholecystitis in the past.

Symptoms and signs Nausea, fever, vomiting. RUQ pain radiating under ribs to right scapula. Tender with guarding R hypochondrium. Positive Murphy's sign.

Investigations • Haemoglobin • WCC • LFTs • USS.

Treatment Nil orally. i.v. fluids. NG suction. Analgesia (usually pethidine). Antibiotic (usually cefuroxime i.v.). Symptoms usually settle in 48–72 hours. Elective cholecystectomy is usually carried out 3 months later. Emergency cholecystectomy may be required if symptoms do not settle on conservative management.

Chronic cholecystitis

Virtually always associated with gallstones. Repeated episodes of infection cause chronic thickening and fibrosis.

Symptoms and signs Flatulent dyspepsia. The classical case is the middle-aged obese female who gets upper abdominal discomfort and distension relieved by belching. Intolerance of fatty food. Often little to find on clinical examination.

Investigations • USS.

Treatment Cholecystectomy. This may be by the open or laparoscopic technique. Unfit patients may be placed on a low-fat diet to control symptoms or treated by extracorporeal shock wave lithotripsy if suitable. Dissolution of stones which are small and non-radio-opaque in a functioning gall bladder may be attempted with chenodeoxycholic acid given orally.

Biliary colic

This is a symptom rather than a complication of gallstones. It is produced by impaction of a stone in the neck of the gall bladder or in the cystic duct. The stone may either fall back into the gall bladder or pass through the cystic duct into the CBD, whence the pain abates.

Symptoms and signs Sudden onset of severe pain across the epigastrium (it is not confined to the RUQ). Severe spasms of colic against the background of continuous severe pain. The patient rolls around in agony and cannot get into a comfortable position. Tachycardia, sweating, and vomiting. Examination may reveal rigidity in the upper abdomen (beware making a diagnosis of peritonitis – in peritonitis the patient does not roll around but remains still). An attack may last 2–4 hours. Following an attack jaundice may occur owing to the passed stone impacting in the CBD.

Treatment Pethidine i.m. Subsequent investigations for gall bladder disease and cholecystectomy if appropriate.

Mucocele

This may follow an attack of biliary colic. Stone impacts in neck of gall bladder. Bile absorbed. Mucus secretion continues.

Symptoms and signs Previous history of biliary colic. RUQ discomfort. Occasionally patient feels lump. Large, tense globular mass in RUQ.

Investigations • USS.

Treatment Cholecystectomy.

Empyema

This follows an attack of cholecystitis. Infection develops after impaction of a stone in the neck of the gall bladder. Obstruction leads to stasis, overgrowth of bacteria and the gall bladder fills with pus.

Symptoms and signs Attack of acute cholecystitis or biliary colic. Fever, toxicity. RUQ pain. Tender mass in RUQ.

Investigations • WCC • USS.

Treatment i.v. fluids. NG suction. Antibiotics – cefuroxime and metronidazole. Cholecystectomy. Occasionally there is so much inflammation that it is impossible to safely carry out cholecystectomy. Drainage of the gall bladder with formation of a cholecystotomy may be appropriate in these circumstances. Cholecystectomy may be undertaken at a later date.

Perforation of the gall bladder

This is rare and usually presents either as generalized biliary peritonitis or leakage of pus from a perforated empyema. Infected biliary peritonitis has a high mortality especially as this condition is most common in the elderly. Treatment involves laparotomy, peritoneal lavage, cholecystectomy and antibiotics (usually gentamicin and metronidazole).

Carcinoma

It is associated with long-standing gallstone disease and is commoner in females. Local invasion of the liver and bile ducts occurs. Jaundice occurs owing to direct extension into the bile duct together with secondaries in the nodes at the porta hepatis. Small tumours may be an incidental finding at cholecystectomy for gallstones. In the latter case, long-term survival may be expected. Many cases present late when local spread and lymph node metastases have occurred. In this case, prognosis is poor – 90% of patients surviving less than 1 year.

Cholangitis

This is a serious condition caused by complete or partial biliary obstruction in association with ascending infection of the biliary tree. It may be complicated by septicaemia and liver abscesses.

Symptoms and signs Fever, rigors, jaundice (Charcot's biliary triad).

Investigations • WCC • Blood cultures • USS.

Treatment Antibiotics – cefuroxime/metronidazole/gentamicin. Acute suppurative cholangitis may occur with pus under tension in the biliary tree. Urgent decompression of the bile ducts via a cannula inserted endoscopically via the ampulla of Vater may be required.

Gallstone ileus

This results from a fistula occurring between the fundus of the gall bladder and the adjacent duodenum. A stone passes through the fistula and may impact in the terminal ileum causing obstruction to the small bowel.

Symptoms and signs Colicky abdominal pain, vomiting and distension. History of flatulent dyspepsia. The diagnosis should be suspected in middle-aged to elderly females with symptoms of small bowel obstruction in the absence of a hernia or previous abdominal surgery to suggest adhesion formation.

Investigations • AXR: dilated loops of small bowel, air in the biliary tree (→ Fig. 14.25).

Treatment Laparotomy. Removal of stone from small bowel lumen by 'milking' through ileocaecal valve or removal by enterotomy. Cholecystectomy at a later date if symptoms referable to gall bladder continue.

Acalculous cholecystitis

Acute cholecystitis without gallstones may occur in a variety of conditions. It may be due to infection, e.g. typhoid, or may occur following sepsis, burns, TPN, multiple injuries, in the puerperium and after unrelated surgery. Treatment is the same as for calculus acute cholecystitis.

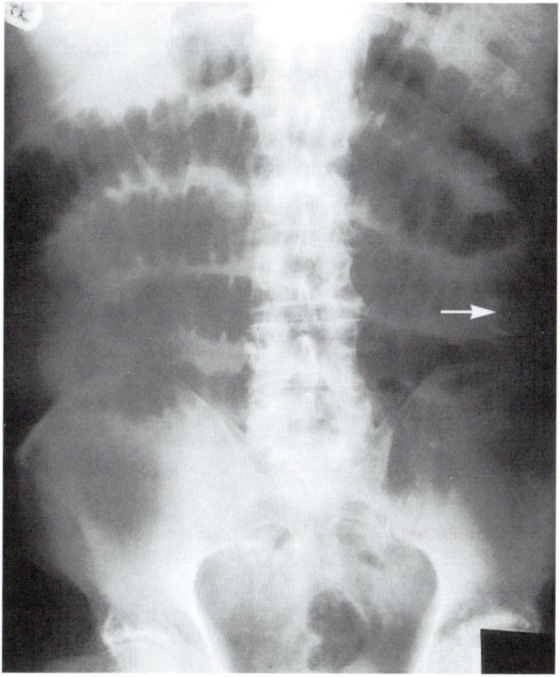

Fig. 14.25 Plain AXR showing gallstone ileus. **A** Dilated loops of small bowel are seen. A gallstone is visible on the left side of the abdomen (arrow).

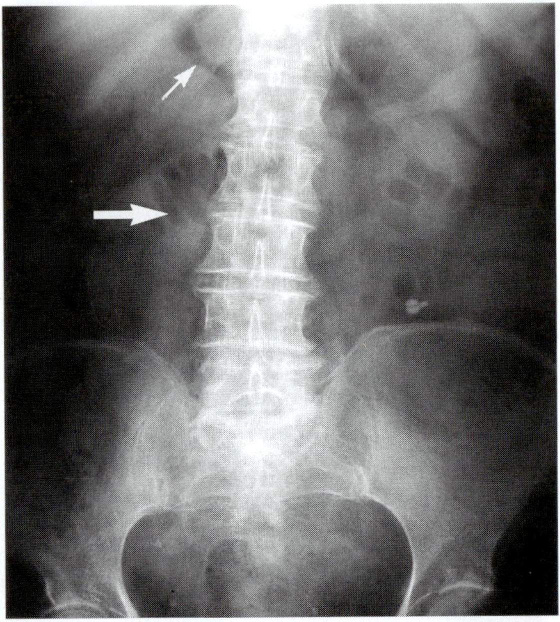

B

Fig. 14.25 (*Contd*) **B.** In this case a large non-radio-opaque stone was obstructing the upper jejunum. Only one small loop of distended bowel is seen in the abdomen (large arrow). In this case, gas is clearly seen in the biliary tree (small arrow) demonstrating the presence of a cholecystoduodenal fistula.

Non-surgical treatment of gallstones

Oral dissolution therapy Suitable for small radiolucent stones in a functioning gall bladder. A combination of chenodeoxycholic acid and ursodeoxycholic acid are given orally. Side-effects include diarrhoea, pruritus and transient rise in serum transaminases. Treatment must be continued for months. Recurrence rates are high.

Extracorporeal shock wave lithotripsy Suitable for medium-sized, radiolucent stones in a functioning gall bladder. Concurrent treatment with chenodeoxycholic acid and ursodeoxycholic acid is required. Treatment by this method requires further evaluation. Biliary colic may occur as fragments are passed through the cystic duct.

→

Endoscopy Stones in the CBD may be treated by endoscopic sphincterotomy and stone extraction. This treatment is suitable for the elderly, unfit patient with a gallstone impacted in the CBD. It allows jaundice to settle even if there are residual stones in the gall bladder; no further treatment is required if they remain asymptomatic. It is useful also for removing retained stones missed at cholecystectomy and exploration of the common bile duct, or recurrent stones forming in the CBD.

Treatment of asymptomatic gallstones

These may be seen on AXR or USS carried out for other conditions, or they may be discovered at laparotomy for another condition. In the younger patient, cholecystectomy is advisable to prevent the complications and to offset the long-term complication of carcinoma. In the elderly and unfit, no treatment is advised.

OBSTRUCTIVE JAUNDICE

Jaundice occurs when the serum bilirubin exceeds 40 μmol/l. Posthepatic obstructive jaundice occurs because of obstruction of the extrahepatic biliary tree.

Causes

In the lumen Gallstones (common), roundworms (rare), blood clots in haemobilia.

In the wall Congenital biliary atresia, traumatic stricture, sclerosing cholangitis, cholangiocarcinoma, choledochal cysts.

Outside the wall Carcinoma of the head of the pancreas, carcinoma of the ampulla of Vater, malignant nodes in the porta hepatis.

Symptoms and signs Previous history of cholecystectomy. Previous history of malignancy. Painless jaundice suggests malignancy. Jaundice preceded by severe upper abdominal pain suggests gallstones. Gradual onset of jaundice associated with dark urine and pale stools. Pruritus. Smooth palpable liver. Palpable gall bladder (carcinoma of pancreas or ampulla of Vater – Courvoisier's law states that 'if in the presence of jaundice the gall bladder is palpable, the cause of the jaundice is unlikely to be due to stones'). The reason for this is that with gallstone disease the gall bladder is usually fibrotic and unable to distend and thus become palpable.

Investigations • Hb • FBC • ESR • U&Es • LFTs: bilirubin and alkaline phosphatase markedly raised • PT: may be clotting defect due to poor absorption of vitamin K • USS: may show dilated ducts and site of obstruction, gallstones in gall bladder. The technique is poor for the lower end of the bile duct and head of pancreas as gas may obscure view • CT: shows intrahepatic lesions, demonstrates invasion of adjacent structures • MRI cholangiography • ERCP (→ Fig. 14.26): possible to carry out biopsy, defines level of lesion, allows stenting and relief of jaundice • PTC (→ Fig. 14.27) if ERCP impossible • Liver biopsy.

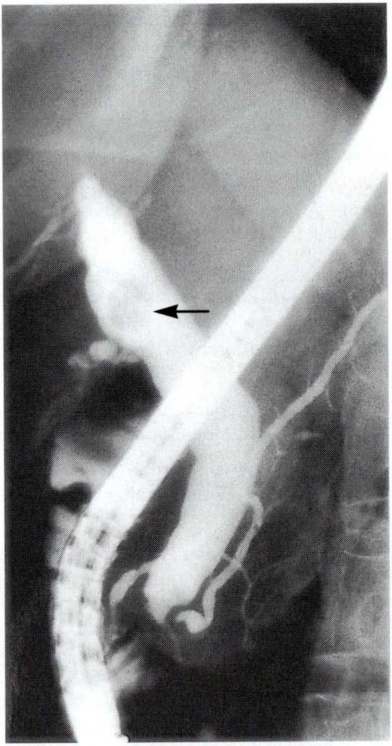

Fig. 14.26 ERCP. A gallstone (arrow) is seen in the dilated bile duct.

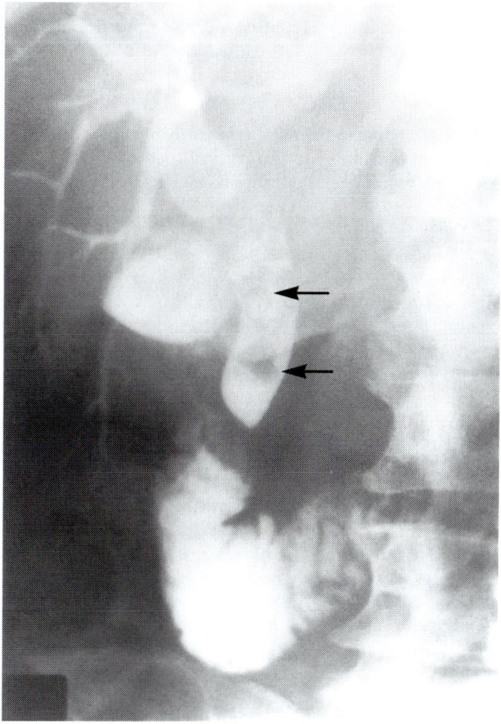

Fig. 14.27 A percutaneous transhepatic cholangiogram. At least two stones (arrows) are seen within a grossly dilated bile duct. There is free flow of contrast into the duodenum.

Treatment Check PT. Correct any clotting problem with parenteral vitamin K. Give mannitol and i.v. fluids preoperatively to prevent hepatorenal syndrome. Prophylactic antibiotics. Subsequent treatment depends on the cause of jaundice:

Gallstone in CBD Explore duct at time of cholecystectomy or remove at ERCP and sphincterotomy.

Congenital biliary atresia (→ Ch. 20).

Traumatic stricture Needs bypass via Roux loop of intestine anastomosed to the proximal dilated duct.

→

Sclerosing cholangitis Hepaticojejunostomy, i.e. anastomose a loop of jejunum to a dilated duct at the hilum of the liver. Stenting by endoscopic retrograde route or percutaneous transhepatic route may be of benefit. The prognosis is poor.

Cholangiocarcinoma Primary resection is rarely possible and has a high mortality. Stenting combined with radiotherapy produces a few long-term survivors.

Choledochal cyst Excision of cyst with Roux-en-Y choledochojejunostomy.

Carcinoma of the head of the pancreas or ampulla of Vater Attempted curative resection may be carried out via a pancreaticoduodenectomy (Whipple's operation). Relatively few tumours are curable. Recurrence rates are high. If the tumour is inoperable as judged by invasion of adjacent structures on CT, or because of liver metastases, stenting may be carried out. If the tumour is found to be inoperable at laparotomy a 'triple bypass' is carried out (→ section on pancreas).

Nodes at the porta hepatis Stenting is the treatment of choice. Adjuvant radiotherapy may help depending upon the type of tumour invading the nodes.

Complications of surgery on the jaundiced patient Coagulation disorders. Renal failure. GI tract haemorrhage (stress ulcers). Delayed wound healing.

PANCREAS

PANCREATITIS

Inflammation of the pancreas may be divided into acute and chronic. Acute pancreatitis is a condition presenting with acute onset of abdominal pain associated with raised levels of pancreatic enzymes in the blood and urine. The gland normally returns to functional and anatomical normality after the cause is treated. Recurrent attacks may occur (relapsing acute pancreatitis). Chronic pancreatitis is a continuing inflammatory disease characterized by irreversible functional and anatomical abnormalities in the gland, resulting in fibrosis of the gland and pancreatic insufficiency.

Acute pancreatitis

Aetiological factors include biliary tract disease (60%), alcohol (20%). Other causes include hyperlipidaemia, hyperparathyroidisim, viral infections (mumps, Coxsackie virus), hypothermia, trauma, postoperative, drugs (steroids, oestrogen-containing contraceptives, azathioprine, thiazide diuretics), familial, scorpion bites, idiopathic, autoimmune (polyarteritis nodosa), post-ERCP, pancreatic carcinoma.

Symptoms and signs Severe epigastric pain radiating through to back. Nausea, vomiting, shock. Tender in epigastrium initially spreading to whole abdomen. Abdominal distension. Absent bowel sounds. Bluish discoloration in flank (Grey Turner's sign) or periumbilical area (Cullen's sign) – due to haemorrhagic pancreatitis with spread of blood retroperitoneally to these areas.

Investigations • Hb • PCV • WCC↑ • U&Es • LFTs: bilirubin↑, mild derangement of others • Amylase raised >1000 u/l • Ca↓ • Blood sugar↑ • ABG • Po_2↓ • ECG changes may occur, diminished T waves. Beware the patient with haemorrhagic pancreatitis who presents late and in whom the amylase is normal because of extensive destruction of the pancreas • AXR: absent psoas shadows, 'sentinel loop' adjacent to pancreas because of local ileus • CXR: small pleural effusions.

Complications ARF. ARDS. Gastric erosions (haematemesis and melaena). DIC. Psychosis. Diabetes. Local complications include pancreatic necrosis, abscess formation, pseudocyst formation. Relapsing acute pancreatitis. Chronic pancreatitis.

Differential diagnosis Perforated peptic ulcer. Acute exacerbation of peptic ulcer. Cholecystitis. Mesenteric infarction. MI.

Treatment

Mild case N/G suction. i.v. fluids. Nil orally. Analgesia (pethidine), antibiotics (cefuroxime and metronidazole). Careful monitoring of urine output. Monitor WCC, blood sugar, U&Es, LFTs, calcium, ABG.

Severe case Best treated in ITU. Severity is indicated by Ranson's criteria, i.e.:

- at presentation, age >55, WCC $>16 \times 10^9$/l, Glucose >11 mmol/l, LDH >350 iu/l, AST >200 iu/l
- during first 48 hours: PCV: fall >10%, urea >16 mmol/l, Ca^{2+} <2 mmol/l, Pao_2 <8 kPa, base deficit <4. The more criteria present the greater the mortality.

Treatment involves nil orally, NG suction. i.v. fluids (crystalloid, colloid, blood), catheterize and measure urine →

output hourly, analgesia (pethidine), antibiotics (i.v. cefuroxime and metronidazole or i.v. imipenem), early enteral feeding (in severe cases this may reduce mortality), peritoneal lavage ('prune juice' peritoneal fluid indicates severe haemorrhagic pancreatitis), H_2 receptor antagonists as prophylaxis against gastric erosions, inotropic support (dopamine, dobutamine), calcium gluconate for hypocalcaemia, O_2 by mask, ventilation if ARDS, dialysis if ARF. ERCP if common bile duct stones, i.e. jaundice with deranged liver function tests and dilated common bile duct.

Indications for surgery

- Uncertainty of diagnosis.
- Deterioration of patient's condition. Drainage of abscesses or removal of necrotic pancreas may be required. Fat necrosis may be seen at laparotomy. Drainage of pseudocyst. Early cholecystectomy if gallstones are the cause.

Prognosis Mortality rate overall is about 10%. With acute haemorrhagic pancreatitis it exceeds 30%.

Chronic pancreatitis

Chronic alcoholism is responsible for most cases. A few cases result from hypercalcaemia, hyperlipidaemia or familial predisposition. Direct trauma with subsequent duct stricture is responsible for a few cases. Damage to acini occurs with destruction of the parenchyma, fibrosis and ductal stenoses with dilatation beyond.

Symptoms and signs Upper abdominal pain often radiating through to the back. Weight loss. Nausea, vomiting, steatorrhoea. 30–40% develop diabetes. A few patients may become addicted to narcotic analgesics because of the severity of the pain. Upper abdominal tenderness. Occasionally jaundice if CBD obstructed.

Investigations • AXR: speckled pancreatic calcification • Blood glucose may be raised • Ca may be raised • Lipid profile (hyperlipidaemia) • Amylase elevated during exacerbations • USS: cystic change and duct dilatation • CT • ERCP: assess duct dilatation and stenoses.

Treatment

Medical Stop alcohol. Low-fat diet. Pancreatic extracts given orally (Pancrex or Creon). Treat diabetes mellitus. Fat-soluble vitamins. Adequate analgesia. Coeliac plexus blockade may be necessary.

→

Surgical Largely carried out for pain. Decompression of the duct by endoscopic sphincterotomy and insertion of pancreatic duct stent at ERCP. Longitudinal pancreaticojejunostomy may be carried out. Other operations include resection of the head, body, and tail or whole gland. If total pancreatectomy is required, brittle diabetes results and therefore one should consider isolating the islets cells from the pancreas and carrying out autotransplantation.

Prognosis Depends upon ability to abstain from alcohol. 25% of patients die within 15 years. Some patients have a miserable life with narcotic addiction, diabetes mellitus and malnutrition.

Pancreatic cysts

True cysts are rare, and may be associated with congenital polycystic disease, retention cysts, hydatid disease and tumour (cystadenoma and cystadenocarcinoma). Pseudocysts are more common and are a consequence of acute pancreatitis, pancreatic trauma or, rarely, posterior perforation of a gastric ulcer.

Pancreatic pseudocyst

This is a collection of fluid in the lesses sac.

Symptoms and signs Pancreatic trauma. Acute pancreatitis. Perforated posterior GU. Rarely no history. Development of a tender epigastric mass. Fever, weight loss, nausea and vomiting.

Investigation • WCC • Amylase • Bilirubin occasionally elevated • USS • CT: collection of fluid in lesser sac.

Complications If left, some cysts may absorb spontaneously. Rarely infection, rupture, or haemorrhage into the cyst may occur.

Treatment Drainage under USS control. If it recurs, laparotomy with drainage of the cyst into the posterior wall of the stomach may be required (cystogastrostomy).

TUMOURS OF THE PANCREAS

Carcinoma of the pancreas

Adenocarcinoma of the pancreas is increasing in frequency in the age range of 40–60 years. It is rarely curable because of local invasion or lymph node metastases before it has been detected. Early diagnosis is difficult. 60% occur in the head of the pancreas, 25% in the body and the remainder in the tail. Risk factors include diabetes mellitus, alcoholism, cigarette smoking. It is more common in workers in the chemical industry.

Symptoms and signs Epigastric pain. Deep boring back pain. Jaundice (head of pancreas, secondaries in porta hepatis). Weight loss, fatigue, malaise, indigestion, pruritus. Palpable epigastric mass. Palpable gall bladder (Courvoisier's law – 'if in the presence of jaundice the gall bladder is palpable, the cause of the jaundice is unlikely to be stones'). Hepatomegaly. Thrombophlebitis migrans. Rarely splenomegaly due to splenic vein thrombosis from direct invasion of latter. Virchow's node.

Investigations • Hb • FBC • ESR • LFTs • Blood sugar • FOBs positive • USS: often small mass obscured by bowel gas • CT scan (→ Fig. 14.28) degree of invasion, metastases, guided biopsy • ERCP: duct obstruction and may show tumour.

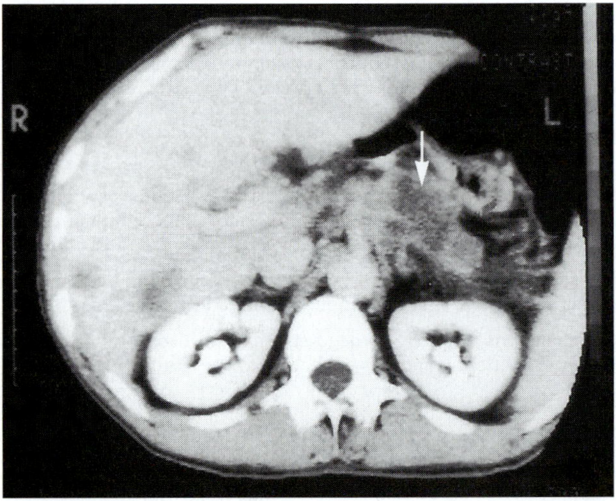

Fig. 14.28 CT scan of the upper abdomen. There is a carcinoma in the pancreas (arrow).

Treatment

- Pancreaticoduodenectomy (Whipple's operation) for carcinoma of the head of the pancreas (→ Fig. 14.29). This involves a partial gastrectomy, partial pancreatectomy, and distal choledochectomy and cholecystectomy. Continuity is re-established via a Roux-en-Y choledochojejunostomy,

→

pancreaticojejunostomy and gastroenterostomy. Operative mortality is high. Relatively few cases are suitable for this operation and the cure rate is very low.
- Total pancreatectomy for extensive tumour.
- Tumours in the tail may be treated by distal pancreatectomy.
- Palliative decompression and relief of jaundice can be treated by 'triple bypass', i.e. cholecystojejunostomy (to drain bile past the obstruction from gall bladder to jejunum), jejunojejunostomy (to prevent food passing up into the gall bladder), and gastrojejunostomy (to ensure adequate drainage of food from the stomach should the tumour invade the duodenum) (→ Fig. 14.30).
- As the prognosis is poor and many cases are inoperable at presentation, endoscopic stenting to relieve the jaundice is becoming the treatment of choice.

Prognosis Many patients are dead within 6 months of presentation. Even with apparently operable lesions only 5–10% of patients survive 5 years.

Endocrine tumours of the pancreas

Rare. Include gastrinomas (Zollinger–Ellison syndrome → p. 231), insulinomas and, more rarely, glucagonomas and vipomas.

Insulinoma

80% are solitary benign tumours of the β cells, 10% are malignant and 10% are multiple. They produce insulin and the symptoms are related to this.

Symptoms and signs

Related to cerebral glucose deprivation These include weakness, sweating, palpitations, memory lapse, bizarre behaviour, coma. Hypoglycaemic episodes are usually precipitated by fasting and relieved by food.

Related to GI tract These are hunger, abdominal pain and diarrhoea. Symptoms relieved by eating. Often excessive appetite with weight gain. The classical diagnostic criteria are 'Whipple's triad':

- the attacks are precipitated by fasting
- the blood sugar is low during an attack
- the symptoms are relieved by the administration of glucose.

Investigations • Fasting blood sugar • Plasma insulin • Glucagon provocation test: infuse glucagon i.v., an elevated insulin level is diagnostic • CT scan to localize tumour

• Rarely, selective angiography may be required. • Intraoperative ultrasound.

Treatment Because of malignant potential, treatment should be surgical exploration and excision.

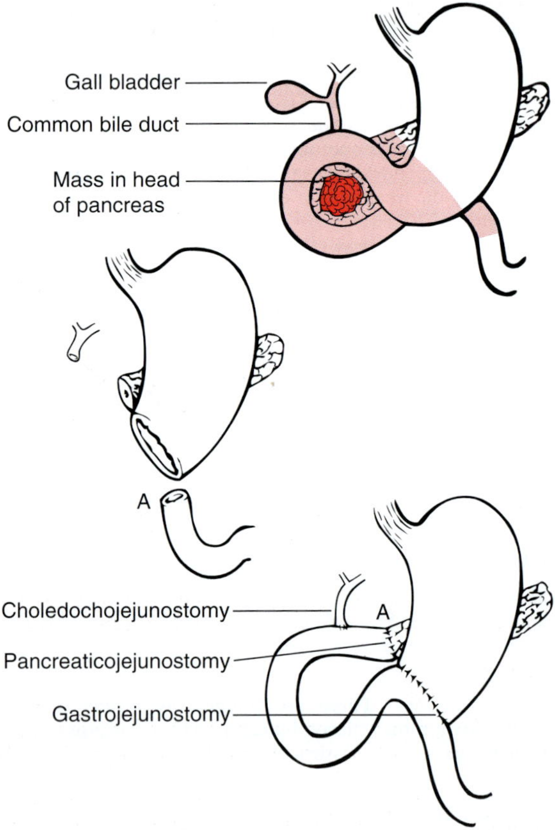

Fig. 14.29 Pancreaticoduodenectomy (Whipple's operation). The shaded area is excised.

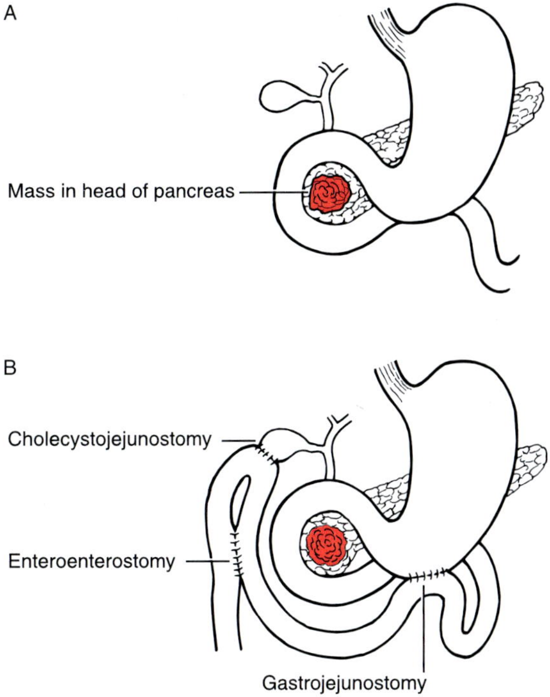

Fig. 14.30 Triple bypass for carcinoma of the head of the pancreas.

SPLEEN

SPLENOMEGALY

The spleen must be enlarged to about three times its normal size before it becomes clinically palpable. The lower margin may feel notched to palpation. It may become so large that it is palpable in the RIF. Massive splenomegaly in the UK is likely to be due to CML, myelofibrosis or lymphoma. Splenomegaly may lead to hypersplenism, i.e. pancytopenia as cells become trapped in an overactive spleen and are destroyed. Anaemia, infection, or haemorrhage may result. (For causes of splenomegaly → Table 14.5.).

Table 14.5
Causes of splenomegaly

Infective		
	Bacterial	Typhoid Typhus Tuberculosis Septicaemia Abscess
	Viral	Glandular fever
	Spirochaetal	Syphilis Leptospirosis
	Protozoal	Malaria
	Parasitic	Hydatid cyst
Inflammatory		Rheumatoid arthritis Sarcoid Lupus Amyloid
Neoplastic		Leukaemia Lymphoma Polycythaemia vera Myelofibrosis Primary tumours Metastases
Haemolytic disease		Spherocytosis Acquired haemolytic anaemia Thrombocytopenic purpura
Storage diseases		Gaucher's disease
Deficiency diseases		Pernicious anaemia Severe iron deficiency anaemia
Splenic vein hypertension		Cirrhosis Splenic vein thrombosis Portal vein thrombosis
Non-parasitic cysts		

Indications for splenectomy These are: trauma; as part of other operative procedures, e.g. radical gastrectomy, splenorenal shunting; haematological disease, e.g. haemolytic anaemia, ITP; tumours; cysts; occasionally for diagnosis.

Complications of splenectomy

Thrombocytosis Platelet counts rise after splenectomy and may reach 1000×10^9/l. Peak rises usually at 7–10 days. There is little evidence to support an increased risk of thromboembolic disease. Full anticoagulation is not indicated although prophylactic aspirin may be given if the platelet count is very high.

Postsplenectomy sepsis Individuals are more susceptible to fulminant septicaemia after splenectomy. Infection with *Streptococcus pneumoniae* is the most common but *Haemophilus influenzae* and meningococci are also possible pathogens. The risk is greatest in young children. In patients in whom splenectomy is a planned procedure, vaccination against pneumococcal infections should be given prior to splenectomy. In children prophylactic penicillin should be given for at least 2 years postsplenectomy and some authorities recommend continuing until 18 years old. In patients having emergency splenectomy the procedure should be covered with penicillin and some authorities recommend that this should be continued for 2 years. Vaccination should be administered postoperatively. A polyvalent pneumococcal vaccine (Pneumovax) is given. Protection lasts 4–5 years after which revaccination is advisable. Vaccination against *H. influenzae* type B (HiB) and meningococci A and C should also be given.

Rupture of the spleen

The spleen may be ruptured by penetrating, non-penetrating, or intraoperative trauma (iatrogenic), or may rupture spontaneously. Rupture of the spleen is the commonest internal injury caused by non-penetrating upper abdominal or lower left chest trauma. RTAs are a common cause, as is a direct blow to the left lower ribs in sports or assault.

Symptoms and signs Death may result from complete disruption of the spleen. There are symptoms and signs of progressive blood loss. Bruising or abrasions over left lower chest and upper abdomen. Tachycardia. Hypotension. Abdominal pain. Signs of peritoneal irritation. Referred pain to shoulder tips because of blood irritating under surface of diaphragm.

Delayed rupture This occurs in about 5% of cases and may occur days to weeks later. A subcapsular haematoma forms slowly and then ruptures through the capsule causing intraperitoneal bleeding.

Spontaneous rupture May occur when the spleen is the site of disease, e.g. infectious mononucleosis, malaria, lymphoma, leukaemia, typhoid. In any disease where there is splenomegaly trivial trauma may cause splenic disruption.

Investigations • CXR: fracture left lower ribs • AXR: displacement of stomach bubble to right, displacement of splenic flexure of colon inferiorly • USS or CT will show tears and free intraperitoneal blood. • Diagnostic peritoneal lavage. The diagnosis is, however, a clinical one and emergency laparotomy is often required.

Treatment Minor capsular tears may be treated by application of local haemostatic agents. The present vogue is to suture lacerations, avoiding splenectomy and thus preserving the spleen's immunological functions. Major injuries with deep lacerations and or disruption require splenectomy.

15 Peripheral vascular disease

ARTERIAL

History

Peripheral vascular disease usually affects the lower limb but may affect the upper limb, GI tract, cerebral vessels and renal vessels.

Risk factors include smoking, hyperlipidaemia (family history), hypertension, and diabetes.

Clinical features

Intermittent claudication is a pain in the muscle due to ischaemia brought on by exercise and relieved by rest. Rest pain is a continuous pain caused by severe ischaemia of the part. Gangrene is tissue necrosis.

The patient should be asked how long the claudication has been present, if there has been any spontaneous improvement, or if there has been rapid deterioration. Questions should also be asked regarding rest pain, particularly if the pain is worse in bed and if it responds to hanging the leg out of bed.

A history should be sought for symptoms involving other areas of the vascular system, e.g. cardiac (MI, angina), GI system (upper to central abdominal cramping pain coming on about 20 minutes after a large meal – 'mesenteric angina'), cerebrovascular (stroke, TIAs, transient blindness, i.e. amaurosis fugax, dizziness, drop attacks) and renal (hypertension).

Examination

The patient's limb should be examined in a warm room.

Inspection Check the colour of the limb. An ischaemic limb may be as white as marble (acute ischaemia) or show varying degrees of pallor, purple/blue cyanosis or a red shiny appearance (chronic ischaemia). The vascular angle (Buerger's angle) is the angle to which the leg must be raised before it becomes white. Normally the straightened leg can be raised to 90° and the toes will stay pink. In a severely ischaemic leg elevation to 15° may cause pallor. Dependent rubor (a purple/red colour to the feet when dependent) denotes severe ischaemia. In a normal limb the veins should be full even when the patient is horizontal. In the ischaemic foot veins will be collapsed and look like pale blue gutters in the subcutaneous tissue. This is the sign of guttering of the veins. Inspect the pressure areas (heel, tips of toes, ball of foot, head of fifth metatarsal) for signs of trophic changes, ulceration or gangrene; inspect between the toes.

Palpation Check the skin temperature. Check the capillary refilling time, i.e. press the tip of the nail or pulp of the toe or finger for 2 seconds and observe the time taken for the blanched area to turn pink. In the normal digit this should occur immediately. Delay will

Table 15.1
Tabulation of pulses

Pulses	**R**	**L**
Radial	++	++
Brachial	++	++
Subclavian	++	++
Carotid	++ (bruit)	++
Femoral	++	++ (bruit)
Popliteal	+	–
Posterior tibial	–	–
Dorsalis pedis	–	–

++ = normal volume
+ = diminished volume
– = absent

occur in the ischaemic digit. Palpate and record all the pulses. This includes not only the pulses in the foot but those in the arm and the carotids. Pulses should be recorded as shown in Table 15.1.

Auscultation Listen along the course of all the major arteries for bruits. Listen to the arteries in the neck, the abdomen and the groin. Measure the BP in both arms to exclude any subclavian disease. The pressure in the lower limb is best measured by Doppler studies. Bruits should be tabulated as shown in Table 15.1.

ARTERIAL OCCLUSIVE DISEASE

Acute arterial occlusion

Causes

Embolus This may come from the heart (e.g. left auricular thrombus in AF, mural thrombus following MI, valvular disease, atrial myxoma) or it may come from proximal atherosclerotic lesions or aneurysms.

Thrombosis This usually occurs in an area of arteriosclerotic narrowing. There is usually a history of claudication prior to the acute event.

Trauma This may be: penetrating trauma; a result of arterial catheterization or angioplasty; following a limb fracture, e.g. popliteal artery damage following supracondylar fracture of the femur; brachial artery damage following a supracondylar fracture of the humerus in a child; accidental intra-arterial injection, e.g. a misplaced injection in an intravenous drug abuser.

Symptoms and signs The classical symptoms are the six 'Ps': pain, pallor, paraesthesia, paralysis and pulselessness and perishing cold. The most reliable of these signs are paralysis and paraesthesia. If neurological symptoms are present then the situation is one of extreme urgency as also is the presence of muscle tenderness. Establish the exact time of onset of symptoms. Symptoms prior to the acute event should be sought, e.g. intermittent claudication. History of previous ischaemic heart disease, valvular heart disease, cardiac surgery, e.g. prosthetic valve or previous vascular surgery.

Investigations • FBC • U&Es, glucose, and cross-match • Clotting screen • CXR • ECG • Urgent arteriography.

Treatment Anticoagulate with heparin. If the likely cause is peripheral arterial embolism on a previously normal arterial tree, embolectomy should be undertaken. If embolism is suspected and the limb is clearly threatened, proceeding to angiography may introduce unnecessary delay and in such a case it may be best to take the patient directly to theatre and attempt embolectomy. 'On-table' angiography may be performed if the diagnosis turns out to be thrombosis.

In acute *in situ* thrombosis either emergency thrombectomy or intra-arterial thrombolytic therapy may be undertaken. In the case of acute or chronic thrombosis in the absence of neurological symptoms, intra-arterial thrombolytic therapy followed by either angioplasty or arterial bypass grafting may be appropriate. Following revascularization, fasciotomy may be appropriate to prevent compartment syndrome.

Prognosis Ideally, surgery should be undertaken within 8 hours of onset of symptoms if a good result is to be obtained. Delay in treatment increases the incidence of amputation and mortality.

CHRONIC ARTERIAL OCCLUSION

Causes Invariably due to arteriosclerosis, usually consequent on smoking. Other causes include multiple recurrent small emboli, arteritis, Buerger's disease and Takayasu's disease (rare).

Aorto-ilio-femoral disease

Arteriosclerosis may involve the arteries of the lower limb singly or in combination. Typical patterns include aortoiliac disease, isolated iliac stenoses and superficial femoral occlusion.

Symptoms and signs Intermittent claudication affecting the calf (block in the superficial femoral artery), the thigh (block in the external iliac artery) or buttock (block in the lower aorta or common and internal iliac arteries). Occlusion of the aortoiliac segment associated with buttock claudication and impotence is known as Leriche's syndrome. Rest pain may develop involving an aching pain in the toes and forefoot which appears when the patient lies horizontal. It is relieved by hanging the foot over the side of the bed. Ischaemic ulcers and gangrene may supervene. Ischaemic ulcers tend to develop at pressure areas, e.g. bunion area, tips of toes, lateral aspect of head of fifth metatarsal and around the heel. The foot may be cold, pale and show venous guttering and dependent rubor. Absent pulses. Palpable thrills. Bruits.

Investigations • Haemoglobin • FBC • ESR • U&Es • Glucose • Lipids • CXR • ECG: treadmill test to assess claudication

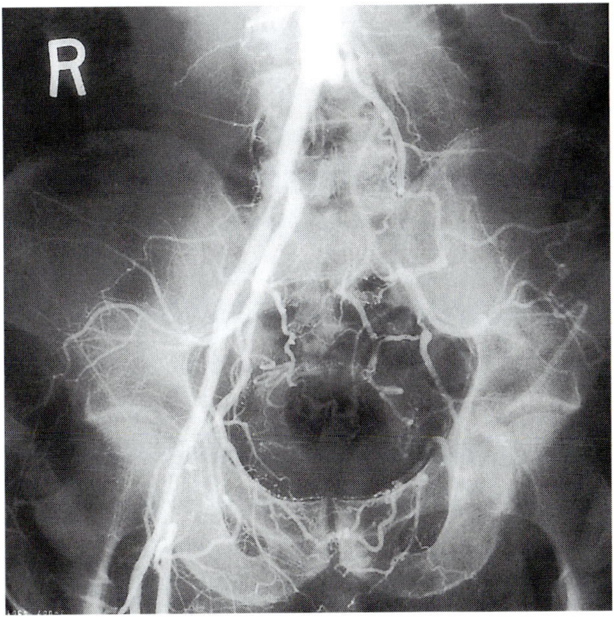

Fig. 15.1 An arteriogram showing complete occlusion of the left common iliac artery. Note the numerous collateral vessels. There is also stenosis in the right external iliac artery as well as in the right internal iliac artery at its origin.

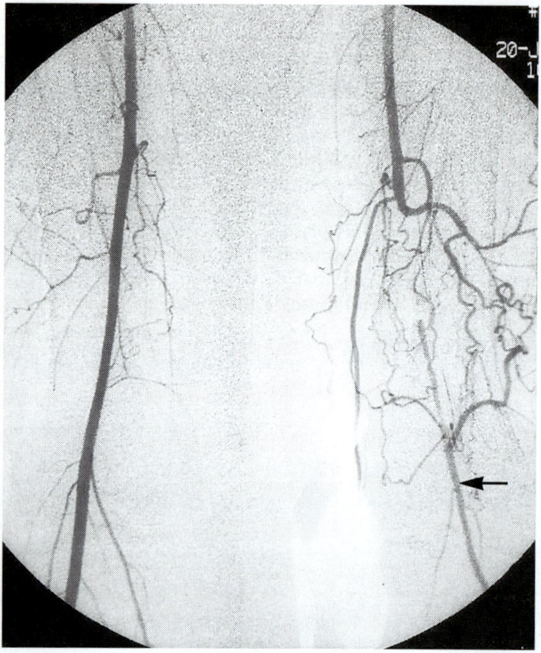

Fig. 15.2 A femoral digital subtraction angiogram. There is a block in the left femoral artery in the adductor canal. The distal femoral artery (arrow) fills via numerous collaterals.

distance • Doppler studies to assess ankle blood pressure as well as areas of stenosis • Pressures measured at the ankle can be related to pressure in the brachial artery, i.e. ankle/brachial ratio. Normally this is between 1 and 1.2. Pressures around 0.8 are compatible with claudication and pressures around 0.4 with rest pain. Pressures below 0.4 indicate severe ischaemia and are usually associated with ulceration and gangrene • Duplex doppler • Arteriography is undertaken if surgery or angioplasty are contemplated (→ Figs 15.1 and 15.2).

Treatment

Medical Mild to moderate claudication which is not disabling does not require surgical treatment. Advice is given to patients to lose weight, stop smoking, exercise regularly →

within their claudication distance. Advice is also given on foot care, particularly chiropody. Antiplatelet agents should be given, usually aspirin, but in patients who will not tolerate aspirin an alternative antiplatelet agent should be prescribed, e.g. clopidogrel. Correct any cholesterol or triglyceride abnormality. There is clear evidence that cardiac events can be reduced by up to one-third by reducing total cholesterol to <5.0 mmol by use of a statin. Control hypertension. Regular follow-up. Patient should be encouraged to seek medical advice if claudication suddenly deteriorates or rest pain develops.

Surgical Surgery is indicated for disabling claudication, rest pain, ulceration, or digital gangrene. Preoperative arteriography should be undertaken to assess the site of the lesion and the 'run off', i.e. to assess the patency of arteries distal to the block and their suitability for grafting. Short segment stenosis may be suitable for balloon angioplasty.

Surgical approaches include endarterectomy (which has largely been superseded by balloon catheter angioplasty) and arterial bypass grafting. In aortoiliac disease, bypass grafting is via a Y graft constituted of woven Dacron. Superficial femoral occlusions are treated by femoropopliteal bypass grafting. This may be either with the great saphenous vein which may be used either reversed or as an in situ graft, the valves having been destroyed with a valve stripper. In the absence of a suitable autogenous vein, prosthetic material is used (expanded polytetrafluoroethylene – ePTFE).

Patients not suitable for bypass grafting may eventually require amputation although other methods have been used to attempt limb salvage. These methods are temporary or ineffective and amputation is usually required. Drug therapies include prostacyclin, a vasodilator, or naftidrofuryl which increases oxygen uptake by muscle.

Cerebrovascular disease

Lesions of the extracranial cerebral vessels account for at least 50% of vascular neurological problems. Arteriosclerosis is the most common cause. This usually affects the internal carotid artery just distal to the common carotid bifurcation. The origin of the vertebral artery is the next most common vessel affected.

Symptoms and signs

- TIA, e.g. paralysis or numbness of the contralateral arm or leg or temporary loss of vision of ipsilateral eye (amaurosis fugax). By definition, all symptoms must resolve in 24 hours but in practice the attacks often last less than 30 minutes.
- Stroke with permanent neurological sequelae.

- Dizziness and fainting due to decreased cerebral perfusion.
- Vertebrobasilar ischaemia, with vertigo, drop attacks, ataxia and visual disturbance. Examination may reveal reduced carotid pulses or bruits over the carotid artery.

Investigations Patients with TIAs and asymptomatic bruits should be investigated initially by non-invasive means. Duplex scanning is the investigation of choice. Surgery may be carried out on the basis of duplex scanning although where there is doubt then digital subtraction imaging may be more appropriate (→ Fig. 15.3). Magnetic resonance or computed tomography angiography is a useful alternative non-invasive assessment.

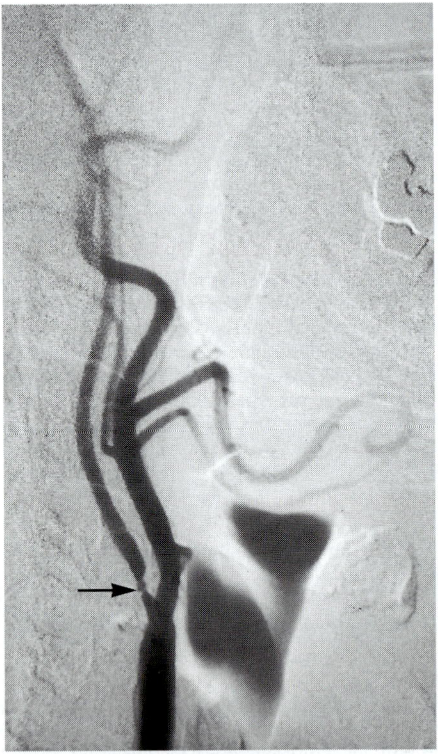

Fig. 15.3 A digital subtraction carotid angiogram. There is a tight stenosis (arrow) at the origin of the internal carotid.

Treatment The object of treatment is to prevent stroke and relieve symptoms. A fixed neurological defect cannot be reversed. Medical management includes taking aspirin 75 mg a day or oral anticoagulation. Recent studies have clearly shown that surgery is indicated for TIAs, amaurosis fugax, and CVA with good recovery if the patient has a stenosis of greater than 70% in the relevant internal carotid artery and is expected to survive for more than 2–3 years. Surgery is not indicated for the vast majority of patients who have a stenoses of less than 70%. Patients who require surgery are treated by carotid endarterectomy. This carries a small risk of stroke.

Renovascular disease

Hypertension may be caused be renal hypoperfusion with release of renin from juxtaglomerular cells with activation of angiotensin. The most common causes are arteriosclerosis and fibromuscular dysplasia of the renal arteries. Arteriosclerosis usually involves the origin of the artery and occurs in the older patient. Fibromuscular dysplasia affects the middle to distal part of the artery and usually occurs in the younger patient.

Renal artery stenosis is an important, and potentially correctable, cause of renal failure in the older patient. The diagnosis of renal artery stenoses is frequently made following a deterioration of renal function in patients commenced on angiotensin-converting enzyme inhibitors.

Symptoms and signs Hypertension – either symptomatic or picked up on routine examination, e.g. insurance medical. Occasionally it is picked up on an IVU when a non-functioning or poorly functioning kidney is noted.

Investigations • Duplex scanning • Arteriography.

Treatment Indications for surgery or angioplasty include:

- A diastolic BP greater than 110 despite management with antihypertensive agents.
- A significant lesion demonstrated angiographically. ACE inhibitors should be avoided in patients with suspected renal artery stenosis. The treatment of choice is angioplasty often with the use of a stent. Surgery should be reserved for those patients who cannot be treated by endovascular means and for those patients in whom there is recurrence. However, many patients undergo successful repeat angioplasties, so avoiding surgery. It is important that renal artery stenosis is diagnosed preoperatively in patients requiring

→

aortic surgery, e.g. aortoiliac bifurcation grafts or repair of aortic aneurysms. Hypotension occurring during surgery for such conditions may precipitate occlusion in the narrowed renal artery.

Chronic visceral occlusion

Visceral occlusion is usually due to arteriosclerosis. In practical terms the superior mesenteric artery is most involved.

Symptoms and signs Cramping upper abdominal pain approximately 30 minutes after a meal ('mesenteric claudication'). This usually lasts 1–3 hours. Weight loss occurs because of 'food fear' due to the pain caused by eating. An upper abdominal bruit may be audible. Occlusive vascular disease is likely elsewhere.

Investigations • Duplex scanning • Arteriography.

Treatment Treatment is surgical. This is achieved by bypass grafting using the saphenous vein from the aorta to the distal superior mesenteric artery beyond the block, or by endarterectomy. However, there is now some experience of percutaneous transluminal angioplasty and stenting and in the high-risk patient this is an attractive alternative.

Acute visceral occlusion

This may be due to arterial occlusion (thrombosis or embolus), venous thrombosis or hypoperfusion which may occur in shock. Massive infarction of the bowel may occur.

Symptoms and signs Sudden onset of severe colicky abdominal pain, vomiting and diarrhoea which may be bloody. There may be a history of atrial fibrillation, sepsis, oral contraceptive, 'mesenteric claudication', portal hypertension. The pain experienced is usually out of proportion to the early physical findings. Subsequently, the patient will develop fever, abdominal tenderness, distension and, ultimately, peritonitis and shock.

Investigations • FBC • WCC↑ • HCO_3↓ • Serum lactate↓ • Plain AXR (air/fluid levels) • Serum amylase may be raised with infarcted bowel (confusion with acute pancreatitis) • Arteriography (duplex ultrasound for the diagnosis of *acute* mesenteric ischaemia is highly unreliable) • Laparotomy provides the diagnosis in most cases.

Treatment Urgent laparotomy. Venous thrombosis without infarction requires anticoagulation. If the patient does not improve within 12 hours a 'second look' laparotomy may be required to assess intestinal viability.

→

In the case of arterial occlusion, if the bowel is not viable it should be resected until healthy bowel is located. If the bowel is considered viable and there is no pulsation in the superior mesenteric artery, Fogarty embolectomy should be undertaken. If a tight stenosis is found to be present at the origin of the superior mesenteric artery, bypass grafting or endarterectomy should be carried out as for chronic mesenteric ischaemia. Acute intestinal ischaemia more frequently occurs in the elderly patient and carries a high mortality rate. Many patients are left with short segments of bowel and consequent metabolic problems.

ANEURYSMS

An aneurysm is an abnormal dilatation of an artery. A true aneurysm contains all layers of the vessel walls and appears as either a fusiform or a saccular dilatation. A false aneurysm is a pulsating haematoma, the cavity of which is in direct continuity with the lumen of an artery. It is contained by a fibrous capsule rather than by the layers of the vessel wall. True aneurysms are commonest in the infrarenal aorta, iliac vessels, common femoral and popliteal arteries. A false aneurysm may occur anywhere and is usually the result of trauma. (For classification of aneurysms → Table 15.2.)

Table 15.2
Aetiology of aneurysms

True	
Congenital	Berry aneurysm of circle of Willis Aneurysmal varix associated with arteriovenous fistula
Acquired	Trauma: irradiation Infection: syphilis, mycotic aneurysm Degeneration: arteriosclerosis, cystic medical necrosis
False	Trauma

Abdominal aneurysms

These usually affect the infrarenal aorta but occasionally extend above. The common iliac vessels are often involved.

Symptoms and signs Often asymptomatic and picked up on abdominal examination for other conditions or ultrasound scanning for other conditions. Symptomatic ones often cause backache by pressure on the adjacent lumbar vertebral bodies or abdominal pain. Examination reveals a pulsatile abdominal mass just above the umbilicus. Look for other peripheral artery aneurysms.

Investigations • USS to assess the maximum diameter of the aneurysm, and relationship to renal arteries.

Complications These include:

- rupture with retroperitoneal haemorrhage or intraperitoneal haemorrhage, or into the IVC (AV fistula)
- distal emboli
- severe back pain due to erosion of the lumbar vertebral bodies
- thrombosis with distal ischaemia.

Treatment Asymptomatic aneurysms under 5.5 cm in diameter may be treated conservatively, especially if the patient is a poor operative risk. Routine follow-up with yearly ultrasound scans should be undertaken. Aneurysms greater than 5.5 cm in diameter should be considered for surgery because of the increased risk of rupture. Treatment is by an inlay Dacron graft or a Dacron Y graft. Mortality for elective surgery should be less than 10%. Mortality rate is related more to MI and CVAs than to direct complications of surgery to the aneurysm.

Ruptured aortic aneurysm (→ Fig. 15.4)

If rupture is suspected immediate surgery is required. Patients with ruptured aneurysm should not be resuscitated with i.v. fluids. Patients with ruptured aneurysms survive to reach hospital because of vasoconstriction, abdominal tamponade, development of a prothrombotic state and the development of 'controlled' hypotension. The infusion of even modest amounts of crystalloid or colloid rapidly upsets that fine balance. If the patient requires significant volumes of fluids to maintain blood pressure on the way to hospital or in the emergency room then it is very unlikely that that patient will survive surgery. The patient is transferred to operating theatre. Undertake emergency repair of the aneurysm once blood is available. The mortality rate for ruptured aneurysm is 30–50%. Postoperative morbidity is high and results from haemorrhage, ARDS, ARF, multiorgan failure, MI and stroke.

Late complications include graft infection often with aorto-duodenal fistula and life-threatening haemorrhage. This requires graft removal and bilateral axillofemoral grafting.

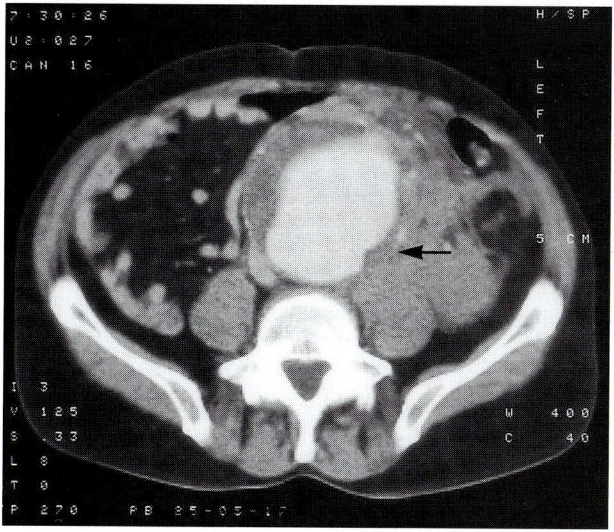

Fig. 15.4 CT scan of the abdomen showing a large leaking abdominal aortic aneurysm. Note the areas of calcification in the wall of the aneurysm. There is evidence of leakage to the left of the aneurysm (arrow).

Femoral aneurysms

These usually involve the common femoral artery.

Symptoms and signs Usually asymptomatic pulsatile mass in the groin. May be associated abdominal aortic aneurysms. False aneurysms are common in the femoral artery and may result from:

- percutaneous catheterization for angiography; stab wounds
- previous surgery especially with prosthetic grafts (infection).

Treatment Small true aneurysms may be treated expectantly. Rapidly expanding true aneurysms require surgery. Iatrogenic false aneurysms are being increasingly treated by compression therapy, usually with an ultrasound scan probe and/or thrombin injection.

Popliteal aneurysm

Symptoms and signs Pulsatile mass in the popliteal fossa. If a medical student can palpate a popliteal pulse easily it may be aneurysmal. Often bilateral and associated with aneurysms elsewhere. Complications include thrombosis with compromise of the distal circulation, and rupture (rare).

Treatment Surgical repair is undertaken in an otherwise fit patient once the aneurysm exceeds 2 cm in diameter, especially if it contains a significant amount of thrombus. Treatment is by resection and grafting. In those patients who are being treated conservatively, repeat examination is required and the patient is normally anticoagulated with warfarin.

Visceral artery aneurysms

Aneurysms may arise form the splenic artery, hepatic artery, superior mesenteric artery or renal arteries.

Symptoms and signs Visceral aneurysms may produce abdominal or flank pain. Renal artery aneurysms may cause haematuria or hypertension. Diagnosis is confirmed by ultrasound scanning and arteriography.

Prognosis Splenic artery aneurysms may affect women during child-bearing years. Rupture is a major complication and tends to occur in the third trimester of pregnancy and is associated with a high mortality rate. The mortality rate for surgery on visceral aneurysms is high, particularly if they rupture.

OTHER VASCULAR PROBLEMS

Thromboangiitis obliterans (Buerger's disease)

This affects small vessels of the extremities. It occurs almost exclusively in young males who are heavy cigarette smokers. It may be associated with migratory thrombophlebitis.

Symptoms and signs Claudication in the muscles of the foot. Digital pain, cyanosis, coldness progressing to necrosis and gangrene. Ankle and wrist pulses disappear first and the proximal pulses remaining normal. Progressive digital ischaemia occurs with eventual loss of feet and hands.

Investigations • Arteriography reveals discrete foci of occlusions alternating with apparently uninvolved arterial segments in the distal circulation.

Treatment It is essential to stop smoking to avoid progression of the disease. Sympathectomy is of benefit but eventually if the patient continues smoking, amputation is necessary for rest pain or gangrene. Reconstructive surgery is rarely possible because the disease involves the small distal vessels. Repeated prostacyclin infusions may be beneficial.

Raynaud's phenomenon

This is a vasospastic condition of diverse aetiology. The following conditions have been implicated:

- systemic diseases or conditions, e.g. collagen diseases (scleroderma), cryoglobulinaemia, myxoedema, macroglobulinaemia
- compression syndromes, e.g. carpal tunnel syndrome, cervical rib, thoracic outlet syndrome
- occupational trauma, e.g. vibration-induced white finger (pneumatic drill, chainsaw, grinders), piano playing, typing, cricket.

Symptoms and signs Sequential changes of pallor, cyanosis and rubor particularly after exposure to cold. This represents vasoconstriction followed by reflex vasodilatation. In severe long-standing cases tissue necrosis may occur involving non-healing ulcers and gangrene of the extremities. Tissue necrosis always denotes underlying pathology, i.e. the patient has secondary Raynaud's as opposed to primary Raynaud's disease.

Investigations • FBC • Platelets • ESR • CXR (cervical rib) • Cold agglutinins • Serum protein electrophoresis • Autoantibody screen • Rheumatoid factor • LE cells • Arteriography.

Treatment

- Treatment of underlying disorder, e.g. excise cervical rib.
- Avoidance of cold exposure – heated gloves and boots.
- Stop smoking.
- Advice from Raynaud's and Scleroderma Association.
- Drugs, e.g. nifedipine, i.v. prostacyclin.
- Plasmapheresis.
- Sympathectomy.

Diabetic foot

Contributory factors include microangiopathy, peripheral neuropathy, impaired tissue metabolism, and the glucose-rich environment which favours bacterial overgrowth.

Symptoms and signs The patient may present with either a neuropathic foot or an ischaemic foot with signs of both large and small vessel disease. The neuropathic and ischaemic elements frequently coexist.

The neuropathic foot is warm, dry with palpable pulses. Calluses may be present as may painless penetrating ulcers at pressure points and sites of minor injury. Painless necrosis of the toes may occur. Spreading infection can occur along plantar spaces. There is usually general loss of pain and thermal sensation.

The ischaemic foot is cold with absent pulses, absent calluses, painful ulcers, claudication and rest pain.

Treatment

Neuropathic foot

- Control diabetes.
- Stop smoking.
- Lose weight.
- Refer for chiropody to remove calluses.
- Treat infections with antibiotics. Antiseptics and dressings may be required for ulcers.
- Remove necrotic tissue.
- Ray amputations with filleting out of dead tissue until healthy bleeding tissue is obtained.
- Weight-bearing areas should be protected by specialized footwear.

Ischaemic foot

- Control diabetes.
- Stop smoking.
- Lose weight.
- Chiropody.
- Treat infection with antibiotics.
- Arteriography with a view to possible arterial reconstruction and angioplasty.
- Major amputations, e.g. below knee or above knee; minor amputations are rarely successful when the major element is ischaemic.

Thoracic outlet syndrome

This represents a variety of symptoms related to arterial, venous and nerve compression as they exit from the chest. Compression usually occurs in the area bounded by the clavicle, the first rib and the scalenus anterior muscle.

Symptoms and signs

Vascular Claudication or rest pain. Distal arterial disease may be due to embolization from an area of dilatation just beyond subclavian artery compression.

Venous Venous hypertension – compression of subclavian vein or subclavian vein thrombosis.

Nervous Sensory and motor deficit in the distribution of C8/T1.

Investigations • CXR: cervical rib (the CXR should include the thoracic inlet and the total number of ribs on a particular side counted – if there are 13 then a cervical rib is present • Duplex doppler – duplex in positions of provocation, e.g. with the arm raised above the head, will give more functional information about the impingement on the subclavian artery than will angiography • Arteriography: subclavian artery stenosis or constriction by fibrous band • Venography: compression of subclavian vein or subclavian vein thrombosis • Nerve conduction studies to distinguish from carpal tunnel syndrome.

Treatment With minimal neurological symptoms, shoulder girdle exercises may be appropriate. For more severe compression, surgical decompression of the thoracic outlet with removal of the first rib or cervical rib if present. For patients presenting with primary axillary vein thrombosis (Paget–von Schrötter syndrome) thrombolysis is appropriate.

Arteriovenous fistula

Congenital These may present as multiple small lesions. Present from birth. Clinically manifest 10–20 years. May enlarge to involve most of the limb.

Acquired This is due to trauma, e.g. stabbing, arteriography, iatrogenic for dialysis. Usually history of trauma and typically single communication.

Symptoms and signs Pain and swelling in area of fistula. Enlarged tortuous arteries and veins. Increased skin temperature. Elongation of leg. Venous hypertension distally. Ischaemia distally. Palpable thrill. Continuous machinery bruit.

Investigations • CXR for cardiomegaly • Limb radiograph for bone elongation • MRI: this will show the true extent of the lesion which is nearly always more extensive than appears to be the case clinically • Arteriography: this should only be performed if consideration is being given to embolization.

Complications Cosmetic, haemorrhage, thrombosis, distal ischaemia, venous hypertension in limb, high output cardiac failure (Branham's sign – compression of the fistula results in a fall in the heart rate).

Treatment Not all arteriovenous fistulae require treatment. Small peripheral fistulae may be observed and frequently will never cause difficulties. Indications for intervention include haemorrhage, expansion, severe venous or arterial insufficiency, cosmetic deformity and heart failure. Most fistulae are now managed by embolization under radiographic control. Simple ligation of feeding vessels should never be performed. Recurrence is inevitable and when recurrence does occur, previous ligation means that it is difficult to perform angiography and embolization. Embolization and excision may be required for very large lesions.

VENOUS DISEASE

VARICOSE VEINS

These are dilated tortuous veins. They are divided into primary and secondary. Primary veins are the most common and are often familial. They are possibly due to a weakness of the vein wall that allows dilatation of the valve ring.

Secondary varicose veins may be classified as follows:

- obstruction to venous outflow, e.g. pregnancy, fibroids, ovarian cysts, abdominal lymphadenopathy, pelvic cancer, iliac vein thrombosis or retroperitoneal fibrosis
- valve destruction, e.g. DVT
- high flow and pressure, e.g. AV fistulae.

Symptoms and signs Tortuous dilated veins of the long or short saphenous system. Aching discomfort worse towards the end of the day, relieved by sitting with legs elevated. May present with complications. Examine the patient standing up and assess the site and size of the veins. Palpate for defects in the fascia. Check the state of the skin and subcutaneous tissue. Carry out Trendelenburg's test to assess the site of incompetent perforating veins. This is carried out with the patient supine, the leg being elevated and the tourniquet applied just below the saphenofemoral junction. The patient then stands erect for 30 seconds. If the saphenous vein fills rapidly from below with the tourniquet in place, the perforators lower down the legs are incompetent. If the long saphenous vein fills rapidly from above following removal of the tourniquet, the valve at the saphenofemoral junction is incompetent. Repeat at different levels down the leg to determine the level of incompetent perforators. If a swelling is apparent over the saphenofemoral junction (saphena varix), the diagnosis should be confirmed by placing the hand over the swelling and tapping the varicose veins lower down the legs. A palpable thrill at the groin will confirm the presence of a saphena varix. Auscultation over the veins should be carried out to exclude arteriovenous fistulae.

Complications Superficial thrombophlebitis. Haemorrhage. Varicose eczema. Varicose pigmentation due to haemosiderin deposition. Lipodermatosclerosis. Chronic venous ulceration. Long-standing venous stasis ulcers may become malignant (Marjolin's ulcer).

Treatment Mild varicosities – compression stockings and periodic elevation of the legs. Small varicosities below the knee are suitable for injection with a sclerosing agent and compression bandaging worn for 2 weeks. If the patient is on the contraceptive pill this should be either stopped 6 weeks prior to injection or the patient should be treated prophylactically with heparin. Surgery is indicated for saphenofemoral incompetence, saphenopopliteal incompetence, or thigh perforators. Mark out the varicose veins prior to surgery. Surgery includes high ligation of the long saphenous vein at the saphenofemoral junction together with ligation of all tributaries. The great saphenous vein should be stripped to the knee. Previously marked veins should be avulsed. Compression bandaging postoperatively. Encourage early mobilization. Walk at least 3 miles a day. Sit with legs elevated.

DEEP VEIN THROMBOSIS (DVT)

This is a major cause of morbidity and mortality after surgery and trauma. It may occur spontaneously with high oestrogen contraceptive pill. HRT may be an aetiological factor. Only about 25% of DVTs cause symptoms and signs, others being silent. Pathological features (Virchow's triad) leading to DVT include:

- changes in the constituents of the blood
- changes in the blood flow
- changes in the vessel wall

Predisposing factors include trauma and surgery, previous DVT, malignant disease, prolonged bed rest, cardiac failure, oestrogen-containing oral contraceptive pill, pregnancy, pelvic masses, obesity, dehydration, and certain blood disorders, e.g. polycythaemia.

Symptoms and signs Swelling of the leg, tenderness of the calf muscles, increased temperature of the leg, calf pain on passive dorsiflexion the foot (Homan's sign). Occlusion of the iliofemoral segment produces gross swelling of the whole limb which is painful and white (phlegmasia alba dolens). Complete blockage of the iliofemoral segment causes extreme pain with bluish discoloration and impending venous gangrene (phlegmasia caerulea dolens). Diagnosis is confirmed by duplex scanning or venography.

Treatment

Prevention General measures include adequate hydration, avoiding calf pressure, and early postoperative mobilization. Some authorities recommend stopping oral contraceptives at least 6 weeks prior to surgery while others merely recommend heparin prophylaxis. The case for stopping HRT is controversial. Patients at special risk should be treated as follows:

- low-dose subcutaneous heparin: 5000 units b.d. preoperatively and postoperatively until the patient is mobilizing satisfactorily
- calf compression devices used intraoperatively
- graded compression stockings, i.e. thromboembolic deterrent (TED) stockings. These should be worn preoperatively, intraoperatively and postoperatively until the patient is mobilizing satisfactorily.

Therapeutic Start systemic anticoagulation with heparin: 10 000 units i.v. stat. followed by 20–30 000 units by i.v. infusion in 24 hours. Keep APTT at 2.5 times normal. Uncomplicated DVT may be treated as an outpatient with low molecular weight heparin initially and early mobilization converting to oral anticoagulants. Thrombolytic therapy may be appropriate in selected cases. Phlegmasia caerulea dolens may be treated with thrombolysis which may be given into a vein but perhaps more effective intra-arterially to clear the arterial side of the microcirculation. Occasionally, phlegmasia caerulea dolens requires venous thrombectomy.

POSTPHLEBITIC LIMB

This occurs as a consequence of DVT. The deep venous system remains obstructed, the valves destroyed and reflux of blood through incompetent perforators results in high pressure in the superficial veins.

Symptoms and signs

- Peripheral oedema. This gets worse towards the end of the day and tends to settle with elevation.
- Venous eczema and brawny induration of the skin.
- Venous pigmentation associated with haemosiderin deposits in the tissues.
- Venous stasis ulceration which is common in the area of the medial malleolus.
- There is often severe pain associated with the swelling and ulceration.

Treatment Difficult to treat and patient rarely gets complete relief. Advise patient to avoid long periods of standing and to sit with legs elevated. Graded compression stockings. Treat venous stasis ulcers by reducing swelling of the leg by bandaging, excision of necrotic tissue and control of any cellulitis. Antibiotics for cellulitis. Clean ulcers with normal saline, osmotic preparations, or enzymatic preparations. Apply compression stockings until ulcers are healed. However, compression stockings should not be applied to patients until the arterial status has been confirmed. If pulses are not palpable then the ankle/brachial pressure index should be measured and compression applied only if it is greater than 0.8.

SUPERFICIAL THROMBOPHLEBITIS

The causes are show in Table 15.3. Treatment is usually symptomatic and depends on the underlying cause.

LYMPHOEDEMA

This is due to hypoplasia or obstruction of lymphatics. It may be primary or secondary.

Primary

Congenital lymphoedema (Milroy's disease) presents at birth or within the first year of life. Lymphoedema praecox occurs at puberty or shortly afterwards. Lymphoedema tarda occurs after the age of 30.

Secondary

Lymphatic obstruction may occur secondary to other disease processes, e.g. secondary neoplasms in lymph nodes, infection in

Table 15.3
Causes of superficial thrombophlebitis

Varicose veins
Occult carcinoma:
- bronchus
- pancreas
- stomach
- breast

Mondor's disease – superficial thombophlebitis on chest wall
Buerger's disease
Polycythaemia
Local bacterial infection
Polyarteritis
Iatrogenic – intravenous infusions
Drug abuse
Idiopathic

lymph nodes, or may occur following surgical removal of lymph glands, i.e. block dissection or radiotherapy.

Symptoms and signs There is progressive swelling of one or both extremities, usually beginning around the ankle but often involving the whole extremity. The scrotum may be involved. Oedema is non-pitting and does not settle with elevation. Often

Table 15.4
Causes of swelling of the leg

Local		
	Acute swelling	Trauma DVT Cellulitis Allergy Rheumatoid
	Chronic swelling	Venous: • varicose veins • obstruction to venous return, e.g. pregnancy, pelvic tumours, IVC obstruction postphlebitic limb Lymphoedema Congenital malformations, e.g. arteriovenous fistulae Paralysis (failure of muscle pump) Dependency

Table 15.4
Causes of swelling of the leg *(Contd)*

General	Congestive cardiac failure Hypoproteinaemia, e.g. liver failure Nephrotic syndrome, malnutrition Renal failure Fluid overload Myxoedema

the leg aches and feels tight but there is no pain. Minor trauma will cause cellulitis. Need to differentiate from other causes of leg swelling (→ Table 15.4).

Investigations • Lymphangiography. Lymphoedema is essentially a clinical diagnosis and no further tests are required in the great majority of patients. Where there is doubt about the diagnosis then lymphoscintigraphy is easy to perform and less traumatic for the patient. In patients presenting with lymphoedema for the first time over the age of 45 it is important to obtain an abdominal or pelvic CT scan to exclude masses especially neoplasia.

Treatment It is important that lymphoedema is differentiated from other causes of lower limb swelling. Treatment is either medical or surgical. The aim of treatment is to control the oedema and to prevent infection. Compression stockings or compression devices (flowtron therapy) may help. If any breaks in the skin occur, e.g. insect bites or minor trauma, antibiotics should be prescribed. Occasionally, surgical treatment is helpful but does very little to improve the cosmetic appearance. Excision of skin and subcutaneous tissue has been tried, as has burying a flap of dermis beneath the skin to improve lymphatic drainage. Complications include recurrent cellulitis and lymphangitis usually caused by streptococci which respond to penicillin. Lymphangiosarcoma may occur. The tendency is for steady progression of the swelling and recurrent infections.

AMPUTATIONS

Indications for amputation

- Vascular, e.g. severe rest pain with arteries unsuitable for reconstruction, gangrene.
- Trauma.
- Infection, e.g. gas gangrene, osteomyelitis.

- Tumour, e.g. osteogenic sarcoma, soft tissue sarcomas, subungual melanoma.
- Useless limb, e.g. poliomyelitis, severe brachial plexus lesions associated with vascular damage.

Principles of amputation

- Select the appropriate level. Must be adequate circulation at that level to ensure healing. Tissues must show healthy bleeding at time of surgery.
- Amputation level must take into account the fitting of a prosthetic limb.
- Assess joints. Contractures or arthritis may influence the amputation level.

Preparation for amputation

Fully explain the operation to the patient who may take a while to accept that it is necessary. Preoperative physiotherapy and occupational therapy should be undertaken and a visit made to the Limb Fitting Centre. Ensure that the patient is pain-free. Epidural anaesthesia may be useful in this context. Give antibiotic (penicillin) with induction of anaesthesia, which is prophylactic against *Clostridium perfringens* (gas gangrene).

Types of amputation

Minor This involves simple amputation of the digits, or 'ray' amputations where, e.g. in the foot, the metatarsal head and tendons are removed. This type of amputation is useful in diabetics, Buerger's disease and severe Raynaud's. Occasionally for ischaemia of all toes, transmetatarsal amputation may be undertaken. This requires a long plantar flap of skin to be successful. The indications are as above.

Major

Below-knee amputation This is suitable in diabetics with a palpable popliteal pulse, Buerger's disease and in some patients with arteriosclerosis. The standard tibial stump is 12.5 cm long and the fibular stump 10 cm. A long posterior flap with muscle is fashioned and this is folded over to cushion the bone end. Function is variable, less than half the patients being independently mobile at 2 years.

Above-knee amputation This is the most common amputation in patients with arteriosclerosis. The stump of the femur is 25 cm long measured from the greater trochanter. Equal anterior and posterior myoplastic flaps sutured over the bone end.

Less-frequently performed amputations These include Syme's amputation (at the ankle), Gritti-Stokes amputation (at the knee) and through-knee amputation. Disarticulation at the hip and hindquarter amputations are usually performed for major trauma or malignancy.

Postoperative care

Pain relief The aim is to prevent breakthrough pain rather than treating pain once it occurs.

Care of the good limb This involves physiotherapy. It is important to avoid pressure ulcers by nursing on sheepskin.

Physiotherapy Build up muscle power and coordination. Start as soon as patient is comfortable and continue in gymnasium. Aim is to prevent contractures and ensure rapid mobilization with prosthesis.

Prosthesis Measure patient as soon as stump shrinks and volume of stump is stable.

Complications

Early These include haemorrhage, haematoma, abscess, gas gangrene, wound dehiscence, ischaemic flaps and fat embolism.

Late These include pain, sinus formation, osteomyelitis, neuroma, phantom limb and ulceration of the skin (pressure from prosthesis or continuing ischaemia).

VASCULAR TRAUMA

This includes penetrating trauma (90%), blunt trauma (RTAs or fractures), and iatrogenic trauma (angiography, angioplasty or accidental intra-arterial injection). Prompt diagnosis and treatment are essential to save life and limb. Complete transection of an artery because of penetrating trauma may stop bleeding, owing to vessel retraction. Partial transection is more serious as the remaining intact wall holds the vessel open, resulting in torrential haemorrhage. Blunt injury usually leads to intimal tear with a resulting intimal dissection flap which may compromise the distal circulation. Venous injuries are usually due to penetrating trauma. Haemorrhage and/or thrombosis may result. High-velocity bullet wounds may cause considerable disruption of vessels.

Symptoms and signs Mechanism of injury, degree of violence, type of weapon, time of incident. Haemorrhage – arterial or venous. Hypotension. Shock. Expanding haematoma. Diminished or absent distal pulses. Associated injuries, e.g. nerve injuries, fractures, head injury.

Investigations There may be no time for investigations as urgent transfer to theatre may be required.

- Plain radiographs if time permits, e.g. fractures, position of bullets or foreign bodies.
- Arteriography is required if there are signs of impaired circulation.

Treatment Principles of treatment include:

- arrest of haemorrhage
- management of airway
- correction of hypovolaemia
- diagnosis of type and degree of injury
- repair of vessels
- management of associated injuries
- rehabilitation.

Emergency measures Arrest of haemorrhage should be by direct pressure. Never use a tourniquet. Insert two wide-bore cannulae. Correct hypovolaemia. Splint any fractures.

Surgery Explore the wound. 'On-table' angiography may be required. Puncture wounds and clean lacerations may be repaired by direct suture, provided it does not narrow the lumen of the vessel. Smaller arteries, e.g. radial and ulnar (but not both), may be ligated. Larger arteries with ragged lacerations or intimal flaps must be repaired with vein patches or bypassed. Long segments of damaged artery may be replaced with autogenous reversed vein. Prosthetic material should be avoided if possible because of the risk of infection and consequent haemorrhage. Small veins may be ligated but large ones must be repaired with autogenous vein if possible. Fasciotomies may be required to prevent compartment syndrome. Amputation may ultimately be required.

Complications Thrombosis. Secondary haemorrhage. False aneurysm. AV fistulae. Compartment syndrome. Lymphatic leaks or lymphocele due to damage of lymphatic vessels. Distal vascular insufficiency. Ischaemic muscular contractures.

16 Urology

CONGENITAL DISORDERS OF THE URINARY TRACT

KIDNEY AND URETER

Congenital absence of one kidney Incidence is 1 : 2500.

Pelvic kidney Incidence is 1 : 800. Often associated with reflux or PUJO. Large pelvic kidney may interfere with childbirth.

Horseshoe kidney Incidence is 1 : 1000 to 1 : 1800. The combined kidney lies lower than normal. Renal pelvis rotated anteriorly and the lower pole medially. Usually associated with reflux, undescended testes.

Congenital hydronephrosis (PUJO) Aetiology unknown. Lower pole vessel may aggravate but rarely responsible for condition. Failure to thrive, recurrent UTI, mass, hypertension. Often discovered on prenatal USS.

Infantile polycystic disease Incidence is 1 : 10 000. Rare, autosomal recessive.

Adult polycystic disease Incidence is 1 : 1500. Autosomal dominant, involving both kidneys. Patients usually present aged 30–40 with hypertension, mass, haematuria, renal failure. May be associated with cysts in the liver. Family screening and genetic counselling.

Medullary sponge kidney Incidence is 1 : 20 000. Characterized by congenital dilatation or cysts of the distal collecting ducts. May be associated with hypercalciuria, impaired urinary concentration.

Ureteric duplication Often bilateral. The upper pole ureter lies medial and inferior to the lower pole ureter at the bladder.

Ureterocele Dilatation of the submucosal portion of the ureter. Filling defect on IVU.

Megaureter Secondary to either dysplastic (non-obstructed) or obstructed ureter. May be associated with stones, UTI, reflux.

Vesicoureteric reflux Reflux is the abnormal passage of urine from bladder to the ureter. Primary reflux is due to a defect of the vesicoureteric junction. Usually resolving spontaneously in 70% of cases. Secondary reflux is usually due to outflow obstruction. 20% of children presenting with recurrent UTI have reflux. Diagnosed: voiding micturating cystourethrogram. Treatment: antibiotics, regular voiding, ureteric reimplantation.

BLADDER

Ectopia vesica (exstrophy of the bladder) This occurs in 1 : 20–40 000. It is more common in the male. The anterior wall of the bladder fails to close. The posterior bladder wall, the trigone and posterior urethra are exposed and urine leaks onto the skin. Associated anomalies include wide separation of the pubic symphysis with waddling gait, epispadias, umbilical and inguinal hernias, imperfectly descended testes, and rectal prolapse. Complications include ureteric dilatation and pyelonephritis. Treatment involves reimplantation of the ureters into an ileal loop conduit with excision of the bladder and repair of the abdominal wall defect. In some cases, bladder reconstruction may be possible.

Urachal abnormalities Defects may result from the primitive urachal connections between bladder and umbilicus. If the tract persists, urine may discharge from the umbilicus. A urachal cyst may occur if part of the urachus persists but is closed off above and below. Infection may occur in a urachal cyst. Treatment is by excision.

URETHRA

The urethra may terminate on the ventral aspect of the penis (hypospadias) or on its dorsal aspect (epispadias). Hypospadias may result in difficulty with intercourse. Plastic reconstruction of the urethra may be required. Epispadias is rare and more disabling and difficult to correct than hypospadias. It may be associated with incontinence. Plastic reconstruction or urinary diversions are possible treatments. In the female, the urethra may open on to the anterior vaginal wall.

Urethral valves may occur in the posterior urethra. The condition is rare occurring with an incidence of 1 : 5000, 50% of cases occurring under 1 year of age. They cause dilatation of the prostatic urethra, bladder, ureters and pelvis. It is often diagnosed on prenatal USS. Rarely there may be uraemia with palpable bladder and kidneys at birth. Milder cases present later in childhood with difficulty in voiding, recurrent UTIs and uraemia. Treatment is by transurethral resection of the valves. With early presentation the prognosis is good. With extensive renal damage, dialysis and transplantation may be required.

HAEMATURIA

Haematuria is the passage of blood in the urine. This may vary from a few red cells detected on 'stix' testing to the passage of frank blood. Haematuria may be noted at the beginning of micturition, throughout micturition or at the end of micturition. Care must be taken to avoid menstrual bleeding being mistaken for haematuria. Other causes of red urine include excessive beetroot ingestion, rifampicin, porphyria, haemoglobinuria and myoglobinuria. (For causes of haematuria → Table 16.1.)

Table 16.1
Causes of haematuria

Kidney	Glomerular disease Polycystic kidneys Carcinoma Stone Trauma (including renal biopsy) Tuberculosis Embolism Renal vein thrombosis Vascular malformation
Ureter	Stone Neoplasm
Bladder	Carcinoma Stone Trauma Inflammatory – cystitis, tuberculosis, bilharzia
Prostate	Benign prostatic hypertrophy Neoplasm
Urethra	Trauma Stone Urethritis Neoplasm
General	Anticoagulants Thrombocytopenia Haemophilia Sickle cell disease Malaria

Symptoms and signs Family history, e.g. polycystic kidney. Painless haematuria is suggestive of neoplasia. Loin pain or ureteric colic suggests stone or clot colic associated with tumour. Suprapubic discomfort suggests bladder stone. Terminal bleeding with pain suggests bladder calculus. Urethral bleeding independent of micturition suggests a urethral lesion. Check the drug history. Spontaneous bruising. Palpable kidney. Palpable bladder. Enlarged prostate on examination PR.

Investigations • Hb, FBC • ESR • U&Es • LFTs • Clotting screen • Urine microscopy: red cells exclude haemoglobinuria and beetroot ingestion, white cells suggest infection, granular casts suggest nephritis • Urine cytology • CXR: secondaries, TB • KUB • IVU • USS • CT/MRI scan • Flexible cystoscopy under LA: intravesical lesion, bleeding from prostate • Ultrasound-guided renal or prostatic biopsy.

Treatment Appropriate to the underlying condition.

OBSTRUCTIVE UROPATHY

Hydronephrosis is the distension of the calyces and pelvis of the kidney owing to obstruction to the outflow of urine. It may be bilateral or unilateral. (For causes of hydronephrosis → Table 16.2.)

Table 16.2
Causes of hydronephrosis

Unilateral
- Pelviureteric junction obstruction
  - Congenital pelviureteric junction obstruction
  - Aberrant renal vessels
  - Calculus
  - Tumours of the renal pelvis
- Ureteric obstruction
  - Calculus
  - Ureteric invasion, e.g. cervical, rectal or colonic tumours
  - Iatrogenic – damage at surgery

Bilateral
- Urethral valves
- Urethral or meatal stenosis
- Prostatic enlargement
- Extensive bladder tumours
- Retroperitoneal fibrosis

Symptoms and signs Loin pain. Upper abdominal pain. Fever. Rigors – if infection. Ureteric colic. Hesitancy, poor stream, frequency, distended bladder with suprapubic discomfort. Uraemia may be presenting complaint. Palpable kidney. Palpable prostate.

Investigations • Hb, FBC • ESR • U&Es • LFTs • MSU • KUB: enlarged renal outline, opaque calculi • USS: confirms diagnosis and may demonstrate lesion • IVU (→ Fig. 16.1): early stages show pelvic dilatation with clubbing of the calyces, site of obstruction, function of kidney, trabeculation of bladder, residual urine (if bilateral hydronephrosis and uraemia, no further information would be obtained from an IVU) • CT scan

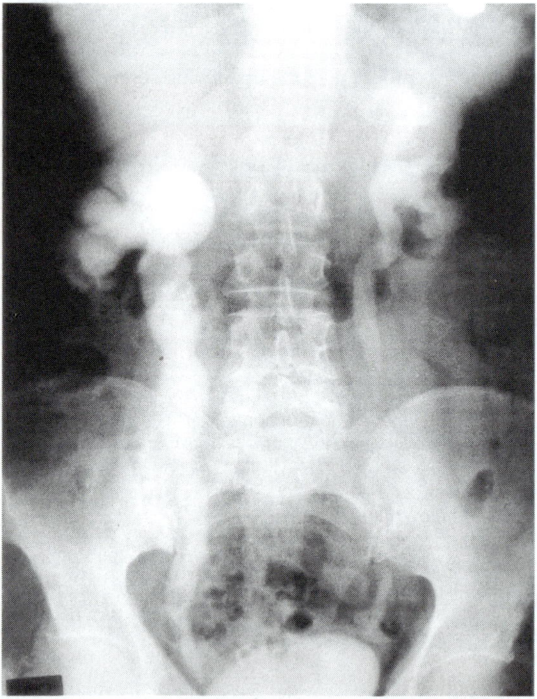

Fig. 16.1 Intravenous urogram. There is a right-sided hydronephrosis and hydroureter. Note the dilatation of the pelvis with clubbing of the calyces and also dilatation of the ureter down to its entry into the bladder.

• Cystoscopy: cause of bladder outlet obstruction or bladder tumour • Retrograde pyelogram defines exact site of obstruction.

Treatment Directed at the underlying cause. With a small ureteric stone the obstruction may be relieved with the passage of the stone. The presence of acute infection or marked renal impairment requires urgent decompression of the urinary tract under antibiotic cover. This may be done by percutaneous nephrostomy, suprapubic cystostomy, ureteric catheter drainage or urethral catheter drainage. A non-functioning kidney especially if infected should be removed.

Complications Infection: pyonephrosis. Stone formation in stagnant urine. Hypertension due to renal ischaemia. Traumatic rupture of a hydronephrotic kidney. Uraemia.

CALCULOUS DISEASE

Urinary calculi are often idiopathic. They also arise secondary to stasis and infection and also in association with metabolic disorders, e.g. cystinuria. Stones may form in the kidney or bladder. Ureteric calculi are in transit from the kidney to bladder. Stones occur in about 1% of the population. The majority are composed of calcium, magnesium ammonium phosphate, or urate.

Types of calculi

Calcium oxalate (75%) 'Mulberry' stones covered with sharp projections. They cause bleeding and are often black owing to altered blood on their surface. Because of their sharp surface they give symptoms when comparatively small. Occur in alkaline urine.

Phosphate (15%) Usually compound of calcium, magnesium and ammonium phosphate. Smooth and dirty white. They may enlarge rapidly and fill the calyces taking on their shape, i.e. staghorn calculus. Occur in strongly alkaline urine.

Urate (5%) Arise in acid urine. Hard, smooth, faceted and light brown in colour.

Cystine (2%) Usually multiple. Arise in acid urine and are of metabolic origin owing to decreased reabsorption of cystine from the renal tubules. White and translucent.

Xanthine and pyruvate stones Rare. Due to inborn error of metabolism.

90% of calculi are radio-opaque. Usually only urates are radiolucent, cystine stones being radio-opaque because of their sulphur content. Precipitating factors include: diet, dehydration, stasis, infection, hyperparathyroidism, idiopathic hypercalciuria, milk–alkali syndrome, hypervitaminosis D, cystinuria, inborn errors of purine metabolism, gout, and chemotherapy (excess uric acid following treatment of leukaemia or polycythaemia).

Symptoms and signs Renal calculi – may be asymptomatic even with large stone. Loin pain. Haematuria. Dysuria. Signs of uraemia. Colic if stone impacts in pelviureteric junction. Ureteric calculi – severe colicky pain radiating from loin to groin. Sweating. Nausea. Vomiting. Bladder calculi – dull suprapubic discomfort, terminal haematuria, dysuria, strangury. Patient may have loin tenderness, pyrexia if infection, kidney may be palpable with gross hydronephrosis or pyonephrosis.

Investigations Emergency for severe renal pain or ureteric colic: • Urine microscopy • MSU • U&Es • KUB: 90% of calculi are radio-opaque • Emergency IVU: site of obstruction, function of other kidney.

Following acute attack or routine for urinary symptoms or incidental finding of stone: • Hb, FBC • ESR • U&Es • Creatinine • Calcium • Phosphorous • Uric acid • 24-hour urine for calcium, phosphorous, oxalate, urate, cystine • Creatinine clearance • KUB • IVU • USS • Isotope renography to establish functional contribution of each kidney • Cystoscopy • Retrograde pyelogram.

Treatment Acute symptoms – ureteric colic:

- Relieve pain – diclofenac sodium i.m. or PR; or pethidine.
- Admit to hospital.
- Bed rest.
- Intravenous fluids or increased oral fluids.
- Collect and sieve all urine to retrieve calculus for analysis.
- Check radiographs to assess progress of stone.
- Stones less than 4 mm will usually pass spontaneously. 50% of stones between 4 and 6 mm will pass spontaneously. Stones greater than 6 mm usually require removal.
- Obstruction and infection require removal of stone.
- Stone removal may be carried out by: ureteroscopy with destruction of stone by lithoclast or electrohydraulic lithotripsy; ureterolithotomy (stones >5 mm and anywhere in the ureter); percutaneous nephrolithotomy after the stone has been pushed into the renal pelvis with a ureteric catheter (for small stones in the upper ureter). Stones may be visualized via a ureteroscope passed directly into the ureter, and then grasped or fragmented for removal.

→

Routine treatment of established urinary calculus Any renal or bladder calculus can be removed by open surgical techniques. However, in recent years there has been a move to minimally invasive surgery using endoscopic techniques or extracorporeal shockwave lithotripsy.

Percutaneous nephrolithotomy A nephroscope is inserted into the kidney under radiographic control via a previously dilated track. The stone is then removed by grasping forceps (if small), ultrasonically disintegrated and removed by suction or disrupted into small fragments by electrohydraulic or laser lithotriptors.

Extracorporeal shockwave lithotripsy This consists of an external energy source which is focused to provide a high-pressure zone that is directed to fragment the calculus. The calculus is fragmented into small particles which pass in the urine.

Open surgery This is used less often. A stone may be removed through the kidney substance (nephrolithotomy), or through the renal pelvis (pyelolithotomy). Surgery may be needed to correct hydronephrosis associated with a stone. If the kidney is irreparably damaged, nephrectomy is required.

Bladder calculi Small stones may be removed cystoscopically after crushing with a lithotrite or disintegration using an electrohydraulic lithotriptor. Large stones > 5 cm are removed by suprapubic cystostomy.

The stone must be analysed. The underlying cause must be treated if possible, e.g. parathyroidectomy or correction of an obstructive lesion. Attempts should be made to prevent recurrence.

Prevention of recurrence Up to 50% of patients may have recurrence within 5 years. Prevention involves: (i) high fluid intake especially in hot weather; (ii) reduce milk intake; (iii) prompt treatment of urinary tract infections; (iv) calcium stones, low-calcium diet, thiazide diuretics, acidify urine; (v) oxalate stones – reduce oxalate intake – exclude rhubarb, spinach, tomatoes, strawberries, tea and chocolate; (vi) urate stones – allopurinol, urinary alkalinization.

TUMOURS OF THE RENAL TRACT

KIDNEY

Benign tumours are rare. Adenocarcinoma accounts for 80% of

renal tumours. Transitional cell tumours occur in the renal pelvis. Squamous cell carcinomas may occur in the renal pelvis and are associated with squamous metaplasia due to chronic irritation caused by stone or infection.

Hypernephroma (renal adenocarcinoma)

This arises from renal tubular epithelium. Males are affected twice as commonly as females. It usually occurs over the age of 40. There is increased incidence in smokers, coffee drinkers, industrial exposure to cadmium, lead, asbestos, aromatic hydrocarbons; renal cysts in dialysis patients; von Hippel–Lindau disease. Spread is by direct extension into perinephric tissues, by lymphatics to the para-aortic nodes, by the blood, along the renal vein which may contain tumour, to bone, liver, brain and lung (cannon ball metastases).

Symptoms and signs Haematuria, loin pain, PUO. Palpable mass, anaemia, polycythaemia. Symptoms and signs due to secondaries – hepatomegaly, breathlessness, pathological fractures.

Investigations • Urinalysis • Hb, FBC • ESR: anaemia, ESR raised, occasionally polycythaemia • USS • IVU: distortion of

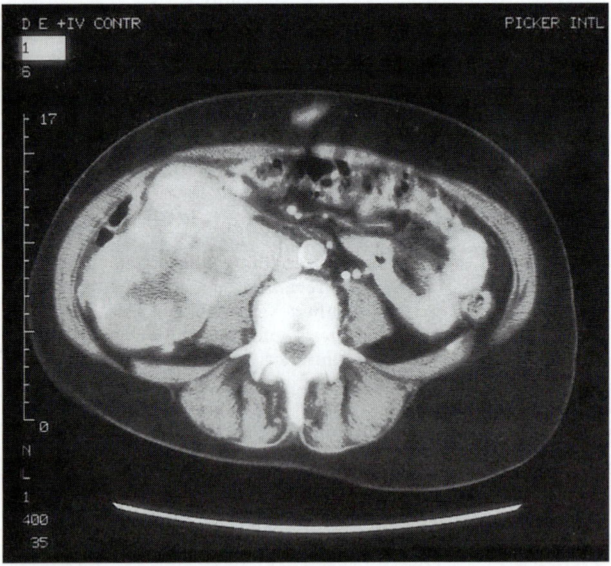

Fig. 16.2 Abdominal CT scan. There is a hypernephroma of the right kidney.

calyces and calcification • CT/MRI scan (→ Fig. 16.2) • CXR: metastases.

Treatment Nephrectomy if no evidence of metastases. Occasionally solitary metastases may be treated by surgery. Radiotherapy is palliative for pain due to metastases. Progesterone therapy induces remission in about 15% of patients. Biological modifiers such as interferon and interleukins for metastatic disease.

Prognosis If the tumour is localized to the kidney, nephrectomy offers a 5-year survival of 70%.

RENAL PELVIS AND URETER

These are either transitional cell tumours or squamous cell carcinoma in areas of squamous metaplasia. The tumour may seed down the ureter and involve the bladder.

Symptoms and signs Haematuria. Infection secondary to hydronephrosis. Ureteric colic due to obstruction or clot.

Investigations • Urinalysis • IVU • Cystoscopy to check for bladder seeding.

Treatment Nephroureterectomy with excision of a cuff of bladder wall. Chemotherapy – as for bladder cancer.

BLADDER

This is the commonest form of urological cancer. 80% are transitional cell carcinomas but chronic irritation from stones or infection may result in squamous cell metaplasia giving rise to squamous cell carcinoma. Adenocarcinomas are rare. Aetiological factors include smoking, aromatic hydrocarbons (rubber and dye industry), bladder diverticulae, bilharzia. What were formally regarded as transitional cell papillomas are recognized as well-differentiated transitional cell carcinomas. True transitional cell papillomas are now considered to be extremely rare. Tumours are more frequent in the middle-aged and elderly and occur more frequently in males. Spread occurs by direct invasion into the prostate, urethra, sigmoid colon, rectum or, in the female, to the uterus and vagina. The ureteric orifices may be occluded giving rise to hydronephrosis and renal failure. Lymphatic spread is to the iliac and para-aortic nodes and blood spread occurs late to the liver and lungs.

Symptoms and signs Painless haematuria. Dysuria, frequency, and urgency. Hydronephrosis. CRF. Pain from pelvic invasion. Examination is usually negative in the early stages. The tumour may be palpable by manual examination under anaesthesia.

T1: Confined to mucosa or submucosa – impalpable
T2: Superficial muscle involved – localized rubbery thickening
T3: Deep muscle involved – mobile mass
T4: Invasion beyond bladder to adjacent structures – fixed mass

Investigations • Hb, FBC • ESR • U&Es • Creatinine • MSU • Urine cytology • IVU: filling defects, hydronephrosis • USS • EUA to assess tumour spread • Cystoscopy and biopsy • CXR • CT scan: to determine spread • Bone scan for metastases.

Treatment of transitional cell carcinoma

T1: Transurethral resection or cystodiathermy. For multiple small tumours, intravesical chemotherapy with epodyl, thiotepa, mitomycin, BCG, or adriamycin.

T2: T2 tumours and above invade the detrusor muscle by definition and should not be managed by transurethral resection alone. A radical cystectomy is the 'gold standard' treatment but radiotherapy may be effective in those not fit for surgery.

For T1 tumours there is a 70% chance of recurrence at 5 years and a 10% chance of developing invasive disease. Check cystoscopy should be carried out at regular intervals (6 months to a year) for life.

T3: This may be treated by radiotherapy, cystectomy or a combination of both. Cystectomy requires urinary diversion by implantation of the ureters into an ileal loop or reconstruction using bowel to fashion a 'neobladder'. The latter can be drained by self-catheterization through a 'continent' stoma, or anastomosed to the urethra to allow normal voiding per urethrum.

T4: Palliative radiotherapy – chemotherapy with cisplatin, vinblastine, methotrexate, may produce remissions.

Prognosis Early tumours are curable. T1 tumours have an 85%, 5-year survival rate falling to 60% with T2. Approximately 40% of patients with T3 tumours are alive at 5 years. Patients with T4 tumours rarely survive for more than 1 year.

URINARY TRACT INFECTIONS (UTIs)

These may be divided into those affecting the kidney (pyelonephritis) and those affecting the bladder (cystitis). UTIs are more common in women and the majority of women will have a UTI some time during their life. Risk factors include pregnancy, urinary tract malformations, urinary tract obstruction, calculus, prostatic obstruction, bladder diverticulum, spinal injury, trauma, urinary tract tumour, diabetes mellitus, immunosuppression.

Symptoms and signs

Acute pyelonephritis This includes loin pain, dysuria, frequency, fever, rigors, cloudy or blood-stained urine. Tender in loin and flank.

Cystitis Frequency, urgency, dysuria, haematuria, often no fever. Tenderness suprapubically or on examination PR or PV.

Investigations • Urinalysis • Microscopy • Culture • Hb, FBC • U&Es • Creatinine. May be haematuria and proteinuria. Colony count of greater than 100 000 organisms/ml of a fresh MSU is significant. Microscopy shows pus cells and organisms (usually Gram-negative rods). Common organisms include *Escherichia coli*, *Proteus*, *Klebsiella*, *Pseudomonas*, and faecal streptococci.

Treatment Drink plenty. Antibiotics – amoxycillin 250 mg t.d.s. or trimethoprim 200 mg b.d. are appropriate initial treatments. Change antibiotic according to organism and sensitivities. Avoid sexual intercourse while infected. If the infection fails to settle on appropriate antibiotics or recurs rapidly after stopping antibiotics, further investigation is required. Two or more UTIs in a female appropriately treated require further investigation. Failure to respond to treatment suggests inappropriate antibiotics, failure to complete the course of antibiotics, resistant organisms, underlying obstruction, calculus, tumour, urinary retention, or specific infection, e.g. TB. Further investigation of recurrent attacks includes IVU, ultrasound, cystoscopy.

Sterile pyuria

Pus cells are apparent on microscopy but there is no growth on culture. Causes include inadequately treated UTI, TB, tumour, stone, prostatitis, polycystic kidneys, appendicitis, diverticulitis or analgesic abuse.

Urinary tract tuberculosis

This has shown a decline in the past 30 years but it remains a problem in the Third World and the immigrant population in the UK. Genitourinary tuberculosis is always secondary to TB elsewhere. The urinary tract is involved by haematogenous spread. The kidney is affected most frequently, the lower urinary tract being secondarily infected by descending infection giving rise to cystitis or infection of the epididymis or seminal vesicles.

Symptoms and signs The renal lesion is often silent. Repeated UTIs with frequency, dysuria, haematuria. Occasionally dull loin pain. Weight loss, fever, night sweats. Symptoms of uraemia may occur. Epididymitis. Scrotal sinuses.

Investigation • Hb, FBC • ESR • Urinalysis: pus cells, protein, red cells • MSU: sterile pyuria • Urine microscopy and ZN staining of early morning specimen of urine may demonstrate acid-fast bacilli • Culture of tubercle bacilli positive (takes up to 6 weeks) • CXR: may show primary lesion • IVU: plain film may show calcification in the renal parenchyma; contrast film may show irregularity of the calyces, obliterated calyces, contractures of ureter or bladder, vesicoureteric reflux • Cystoscopy: small-capacity bladder with tubercles • Biopsy.

Treatment Antituberculous drugs. Surgery may be needed to remove a totally destroyed kidney or to deal with complications, e.g. repair of ureteric stricture or enlargement of small fibrotic bladder (ileocystoplasty, i.e. enlargement of the bladder with a cuff of ileum).

PROSTATE

The three commonest conditions of the prostate are: bladder outflow obstruction due to benign prostatic hypertrophy (over 50s); prostatic cancer (over 65s); and prostatitis in young adults.

BLADDER OUTFLOW OBSTRUCTION

Benign prostatic hypertrophy

This affects most men over the age of 50 but only 10% present with symptoms. The size of the prostate does not correlate with the degree of obstruction. The severity of symptoms depends on the degree of encroachment on the prostatic urethra. Obstruction to outflow occurs and the bladder hypertrophies. Diverticulae of the bladder, urinary infection, hydronephrosis and renal failure may ensue.

Symptoms and signs The cardinal symptoms are difficulty in starting and a poor stream. Other symptoms are nocturia, frequency, dribbling, incontinence, acute retention. Haematuria from ruptured dilated bladder neck veins. Palpable bladder occasionally. Smell of stale urine on patient. Enlargement of kidney (hydronephrosis). Examination PR – smooth enlarged prostate, median sulcus, enlarged lateral lobes. Signs of uraemia.

Investigations • Hb, FBC • ESR • U&Es • Creatinine • PAP and PSA to exclude malignancy • MSU • USS: assess upper urinary tract (hydronephrosis), bladder, residual urine

Treatment Treatment of acute retention (see below). TURP with cystoscopy to check for diverticulae, tumour or stone. The resected prostate should be submitted to histology – unsuspected foci of carcinoma may be present.

Prostatic carcinoma

This is the second commonest cause of death from cancer in men. It is rare below the age of 50. Two-thirds of patients with prostatic cancer in the UK present with advanced disease, when potentially curative treatment is not possible. Early asymptomatic disease can be detected by screening for prostate-specific antigen (PSA); transrectal ultrasound scanning with guided biopsy. Foci of carcinoma may be found incidentally in specimens resected for benign prostatic hypertrophy. Spread occurs to adjacent organs, e.g. bladder, urethra and seminal vesicles. Spread to the rectum is rare. Lymphatic spread is to iliac and para-aortic nodes. Blood spread occurs early, especially to the pelvis, spine and skull (osteosclerotic lesions).

Symptoms and signs Asymptomatic. Hard craggy mass on routine rectal examination. Incontinence, dysuria, haematuria, hesitancy, dribbling, retention. Bone pain, pathological fractures, sciatica, anaemia, weight loss. Rectal examination may reveal nodule in prostate or hard craggy mass involving whole prostate. The median sulcus between the lobes may be obliterated. Palpable bladder. Tenderness over bones. Hepatomegaly.

Investigations • Hb, FBC • ESR • U&Es • Creatinine • PSA: to facilitate early detection and evaluate response to treatment • CXR: metastases in lungs or ribs • Bone radiograph: sclerotic deposits in pelvis, spine, or skull • Bone scan is sensitive indicator of early metastases • USS: residual urine, upper urinary tract obstruction • Transrectal prostatic biopsy • If urinary obstruction, specimens may be obtained at TURP for histology.

Treatment TURP for obstruction. A localized prostatic carcinoma may be completely removed by radical prostatectomy. Most tumours are usually discovered when some spread has occurred. Hormonal manipulation for metastatic disease. Subcapsular orchidectomy slows tumour growth. Other techniques of hormonal manipulation include; luteinizing hormone releasing hormone (LHRH) agonists which produce a fall of luteinizing hormone (LH) from the anterior pituitary with consequent reduction of testicular secretion of testosterone, e.g. cyproterone acetate or bicalutamide. Stilboestrol is rarely used nowadays as it causes gynaecomastia, fluid retention and possible thromboembolic complications. Local radiotherapy especially for bony metastatic pain.

Prognosis Variable. Dependent on stage at presentation. Patients with clinically localized tumours treated radically may expect a normal life expectancy. Those with metastatic disease at presentation have a median 3-year survival.

Prostatitis

This occurs most commonly in young adults. Acute bacterial prostatitis usually presents as an acute febrile illness. Chronic prostatitis presents with recurrent UTIs. If there is a past history of TB anywhere in the body, suspect tuberculous prostatitis.

Symptoms and signs

Acute bacterial prostatitis Fever, low back pain, perineal pain, bladder irritation, outflow obstruction. Enlarged tender prostate.

Chronic prostatitis Symptoms of UTI. Dull perineal ache. Normal or indurated irregular prostate.

Investigations In acute prostatitis: • WBC raised • MSU usually shows growth • Blood culture may be positive. In chronic prostatitis: • Prostatic massage may yield secretions containing white cells and occasionally organisms • Culture for TB in chronic prostatitis.

Treatment Acute prostatitis is treated with bed rest, antibiotics (often i.v.) and analgesia. Prostatic abscess or chronic prostatitis may occur as a complication. Chronic prostatitis is treated with long-term antibiotics, e.g. trimethoprim for 12 weeks. Prostatic massage may be effective. Tuberculous prostatitis is treated with antituberculous therapy.

Urethral strictures

The causes include infection, trauma, foreign bodies, stones, iatrogenic, i.e. postcatheterization or instrumentation, and tumours.

Symptoms and signs Weak stream, dribbling, acute or chronic retention, UTI.

Investigations • Flexible cystoscopy under local anaesthetic • Retrograde or antegrade cystourethrogram.

Treatment Optical urethrotomy. Intermittent self-dilatation with Loferic catheters. Surgical reconstruction with skin flaps.

URINARY RETENTION

The retention of urine may be acute, chronic or acute-on-chronic. Patients with acute retention present as surgical emergencies. (For causes of urinary retention → Table 16.3.)

Table 16.3
Causes of urinary retention

Local	
Urethral lumen or bladder neck	Urethral valves Tumours Stones Blood clot Meatal ulcer or stenosis
Urethral or bladder wall	Urethral trauma Urethral stricture Urethral tumour
Outside the wall	Prostatic enlargement Faecal impaction Pelvic tumour Pregnant uterus
General	
Postoperative	
Neurogenic	Spinal cord injuries Spinal cord disease, e.g. tabes dorsalis, spinal tumour, multiple sclerosis, diabetic autonomic neuropathy
Drugs	Anticholinergics, antidepressants, alcohol

Symptoms and signs Previous history of chronic retention. Poor urinary stream, frequency, UTI, urethritis, ureteric colic, haematuria. Backache. Neurological illness. Palpable bladder. Examination PR – prostatic enlargement. Palpate for urethral stone or stricture. Urethral meatus for ulcer. Signs of uraemia. Neurological signs.

Treatment Attempt catheterization after giving analgesia. If the catheter will not pass, carry out a suprapubic catheterization.

Investigations • Urine microscopy • MSU • Hb, FBC • ESR • PAP • PSA • U&Es • LFTs • CXR • USS: to check for upper urinary tract obstruction due to back pressure, bladder tumour, stone • Cystoscopy: urethral stricture or bladder tumour.

Postoperative retention may be due to anxiety, embarrassment, supine posture, pain, drugs, fluid overload, previous unrecognized prostatism with minimal symptoms. After urological procedures it may be due to blood clot in the bladder. Before catheterizing a patient in the postoperative period, other attempts should be made to allow the patient to pass urine, e.g. standing up in a warm room relaxed, running tap or bathing in warm water. A short period of intermittent self-catheterization often allows full recovery of bladder function and normal voiding within a few days.

Chronic retention

Chronic retention is painless retention of urine of more than 1000 ml urine.

Symptoms and signs Overflow incontinence. Uraemia. Painless palpable bladder.

Treatment Bladder decompression with urethral, suprapubic or intermittent self-catheterization. Watch out for secondary diuresis. Patients often need fluid replacement in the first 48 hours after decompression. Videourodynamic assessment of detrusor muscle is important to rule out detrusor failure as a cause. Treatment is that of the cause of bladder outlet obstruction.

TESTES AND EPIDIDYMIS

Imperfectly descended testes

About 5% of full-term babies do not have one or both testes in the scrotum at birth. In the first year of life many descend leaving only 0.3% undescended at 1 year. When the testes cannot be found in the scrotum it may be because they are:

- retractile
- ectopic
- incompletely descended.

A retractile testis is a normal testis associated with an active cremasteric reflex, the testis being drawn up to the superficial inguinal ring. An ectopic testis is one which has descended to an abnormal site and may be found in the superficial inguinal pouch, the perineum, the femoral triangle or at the root of the penis. An incompletely descended testis lies in the normal course of descent lying anywhere from the posterior abdominal wall to the top of the scrotum.

Symptoms and signs The mother may have noticed that the testes are absent from the scrotum. In later life it may be noticed at a routine medical examination. A retractile testis may be brought down into the scrotum by applying gentle traction with a child relaxed in a warm room. The mother may have noticed that the testes are only present when the child is warm and relaxed, e.g. in the bath. The parents can be reassured that the testes are normal and will eventually take up permanent scrotal residence. An incompletely descended testis cannot be palpated in the inguinal canal because of the tough overlying external oblique aponeurosis. If the testis is palpable easily along the line of the inguinal canal it is almost certainly superficial to the external oblique aponeurosis and therefore ectopic. Absence of both testicles from the scrotum is called cryptorchidism. 90% of imperfectly descended testes have an associated inguinal hernia.

Treatment Retractile testes are normal. Parental reassurance is all that is required. An ectopic or incompletely descended testis must be placed in the scrotum. This should be carried out between 3 and 5 years. The testis is mobilized on the cord, any coexisting hernia repaired and the testis fixed in the scrotum. This is usually done by placing it in a pouch fashioned between the dartos muscle and the skin, i.e. orchidopexy.

Complications of imperfect descent Defective spermatogenesis with infertility in bilateral cases, risk of torsion, risk of tumour or trauma.

Hydrocele A hydrocele is a collection of fluid in the tunica vaginalis. A primary or idiopathic hydrocele develops slowly and becomes large and tense. It usually occurs in the over 40s. A secondary hydrocele tends to be small and lax and occurs secondary to inflammation or tumour of the underlying testes. It tends to occur in the younger age group. Primary hydroceles may be classified as follows:

Vaginal hydrocele This surrounds the testes in the layers of the tunica vaginalis and does not connect with the peritoneal cavity.

Congenital hydrocele This is associated with a hernial sac. It connects with the peritoneal cavity.

Infantile hydrocele This extends from the testes to the deep inguinal ring. It does not connect with the peritoneal cavity.

Hydrocele of the cord This lies along the cord anywhere from the deep inguinal ring to the upper scrotum. It does not connect with either the peritoneal cavity or the tunica vaginalis. A similar swelling may develop in the female and is known as a hydrocele of the canal of Nuck.

Symptoms and signs Scrotal swelling. Testes cannot be felt separately. Fluctuant. Transilluminates. Can 'get above it'. Congenital hydrocele in infants may fill during the day and empty while lying down at night. A hydrocele of the cord moves downwards when traction is applied to the testis.

Treatment A congenital hydrocele may be associated with a hernia. Treatment is by surgical excision of the peritoneal remnant as in herniotomy. An infantile, non-communicating hydrocele usually resolves spontaneously or needle aspiration may be required. A vaginal hydrocele in an adult may be treated by aspiration or by excision. A primary hydrocele in an elderly and unfit patient may be treated by aspiration. This may need to be done every few months. Surgery involves opening the tunica vaginalis longitudinally, emptying the hydrocele, everting the sac after excising the redundant sac and suturing the sac behind the cord thus obliterating the potential space. Secondary hydroceles require treatment of the underlying condition.

Epididymal cyst

They may be small, large, multiple, unilateral or bilateral. If they contain opalescent milky fluid demonstrated on aspiration, they are called spermatoceles.

Symptoms and signs Usually occur over 40. Scrotal swelling. Slowly enlarges. Painless. Lie above and slightly behind the testes. Testis can be felt separately. Can 'get above it'. Usually smooth and lobulated. Fluctuant. Transilluminates if contains clear fluid.

Treatment None unless large where they may show through the trousers and interfere with walking. Aspiration may help but most cysts are multiloculated. Large cysts require excision, but this will compromise the fertility of that testis. Surgery should be restricted to those who have completed their family.

Varicocele

These are varicosities of the pampiniform plexus. More common on the left side.

Symptoms and signs Varicose veins in the scrotum on standing. Disappear on lying down. Heavy or dragging sensation in scrotum. The patient must be examined standing or the diagnosis will be missed. The veins in the scrotum are often described as feeling like a 'bag of worms' but feeling like a 'plate of lukewarm spaghetti' is probably a better comparison. Bilateral varicoceles may cause subfertility. The affected testis may be smaller. Sudden onset of a left varicocele which does not disappear on lying down in the older patient may be caused by an obstruction of the left renal vein by a renal carcinoma – USS of the kidney is appropriate.

Treatment In the asymptomatic patient, no treatment is required especially if the condition is unilateral. Scrotal support for aching and discomfort. Failure of symptoms to settle with scrotal support or evidence of subfertility are indications for intervention. The majority of varicoceles can be treated by embolization and obliteration under radiological control. If surgery is indicated it is via an inguinal approach, all testicular veins bar one being ligated at the deep inguinal ring.

Infections of the testis and epididymis

Inflammation of the testis and epididymis may be acute or chronic. Acute or chronic orchitis may be due to mumps. Acute epididymo-orchitis may be due to coliform organisms or gonorrhoea. It may follow urethral instrumentation or operations on the prostate. Chronic epididymo-orchitis may follow an acute attack or more commonly is due to TB.

Symptoms and signs Pain, swelling, redness of the scrotum, often associated with pyrexia. In the young patient, the differentiation from torsion is often impossible and the scrotum should be explored. Enlarged exquisitely tender testis and epididymis.

Investigations • FBC • MSU • Early morning urine specimens for TB culture.

Treatment

Acute Bed rest. Analgesia. Scrotal support. Antibiotic – ciprofloxacin until the results of culture are known. If due to gonorrhoea, treat appropriately. The swelling may take as long as 2 months to resolve.

Chronic TB – antituberculous drugs. Orchidectomy if improvement does not occur. Long-term antibiotic therapy for non-tuberculous epididymo-orchitis.

Testicular torsion

This is twisting of the testis with interference to the arterial blood supply. The actual torsion is usually of the spermatic cord. It occurs in a congenitally abnormal situation. It is associated with imperfectly descended testis, or high investment of the tunica vaginalis with a horizontal lie of the testis; or when the epididymis and testis are separated by a mesorchium, in which case the twist occurs at the mesorchium.

Untreated, the testis infarcts. The condition is a surgical emergency and to be sure of testicular salvage, untwisting should be carried out within 6 hours of symptoms. Incidence is highest between 10 and 20 years.

Symptoms and signs Sudden onset of severe pain in the scrotum and groin and radiating to the lower abdomen associated with vomiting. May follow strain, lifting, exercise or masturbation. Always examine the testes in a young male with abdominal pain. Examination reveals a swollen, painful, testis drawn up to the groin. Difficult to differentiate from epididymo-orchitis. In the latter there is usually a fever, leukocytosis and the testis is not drawn up to the groin. Epididymo-orchitis is usually associated with UTI. However, doubt usually exists as to the correct diagnosis, in which case the scrotum must be explored.

Treatment Explore the testis as soon as possible. Untwist the testis. Establish that it is not irreversibly infarcted and fix it to the scrotum usually by anchoring it to the scrotal septum. Since the other testis is likely to have an abnormal position, this should be fixed at the same operation. If the testis is infarcted it should be removed. Leaving behind an infarcted testis may result in the development of sperm autoantibodies with depressed spermatogenesis in the remaining testis.

Testicular trauma

This usually occurs in sports injuries or violence. Trauma may result in bleeding into the layers of the tunica vaginalis resulting in haematocele.

Symptoms and signs Severe pain, scrotal swelling, bruising, tender enlarged testicle.

Investigations • Scrotal ultrasound – beware of an underlying testicular malignancy.

Treatment Bed rest. Scrotal support. Surgical exploration may be required to evacuate the haematocele and repair a split in the tunica albuginea. If swelling and irregularity of the testis persists after allowing adequate time for recovery, suspect a testicular tumour and institute appropriate investigations. Unsuspected pre-existing testicular tumours may be unmasked following trauma.

Testicular tumours

This is the commonest malignancy in young men. 90% arise from germ cells and are either seminomas or teratomas. The other 10% are lymphomas, Sertoli cell tumours or Leydig cell tumours. Seminomas occur between 30 and 40 years; teratomas between 20 and 30 years. Imperfectly descended testes have a 20 to 30 times increased incidence of malignancy.

Symptoms and signs Painless swelling of the testis. Heaviness in the scrotum. Occasionally painful swelling. Small lax hydrocele. May be history of trauma. Palpable abdominal mass. Spread to para-aortic nodes. Lump in left side of neck – spread to left supraclavicular node. Chest symptoms due to lung metastases.

Investigations • USS testis • CXR • Tumour markers: AFP, βHCG • CT scan.

Treatment If there is a reasonable suspicion of tumour, explore the testis through an inguinal incision. Clamp the spermatic cord with a soft clamp to prevent tumour dissemination when the testis is delivered into the wound. Palpate the testis. If obviously malignant, carry out orchidectomy. If not obviously malignant the testis is split ('bi-valve') and examined after packing off the rest of the operative field. If any doubt exists, frozen sections should be carried out. Tumour markers should be repeated after orchidectomy. If they are positive, metastases are likely to be present. CT scan of abdomen and chest are carried out to stage disease. If metastatic disease is present, the following is appropriate treatment.

→

Seminoma Very radiosensitive. Radiotherapy to iliac and para-aortic nodes plus chemotherapy as for teratoma. Survival is 90–95% at 5 years.

Teratoma Combination chemotherapy. Agents used include etoposide, vinblastine, methotrexate, bleomycin, cysplatin, in various combinations of three. Survival is between 60 and 90% at 5 years. Surgery may be used for tumour debulking of retroperitoneal nodes.

PENIS

The majority of surgical conditions of the penis relate to problems with the foreskin and glans and the need for circumcision. Carcinoma of the penis and Peyronie's disease are rare.

CONDITIONS OF THE FORESKIN

Balanoposthitis

This is inflammation of the glans and foreskin. In children, this may be due to faecal organisms or staphylococci. It may result in phimosis from scarring. Recurrent attacks may occur in adults associated with poor hygiene. Exclude diabetes especially if candida is the infecting organism. Treatment – antibiotics or topical application of antifungal agents. Circumcision may be required.

Phimosis

It is usually congenital. The foreskin is tight and will not retract over the glans. It may be acquired as a result of chronic or acute inflammation of the prepuce. It may be secondary to attempts to retract the foreskin at an early age. It is characterized by ballooning of the foreskin on voiding. In the extreme case, retention of urine with hydroureters and hydronephrosis may occur. However, this is more often due to meatal stenosis which may be hidden by the phimosis. In adults, phimosis may interfere with sexual intercourse.

Treatment Circumcision.

Paraphimosis

The foreskin is tight and retracts over the corona glandis and cannot be reduced. It forms a tight constriction around the glans interfering with venous return causing swelling of the glans and foreskin, this further exacerbating the difficulty of reduction. It may occur after masturbation, sexual intercourse, bathing glans or after catheterization when the foreskin is not pulled forwards afterwards (iatrogenic).

Treatment Apply local anaesthetic jelly. Administer strong analgesic and attempt manual reduction. If the latter is unsuccessful a 'dorsal slit' under local anaesthetic should be carried out. This divides the tight constriction ring and allows the foreskin to reduce. Formal circumcision should be carried out when the oedema has subsided.

Balanitis xerotica obliterans

This is a condition of the foreskin characterized by loss of skin elasticity and fibrosis, resulting in phimosis. Treatment is by circumcision.

Carcinoma of the penis

This is rare. It occurs between 60 and 80 years and is almost unknown in circumcised males. Poor hygiene and accumulation of smegma may be aetiological factors. Histologically the tumour is a squamous cell carcinoma. The tumour starts in the sulcus between the glans and the foreskin. Spread is to the inguinal nodes. Blood spread to the lungs or bone is rare.

Symptoms and signs Firm ulcerated painless lesion. Offensive bloodstained discharge from under foreskin. Inguinal lymphadenopathy. A red velvety lesion on the glans (erythroplasia of Queyrat) is a premalignant condition.

Treatment If the urethra is not involved, radiotherapy may be used. If the urethra is involved, amputation of the penis is required. If lymph nodes are involved, block dissection of the groin should be carried out or radiotherapy may be given as a palliative measure.

Circumcision

The indications for circumcision are shown in Table 16.4.

Peyronie's disease

The aetiology is unknown. Ages 40–60 years. Fibrotic plaques occur in the corpora cavernosa. Discomfort, pain and deformity occur on erection. The fibrous plaques are palpable in the shaft of the penis. They may become calcified. Spontaneous resolution may occasionally occur. Treatment is unsatisfactory. Steroids may help but surgical incision of fibrous plaques may be necessary but further deformity may result.

Table 16.4
Indications for circumcision

Religious
Phimosis
Paraphimosis
Recurrent balanoposthitis
Diagnosis of underlying penile tumours
Trauma and tumour of foreskin

Priapism

This is persistent, painful erection unassociated with sexual desire. Causes include idiopathic, leukaemia, sickle cell disease, disseminated and pelvic malignancy, and patients on haemodialysis. Treatment includes:

- aspiration of blood from the corpora cavernosa with a wide-bore needle and irrigation with heparinized saline
- anastomosis of the great saphenous vein to the engorged corpora cavernosa thus establishing venous drainage of the corpora.

17
Orthopaedics

FRACTURES

A fracture is a complete or partial break in the continuity of a bone. There are several ways of classifying fractures, e.g. according to causation, according to configuration of fracture or according to their relation to surrounding tissues.

Causation

Trauma The fracture occurs in a normal bone as a result of trauma. The pattern depends upon the direction of the violence. Direct violence usually results in a transverse fracture. Indirect violence, e.g. a twisting injury, usually results in a spiral or oblique fracture. Axial compression results in a comminuted, crush or burst fracture. An avulsion fracture is caused by traction, usually a tendon or ligament tearing off a bony fragment, e.g. patellar fracture with a sudden contraction of quadriceps.

Stress fractures The bone is fatigued by repetitive stress and resembles the fatigue fractures which occur in metals. This type of fracture occurs in individuals undertaking increased amounts of often unaccustomed exercise, e.g. 'march' metatarsal fractures in soldiers.

Pathological fractures These occur in bones already compromised by underlying disease. The trauma may be quite minimal. Common underlying causes include osteoporosis and metastases.

Pattern (→ Fig. 17.1)

Transverse fracture This is caused by direct violence.

Spiral or oblique fracture This is caused by violence transmitted from a distance.

Crush fracture This is caused by direct compression in cancellous bone.

Burst fracture This is caused by strong axial compression of a short bone, e.g. vertebrae.

Avulsion fracture This is caused by sudden, strong traction by a tendon or ligament avulsing a bony fragment.

Fracture-dislocation This occurs when there is fracture of a bone involved in a joint with complete loss of congruity of the joint surfaces.

Greenstick fracture A fracture occurring in children in which the bone buckles and does not fracture completely across.

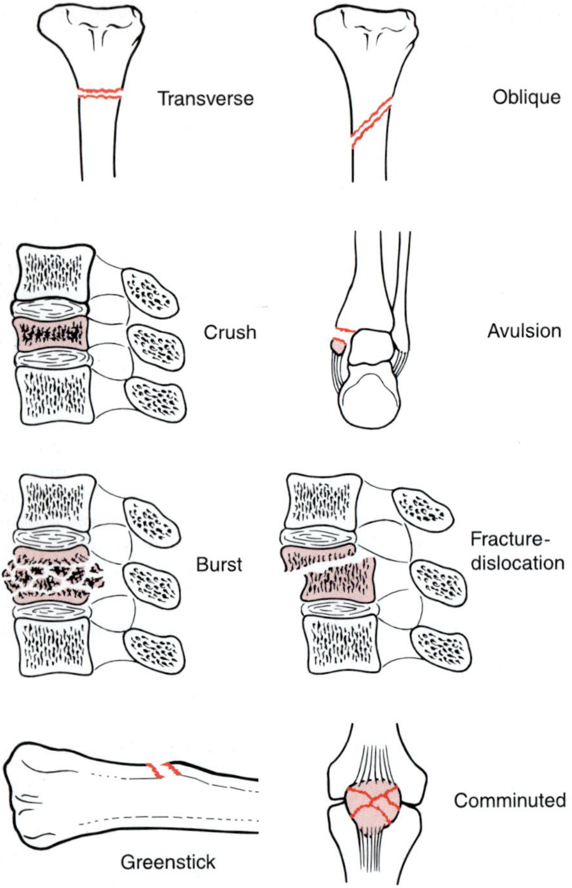

Fig. 17.1 Types of fracture.

Comminuted fracture One in which the bone is broken into more than two fragments.

Relation to surrounding structures

Simple fracture There is no skin or body cavity wound communicating with the site of fracture.

Compound fracture There is communication between the site of fracture and the skin or body cavity wound, e.g. skull fracture communicating with the air sinuses.

Intra-articular fracture The fracture involves an articular surface.

Complicated fracture There is associated damage to nerves, blood vessels or internal organs.

Symptoms and signs History to assess mechanism of injury. Pain. Loss of function. Loss of sensation or paralysis. Tenderness. Deformity. Swelling. Crepitus. Abnormal mobility. Discrepancy in length of limbs, associated nerve and vascular injuries. Examine for any associated injuries. Wound associated with compound fracture.

Investigations Radiographs: in two planes at right angles. With long bones include joints at either end. Normal side for comparison. Radiograph – confirms the diagnosis, accurately localizes it, demonstrates the type, e.g. spiral, comminuted, etc., shows any displacement, shows any pre-existing disease, e.g. pathological fracture through a metastasis, may show foreign body in compound fracture, may show associated joint problem. Occasionally a fracture may not be apparent on initial radiograph (e.g. stress fracture) and further radiographs may be required later when callus associated with healing is apparent. Radiograph may be required to assess associated damage, e.g. arteriography.

PRINCIPLES OF FRACTURE TREATMENT

First aid Ensure clear airway. Ensure adequate breathing. Stop bleeding. Splintage to prevent further damage by movement of fragments. Cover compound fractures with clean cloth.

Treatment of shock Considerable blood loss can occur with fractures – 1.5 litres can be lost with a femoral shaft fracture. Multiple fractures can lead to considerable blood loss. Ensure adequate treatment of shock with blood or plasma expanders before investigation and treatment.

The fracture itself

1. Reduction, i.e. the restoration of the displaced fragments to their anatomical position.
2. Hold, i.e. keeping the bony fragments in the reduced position until union occurs.
3. Rehabilitation starts as soon as possible after the injury. It is aimed initially at maintaining the function of the uninjured parts and, once the fracture is united, restoring function of the injured parts.

Reduction

Is reduction necessary? Small displacements in extra-articular fractures may be acceptable although joint surfaces should be anatomically reduced. Indications for reduction include functional impairment if not reduced, deformity, interference with blood supply, and interposition of soft tissue between bone ends.

How should it be done? Reduction may be either closed or open.

Closed reduction This may be by manipulation or traction, the latter being applied via the skin or skeleton. This must be done under anaesthesia, local, regional or general.

Open reduction This allows accurate alignment of fragments but carries the risk of infection. It is carried out in the following circumstances:

- reduction cannot be obtained by closed manipulation, e.g. because of soft tissue interposition
- there is inability to maintain reduction
- where early mobilization may be appropriate, encouraging rehabilitation and avoiding joint stiffness.

How is reduction held? Some fractures are intrinsically stable and require no additional stabilization. Others require either external or internal fixation.

Methods of holding a fracture

External

Plaster of Paris (or synthetic materials) This may be used for splints, casts or jointed casts. It is usually applied over a layer of wool. Where there is excessive swelling a slab may be used initially, a full cast being applied at a later date. The cast is radiolucent and the position of the bone should be checked by radiograph after the plaster has been applied. The distal circulation should be observed because a tight plaster may interfere with blood flow. All plasters should be checked 24 hours after application. Cast-bracing involves the use of hinged and jointed casts. Various segments are connected by specially designed hinges. This allows joint mobility as well as patient mobility.

Traction This is used to overcome the powerful pull of muscles which may cause shortening or angulation. Traction may be fixed, e.g. a Thomas splint for femoral shaft fractures, or sliding (balanced) where the patient's weight is balanced against an applied load. The patient's weight and friction forces counter the applied traction. The patient can move the limb or can move about the bed while traction continues to act in the desired direction. Traction may be applied to the skin via adhesive tape or to bone via pins or wires. Skull traction can be effected by securing a caliper or a pair of tongs to the skull and applying traction in the longitudinal axis of the neck.

Internal fixation

Wires Encircling wires may be used, e.g. fractures of the olecranon. Kirschner wires are drilled into fragments.

Screws Stainless steel or alloy screws are used. May be used to attach small bony fragment, e.g. fractures of malleoli.

Plating A plate is fastened to both fragments by screws (→ Fig. 17.2). Plates can be designed to compress a fracture giving firmer

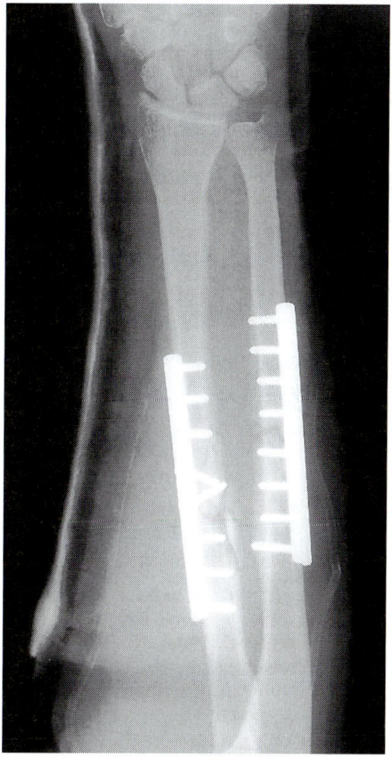

Fig. 17.2 A fracture of the radius and ulna fixed with plates and screws. The radial fracture is comminuted.

fixation allowing good healing without forming much external callus.

Intramedullary nail (Küntscher nail) A rod is passed along the medullary cavity of a long bone across the fracture and locked with transverse locking screws. It is used mainly for long bone fractures, e.g. femoral shaft fractures.

External fixation devices The fragments are transfixed by pins which are then held in an external fixation device to immobilize the fragments. Difficult, comminuted fractures can be reduced and immobilized by this method. The fracture can be held while surgery for associated injuries, e.g. skin, vascular or nerve, is carried out.

Indications for internal fixation

- Failure to maintain adequate reduction by external methods.
- Intra-articular fractures to secure good alignment of joint surfaces and prevent later osteoarthritis.
- Need to avoid long periods of immobilization, e.g. elderly patient with fracture of femoral neck.
- Patients with multiple injuries where internal fixation may facilitate nursing and patient mobility.
- Where damage to other structures, e.g. vessels and nerves, requires stability for good results following repair.
- Pathological fractures.

Compound fractures

Closure of the wound should be carried out as quickly as possible. Principles of management of compound fractures include:

- *First aid*: adequate splintage plus coverage with a clean dressing.
- *Treatment of shock*: bleeding may be external as well as internal.
- *Antibiotic therapy*: as soon as diagnosis is made large doses of antibiotics are given i.v. (benzylpenicillin 1 megaunit 6-hourly and flucloxacillin 500 mg 6-hourly).
- *Tetanus prophylaxis*.
- *Treatment of the wound and fracture*:
  - Clean the wound removing any foreign bodies and all devitalized tissue.
  - Repair any damage to blood vessels.
  - Mark the ends of any nerve that have been severed to facilitate identification for delayed repair.
  - Fracture stabilization, usually by external fixation as internal fixation is associated with increased rates of infection.
  - Clean wounds may be closed primarily.
  - Contaminated wounds older than 6 hours, or dirty wounds are referred for plastic surgery.
  - Massive wounds may require early free tissue flap coverage.
  - If plaster of Paris is applied a window must be cut in it so the wound can be observed and infection excluded.

Rehabilitation

The aims should be the restoration of function of the injured part and rehabilitation of the patient as a whole. Specific advice includes: suitable exercises; active use as much as compatible with fracture healing; active exercises; physiotherapy; occupational therapy; advice from social worker; employment advice.

COMPLICATIONS OF FRACTURES

Immediate (at time of fracture)

- Haemorrhage: this may be internal or external. Internal haemorrhage can be considerable at the fracture site, i.e. up to 1.5 litres with a fractured femoral shaft.
- Injury to nerves and vessels.
- Injury to underlying structures, e.g. brain damage with skull fractures, splenic rupture with left lower rib fractures, urethral trauma with pelvic fractures.

Early (during the period of initial treatment)

Local

- Gangrene due to vessel damage or tight plasters.
- Nerve palsies from tight plasters or involved in callus.
- Wound infection or wound dehiscence.
- Loss of position.
- Tetanus.
- Gas gangrene.

General

DVT This can occur with fractured neck of femur or generalized immobility in bed. Prophylaxis should be given.

Acute urinary retention Always exclude the possibility of bladder or urethral injury.

Pneumonia

Fat embolism This usually complicates fractures of a major long bone at 3–10 days postinjury. Embolization of the pulmonary and systemic microvasculature with lipid globules occurs. The exact source of the fat is controversial. Originally it was thought to be due to fat release from bone marrow adipocytes at the site of the fracture; it is now thought to be more likely to be an abnormal response of fat metabolism to trauma. The main effects are on the brain and lung. The patient may suddenly become drowsy, pyrexial and tachycardic. A petechial rash may appear on the upper trunk. Coma and death may result. With lung involvement the patient develops confusion, breathing difficulties, cyanosis. PO_2 down. Radiograph appearance is similar to ARDS. Renal problems may occur with excretion of lipid droplets.

Diagnosis may be confirmed by finding lipid globules in urine or sputum. Treatment is by oxygen therapy, ventilation and renal support. Early operative immobilization of fractured long bones may reduce incidence.

Compartment syndrome This may occur with or without arterial injury. Muscle swells and compartment pressure rises. Ischaemia results from pressure on surrounding *small* arteries. Distal pulses may still be palpable and the diagnosis therefore missed. Awareness of the possibility of the diagnosis is important. In the lower limb, the posterior compartment (flexors of the ankle), anterior compartment (extensors) or peroneal compartment (evertors) may be involved. Treatment is by prompt fasciotomy which allows the muscle to expand and relieves the pressure on the vessels.

Crush syndrome This is due to extensive crushing of muscle or extensive muscle necrosis, e.g. with ischaemia due to arterial injury. Myoglobin is released into the circulation. Myoglobinuria and renal failure may ensue. Oliguria with dark brownish red urine should suggest the diagnosis. Prompt treatment with an osmotic diuretic may prevent renal failure. Removal of all dead muscle possibly by amputation of the limb may be required. Dialysis is required for established ARF, which usually recovers.

Late (after the period of initial treatment)

Delayed union The fracture does not heal in the expected time. Absence of callus and mobility at the fracture site are features.

Non-union Attempts at repair by normal body mechanisms have ceased and the fracture remains un-united. Persistent mobility at fracture. Radiographs show no trabeculae cross the fracture line. A pseudarthrosis (false joint) may result. Causes of non-union include: inadequate blood supply; infection; poor immobilization; excessive movement at fracture site; interposition of soft tissue between bone ends; pathological fracture. Treatment is by bone grafting with or without further fixation.

Mal-union Healing has resulted in a deformed position. This may be because of shortening, overlap, or angulation. Treatment depends on the degree of deformity and the age of the patient. In children considerable remodelling may occur resulting in correction of the deformity. In recent fractures, manipulation, or wedging of the plaster cast, may suffice. In older fractures osteotomy may be required. Deformity may put strain on adjacent joints resulting in osteoarthritis.

Sudek's atrophy (reflex sympathetic osteodystrophy) The limb becomes painful, swollen and stiff with a reddened, smooth, shiny appearance to the skin. Radiograph shows patchy porosis of the bone. It may be seen after a Colles' fracture, in which case the symptoms affect the hand and wrist. Physiotherapy is required over a prolonged period of weeks or months. The prognosis is usually good.

Avascular necrosis of bone Part of a bone necroses when its blood supply is interrupted by the fracture. Common sites are:

- the head of the femur in intracapsular fractures where the retinacular vessels supplying the femoral head are disrupted
- the proximal part of the scaphoid bone in fractures across the body; the blood supply enters from the distal end.

Diagnosis is by radiograph, the avascular fragment being more dense. Osteoarthritis may result.

Myositis ossificans Calcification with subsequent ossification occurs in a haematoma associated with stripping of the periosteum and release of osteoblasts into the surrounding muscle and tissue. It is most common in injuries around the elbow and those involving quadriceps femoris. Initially treatment involves strict rest and avoidance of passive movements. When radiographs show that the shadow of calcification has been replaced by a clear outline of ossification, exercise may be reinstituted. Occasionally surgical excision of the ossification is necessary but only when the bone is mature.

Osteoarthritis (OA) This may result from misaligned fractures putting strain on joints, or after intra-articular fractures.

Post-traumatic stress disorder Compensation neurosis and malingering may occur.

SPINAL TRAUMA

The incidence in the UK of spinal injuries is about 15 per million of the population per year. RTAs account for over 50%, the remainder being due to accidents in the home, industrial accidents, sports injuries and assault. Many patients have associated head, chest and abdominal injuries. The correct management of spinal injuries is essential at every stage to prevent the continuing risk to the spinal cord. Ideal management involves immediate evacuation from the scene of the accident to a centre where care can be supervised by specialists in spinal injuries. A wide spectrum of spinal trauma ranging from minor whiplash injuries to cord transection may occur. All patients complaining of neck/back pain must be thoroughly assessed. All unconscious patients must be assumed to have a spinal injury until proved otherwise.

MANAGEMENT OF SPINAL INJURIES

SCENE OF THE ACCIDENT

1. Keep the head and neck in neutral position. Avoid any unnecessary movement. Summon help. Do not remove a crash helmet.
2. Medical, paramedical or ambulance personnel. Ensure a clear airway. Apply a collar in suspected cervical injury or a spinal board with an integral head and neck splint prior to extraction from the scene of the accident.
3. Ventilation may be impaired with cervical and upper thoracic injuries. Therefore, avoid opioid analgesics if possible. Intubate if necessary with extreme care.
4. Avoid oropharyngeal suction in tetraplegic patients. It may stimulate the vagal reflex, aggravate the pre-existing bradycardia and precipitate cardiac arrest.
5. The casualty who is trapped should be carefully removed and if conscious or intubated placed supine on a stretcher. A 'scoop' stretcher may be fitted together around the casualty on the ground. Unconscious patients who are not intubated are at risk of passive gastric regurgitation and aspiration of vomit if they are nursed on their backs. If intubation is not performed, the patient should be 'log rolled' into a modified lateral position supporting the head in the neutral position. Log rolling should be performed by four people in a coordinated manner ensuring that unnecessary movement does not occur in any part of the spine.
6. Keep the patient warm. Hypothermia may occur owing to paralysis of the sympathetic system.

INITIAL MANAGEMENT AT THE RECEIVING HOSPITAL

1. Obtain full history from patient, witnesses, and ambulance personnel.
2. Full systematic examination and resuscitation.
3. Assess the spine. 'Log roll' for a proper and safe examination of the back. Look for localized bruising and tenderness. Spinal deformity – gibbus or interspinous gap. Assess for other injuries.
4. Full neurological examination to assess the level and the extent of cord damage. Record pin-prick sensation (spinothalamic tracts); fine touch and joint position sense (posterior columns); power of muscle groups according to Medical Research Council Scale (corticospinal tracts); reflexes – limbs, abdominal, anal, and bulbocavernous. Cranial nerves. Priapism indicates a high lesion.
5. Radiological investigation: radiographs taken with doctor present to ensure that spinal movement is minimized by

keeping the whole of the spine in the neutral position. Make sure that a clear view is obtained of the lower cervical spine. It may be necessary to depress the shoulders by traction on the arms to get a clear view. Special oblique, flexion and extension views may be necessary. Unstable fractures include: fracture-dislocations of the cervical spine; fracture-dislocations of the thoracic and lumbar spine; burst fractures (sometimes); fractures of atlas and axis. CT scan may give clearer view of the damage. MRI shows cord compression and soft tissue damage more clearly.

6. Initial assessment should define two aspects. Firstly, is there a cord injury and is it complete or incomplete (distal sparing easiest to demonstrate as motor activity)? Secondly, is there a significant spinal injury and is it stable or unstable? Note that these two aspects of the injury can be quite independent (e.g. central cord syndrome after a forced extension injury in a spondylitic patient with no spinal fracture).

WHIPLASH INJURIES

Car struck from behind. Neck extends with sudden acceleration and then flexes forward with sudden deceleration. Usually ligamentous and soft tissue damage only, although there may be pain and paraesthesia in the arms and hands. Radiographs are normal or show mild pre-existing degenerative changes.

Treatment Rest in a collar followed by physiotherapy. Prognosis is variable, some patients recovering while others have prolonged symptoms which may be permanent and require a collar. In some patients symptoms settle miraculously after awards of compensation!

FRACTURES AND DISLOCATIONS OF THE SPINE

Classification by mechanism of injury

- Compression: burst fracture (usually stable).
- Flexion compression: anterior wedge fracture. Possible disruption of posterior ligaments.
- Flexion rotation: shearing of all restraining ligaments. Unifacet or bifacet dislocations. These fractures are the commonest cause of neurological damage.
- Hyperextension: disruption of the anterior structures.

These fractures may cause momentary cord compression leading to ‘central cord syndrome’.

Cervical spine fractures and dislocations

Injuries most often occur because of RTAs or sport. A fall on the head with the neck forcibly bent, e.g. flexion and rotation. Subluxation or dislocation occurs with disruption of disc. Forced extension, e.g. a fall on the face or forehead may occur resulting in cervical spine injury. If a cervical spine injury is suspected the first move should be to safeguard the cord by controlling neck movements. Do not allow the head to flex forward, and do not hyperextend the neck. Keep in a neutral position.

Symptoms and signs Often associated head injury so patient may be unconscious. Assume cervical spine injury. Conscious patient may have pain, muscle spasm and localized tenderness. Pain may radiate down arms. Look for neurological signs. The patient with damage above C4 is unlikely to survive because of paralysis of all respiratory muscles. Transection above sympathetic outflow causes bradycardia and hypotension.

Investigations

Radiographs • Lateral to show the 7th cervical and first thoracic vertebrae: may need to draw shoulders down • AP through open mouth to show odontoid • 30° oblique for facet joints • Flexion and extension views to assess stability.

Treatment

Fractures of the atlas These are usually fractured as a result of vertical compression force breaking the ring into four pieces. Inherently unstable requiring halo jacket immobilization and fusion if non-union occurs.

C1–C2 subluxation This is due to failure of the transverse ligament. Treatment is by initial traction in extension then posterior fusion.

Odontoid peg fracture It is uncommon and easily missed. All but the rare apical avulsion type require traction followed by a halo jacket with posterior fusion for non-union.

Crush fractures These may be stable in which case treatment is by halo jacket. If unstable, traction followed by a halo jacket is required. Decompression of the cord and fusion may be necessary.

Anterior wedge fractures These may be stable (treatment in a collar) or unstable with opening of the posterior elements (halo jacket).

→

Facet joint dislocations They are always unstable. Treatment is by reduction and posterior fusion.

Isolated spinous process avulsion These are stable and require treatment in a collar.

Thoracic spine

Flexion injuries result in crush or wedge fractures which are usually stable. Such fractures may occur with minimal trauma if the vertebral body is weakened, e.g. osteoporosis or secondary deposits. Fracture-dislocations tend to occur at the thoracolumbar junction and are caused by flexion and rotation injuries, e.g. a fall from a height on to the shoulders or a heavy load falling on the flexed back. If the disc and posterior ligaments are disrupted the injury is unstable. Paraplegia is common in fracture-dislocations.

Symptoms and signs History of fall from height on shoulder or heavy weight falling on flexed back. Pain over spine. Bruising or abrasions over shoulders. Palpable gap along spinous processus with unstable fracture-dislocations. Associated injuries. Neurological deficit.

Investigations • AP and lateral spine radiographs.

Treatment Simple flexion injuries with crush or wedge fractures are treated by bed rest and analgesia followed by mobilization when pain allows, occasionally in a plaster or polythene jacket. If trauma is minimal an underlying pathological cause should be sought. Fracture-dislocations may be treated conservatively or operatively. Conservative management includes careful nursing with regular turning on a special spinal bed. Spontaneous interbody fusion usually occurs. If there is paraplegia, care is as for the paraplegic patient. To offset the problem of long-term bed rest, operative treatment may be undertaken. The fracture may be stabilized by internal fixation.

Lumbar spine

Compression fractures are the most common and may result from a fall from a height on to the heels. With a burst fracture a fragment of bone may be displaced posteriorly and cause damage to the cord or cauda equina syndrome.

Symptoms and signs History of fall from height on to heels. Pain over lumbar spine. Pain and spasm in paravertebral muscles. Look for associated os calcis fractures or hip injury. Paraplegia.

Investigations • AP and lateral radiograph of lumbar spine (→ Fig. 17.3).

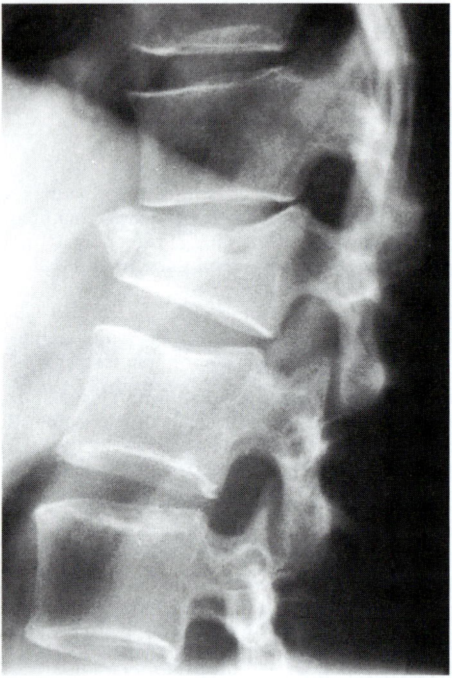

Fig. 17.3 Lateral radiograph of the thoracolumbar spine. There is an anterior wedge fracture of the body of the 1st lumbar vertebra.

Treatment Where there is no neurological damage and the fracture is not comminuted, immobilization in a moulded plastic or plaster jacket will suffice until union occurs. Pathological fractures will require fixation.

Fractures of the transverse processes

The most common are in the lumbar region. It may result from direct violence in a crushing injury or violent muscular contraction. Treatment is symptomatic. There is often severe soft tissue trauma and associated haematoma and prolonged pain may occur.

Fractures of sacrum and coccyx

This may accompany fractures of the pelvis or occur as isolated fractures due to direct violence. Undisplaced linear fractures are treated symptomatically. Displaced fractures may injure sacral nerves with consequent neurological deficit.

Coccydynia

This causes chronic pain in the coccygeal region. It may follow a fall on the buttocks. The pain interferes with sitting. Treatment is by injection of LA and depot steroid or manipulation under anaesthesia (if fracture-dislocation). If conservative management fails excision of the coccyx may be required.

SPINAL CORD INJURY

Types of spinal cord injury

The extent and level of cord damage is very important in determining recovery and final prognosis. Thoracic cord injuries tend to be complete. Incomplete injuries can be identified by the sparing of some tracts and these injuries tend to show much more recovery. The early picture is obscured by 'spinal shock' where all cord function ceases for 24–48 hours.

Anterior cord syndrome The posterior column still functions (proprioception, vibration sensation).

Central cord syndrome Relative sparing of motor supply to legs. Sacral sparing (sensation, anal tone). Brown–Sequard syndrome – hemitransection of the cord. Preserved contralateral motor function, position, and vibration sense. Preserved ipsilateral pain and temperature sensation.

Mixed syndromes These are combinations of the above.

Management and complications of cord injury

Respiratory Impairment of respiratory function is common after injury to the cervical spine. This may relate to partial phrenic nerve palsy, intercostal paralysis, inability to expectorate, and a ventilation–perfusion disorder. Associated chest injuries may be present. Monitor by CXR and ABG. Ventilation and bronchoscopy may be needed.

Cardiovascular Bradycardia and hypotension may occur owing to damage to sympathetic outflow. Excessive i.v. fluids to attempt to correct hypotension may cause pulmonary oedema. Avoid pharyngeal suction as it may potentiate bradycardia via a vagal reflex and lead to cardiac arrest.

Urinary tract Insert catheter to avoid overdistension of an atonic bladder. Suprapubic or intermittent self-catheterization may be required later. Stasis in the urinary tract combined with hypercalciuria due to immobilization may lead to repeated UTIs and stone formation. Urinary catheter should be changed frequently.

Gastrointestinal Paralytic ileus follows a few days after injury. Avoid oral fluids. i.v. fluids and NG suction will be required until bowel sounds return. Beware stress ulceration with perforation. Signs may be lacking. Shoulder tip referred pain may be the only clinical indication.

Hypothermia Hypothermia may occur owing to paralysis of the sympathetic nervous system. The patient should be kept warm.

Thromboembolism The incidence of DVT and PE is high. Start subcutaneous heparin 24–36 hours after injury. Continue until the patient is mobile in a wheelchair.

Pressure sores These form as a result of pressure ischaemia, particularly over bony prominences. Regularly turning in bed every 2 hours is essential. The patient's bottom should be lifted off a wheelchair seat every 15 minutes for a similar reason. Established sores require aggressive treatment with plastic reconstruction if necessary.

LONG-TERM MANAGEMENT OF SPINAL TRAUMA

Nursing care

Good nursing care is essential and should always be in a specialized spinal unit. Objectives include: prevention of secondary complications; facilitation of maximum functional recovery; support for patients and family in adaptation to changed physical status; education of patients and relatives in all aspects of long-term care.

Physiotherapy

This involves care of both the chest and paralysed limbs initially. Later care involves help with strengthening non-paralysed muscles, adaptation to a wheelchair, relearning ability to balance, transfer from wheelchair to bed, toilet, etc., and bracing and gait training.

Occupational therapy

This helps adjustment to a lifetime of disability. Help is given to reach the highest levels of physical and psychological independence at home and at work. Help is provided with the activities of daily living, home alterations, recreation and work.

Social services

This provides help with finance, adaptation of home and employment.

Others

Long-term help with bladder problems, chronic pain, and sexual problems will be required.

PROGNOSIS

It is important to indicate the probable degree of recovery at an early stage to both patients and relatives. Recovery after a complete cord lesion is unlikely. It is, however, difficult to forecast the degree of recovery in an incomplete lesion as improvement may occur after resolution of oedema and contusion. The most encouraging signs are those of incompleteness of paralysis or early return of cord function. Patients with early recovery usually achieve the most recovery. In incomplete lesions improvement may continue for several years. Death in the first days after injury is likely to be due to respiratory failure with high tetraplegia. The level of cervical transection is crucial to long-term prognosis.

Above C4 the patient usually dies of respiratory failure. At C4, patients are able to use their mouth to control a wheelchair. At C5 with special aids they can feed, wash and move their chair. However, they cannot transfer in and out of the chair or dress themselves. At C6 they can drive a special car and dress the upper body but they are unable to transfer themselves from a chair. At C7 their ability is intermediate between that of C6 and C8, the latter being the ability to lead an independent wheelchair life. The other causes of morbidity and mortality include PE, pressure sores and CRF (late).

PELVIC FRACTURES

The pelvis is a ring of bone and ligaments which includes the innominate bone, sacrum, sacroiliac joints, and the pubic symphysis. When fractures occur, the ring tends to break in two places. If only one fracture is visible on radiograph the possibility of sacroiliac joint disruption should be considered. Pelvic fractures occur in the younger patient in RTAs. Elderly patients may sustain isolated pubic ramus fractures, which respond to analgesics and mobilization. Mortality for pelvic fractures varies between 5 and 15%. The pelvis is very vascular and injuries are associated with considerable blood loss. Pelvic visceral and urethral damage may occur.

Symptoms and signs Fall in the elderly. RTA in young patients (beware of associated injuries). Pelvic pain. Abrasions. Bruising. Shock. Inability to pass urine. Bleeding per urethram. Bleeding PR. Bleeding PV. Perineal bruising. High 'floating' prostate on examination PR.

Investigations • Pelvic radiograph • IVU • Urethrogram • CT scan.

Treatment

Shock Intensive resuscitation as bleeding may be dramatic (3–4 litres). For 'open book' types of fracture, emergency stabilization with an external fixator reduces bleeding. For other fractures, radiological intra-arterial embolization is the best option to slow bleeding.

The fracture itself Acetabular fractures require accurate reduction and fixation. 'Open book' fractures require closing with a fixator or plating of the symphysis. Generally bed rest for 10 weeks is required followed by gradual mobilization.

Urethral trauma Avoid catheterization. If the patient can pass urine and it is clear, all is well. Otherwise consider suprapubic catheterization or cystotomy. Retrograde urethrogram and IVU may be required.

Complications Haemorrhage and shock, urethral or bladder injury, rectal injury, paralytic ileus, DVT, damage to hip joint. Late OA may occur in acetabular injuries. Vaginal injury, sciatic nerve injury, mal-union may lead to obstetric difficulties. Sexual dysfunction.

INJURIES TO THE LOWER LIMB

HIP AND THIGH

TRAUMATIC DISLOCATION OF THE HIP

The majority are posterior and follow impact directed along the femoral shaft when the hip is flexed and adducted, e.g. RTA when the knee strikes the dashboard. Anterior, inferior and central dislocations are rare, the latter being caused by the head of the femur being driven into the acetabulum.

Symptoms and signs Often other severe injuries. Shock. Thigh is flexed, adducted and internally rotated with posterior dislocations. May be associated injury to femur or patella. Sciatic nerve injury.

Investigations • Good-quality radiograph of hip with lateral film • Radiograph of femur and patella.

Treatment Reduction under GA with muscle relaxation. Skeletal traction for 6 weeks until capsule is healed. If a bone fragment is displaced from the posterior acetabulum, open reduction and internal fixation of the fragment may be required.

Complications • Associated fractures. Sciatic nerve damage. Avascular necrosis of femoral head. Late OA of hip.

FRACTURES OF THE PROXIMAL FEMUR

The blood supply to the head of the femur comes from three sources:

- retinacular vessels in the capsule
- medullary vessels in the femoral neck
- via the ligamentum teres.

The main source is via the retinacular vessels and these may be damaged in fractures of the femoral neck. Fractures may be classified as intracapsular (subcapital, transcervical), or extracapsular (basal, intertrochanteric; → Fig. 17.4). Extracapsular fractures do not damage the blood supply to the femoral head and therefore there are no risks of avascular necrosis of the femoral head and non-union. They are most common in the elderly, especially females with osteoporotic bones when the traumatic cause is relatively trivial, e.g. a fall in the house. In the young patient they result from major trauma.

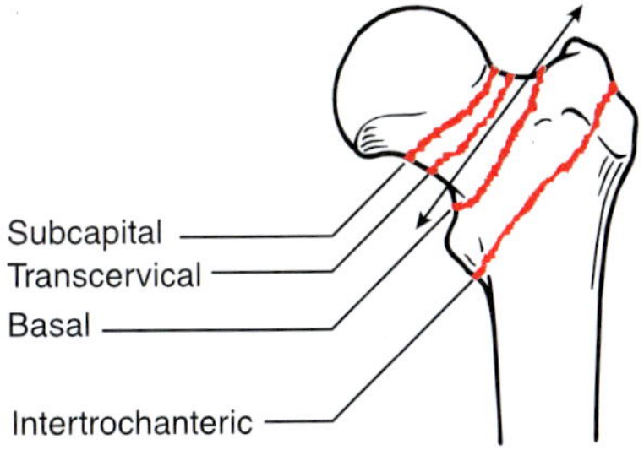

Fig. 17.4 Fractures of the femoral neck. The arrowed line separates intracapsular (to the left) and extracapsular (to the right) fracture sites. Intracapsular fractures are associated with avascular necrosis of the femoral head.

Symptoms and signs Elderly female. Minor trauma. Tripped over carpet. Tripped over pavement. Pain in the hip. Shortening, adduction, external rotation. Movements painful. Weight bearing usually impossible. Beware hypothermia.

Investigations • Radiographs in two planes (→ Fig. 17.5 AP view) • Hb • FBC • U&Es • Blood sugar • CXR • ECG. In the elderly patient there is the possibility of intercurrent disease.

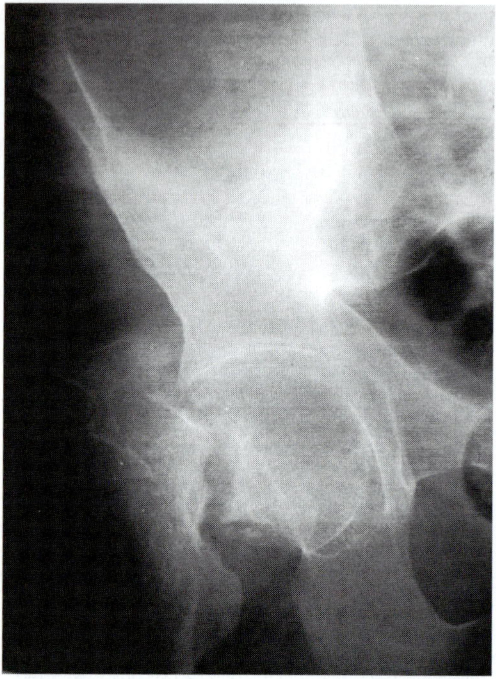

Fig. 17.5 A subcapital fracture of the neck of the femur.

Complications These are of the elderly undergoing surgery, e.g. pneumonia, MI, CVA, DVT and PE. 50% of elderly patients are dead within 6 months of the injury. Avascular necrosis of the femoral head. Non-union. Mal-union with varus angulation and shortening.

Treatment

General Pain relief. Bed rest. Treat intercurrent disease. DVT prophylaxis.

Fracture Surgery to allow nursing, mobilization, and rehabilitation:

- Intracapsular: undisplaced (fixed with screws); displaced – femoral head replacement, e.g. Thompson's prosthesis or primary total hip replacement.

→

- Extracapsular: sliding compression hip screw, allows the nail to slide along a holder which is part of the plate allowing the fracture to compact during weight bearing (Richard's screw).

FRACTURES OF THE FEMORAL SHAFT

Common in younger people and usually result from severe trauma in RTAs. They may occur at any site and be of variable pattern. Treatment is either conservative (traction) or more often operative (internal fixation or external fixator device). There are frequently associated injuries.

Symptoms and signs Severe pain in thigh. Deformity. Shock. Associated injuries. Check head, chest, abdomen, spine. Vascular injury to femoral vessels. Injury to sciatic nerve.

Investigations • Radiographs in two planes • Femoral angiography may be required if vascular injury is suspected.

Treatment Splint leg. Transport to hospital. Pain relief. i.v. Fluids. FBC, U&Es. Crossmatch (blood loss can be 2–4 units). Check if fracture compound. Give tetanus prophylaxis and antibiotics if compound.

Conservative In children, skin traction may be used in association with a Thomas' splint. In children under 3 years old, gallows traction may be used from an overhead beam. In adults a Steinmann pin is inserted through the upper end of the tibia at the level of the tubercle and balanced traction applied through the skeletal pin with the knee flexed on a special knee flexion attachment. Fractures heal quickly in children. In adults cast bracing may be used after 6–8 weeks.

Surgical

- Internal fixation: achieved by a locked intramedullary nail. This allows accurate reduction and ensures early mobilization of the patient. There is a risk of infection and osteomyelitis. This form of treatment is useful for multiple fractures, pathological fractures and when there is associated vascular injury.
- External fixation: used especially for compound fractures where there is soft tissue damage. Pins are inserted above and below the fracture site and reduction and alignment maintained by an external fixator device.

Complications DVT. PE. Fat embolism. Infection. Shortening. Angulation. Non-union.

FRACTURES AND DISLOCATIONS AROUND THE KNEE

Fractures are usually intra-articular causing haemarthrosis, which should be aspirated to decrease pain. They can be caused by a direct blow (car bumper, car dashboard), vertical compression (fall from a height) or excessive strain (forced abduction at the knee). Associated ligamentous and neurovascular injuries are common. Conservative treatment for these injuries involves a long leg cylinder plaster then a hinged cast brace. This type of treatment is also used after open reduction/internal fixation. The knee joint needs accurate repair of the articular surfaces to reduce the risk of post-traumatic OA.

Supracondylar fractures (→ Fig. 17.6)

These are intra-articular or extra-articular. The distal fragment is pulled backwards by the gastrocnemius. The popliteal artery may be damaged by the distal fragment. Conservative treatment is by skeletal traction via the proximal tibia with the knee in about 30° of flexion. Internal fixation is required for all displaced intra-articular fractures (compression screws, blade plates or custom nails).

Isolated femoral condylar fractures

These are usually displaced so internal fixation is advised.

Tibial plateau fractures

In these fractures vertical compression forces or strains drive the femoral condyle through the tibial plateau. Fragments of tibial plateau/condyle may be cleaved off, depressed, or both. Both condyles may be damaged. Displaced or depressed fragments should be reduced and internally fixed, often with support from a bone graft.

Dislocation of the knee

This is an uncommon injury. It is usually associated with damage to the popliteal artery or local nerves. After reduction under anaesthesia any ruptured ligaments should be repaired. Immobilization in plaster then cast brace is required for several months.

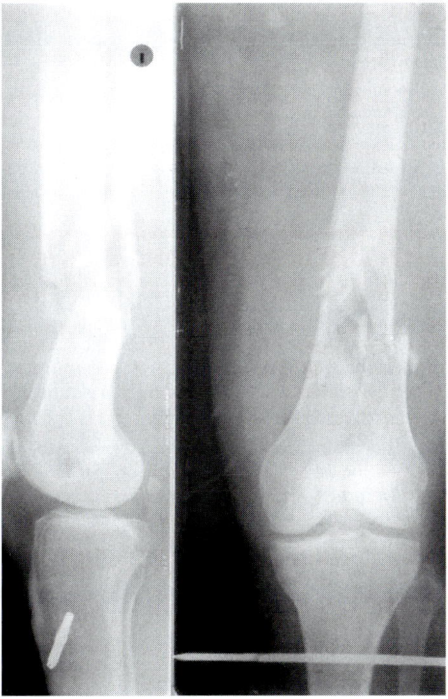

Fig. 17.6 A supracondylar fracture of the femur. In the lateral view, the distal fragment is tilted backwards and may damage the popliteal artery.

INJURIES OF THE EXTENSOR MECHANISM

These involve the following:

- tear of quadriceps insertion into the patella
- transverse fracture of patella with separation
- rupture of the ligamentum patellae, avulsion of tibial tuberosity.

Forced flexion of the knee against a contracting quadriceps causes the extensor mechanism to give way.

Symptoms and signs Pain. Knee cannot be fully actively extended against gravity. Palpable gap and point of maximum tenderness at site of lesion.

Investigations • Radiograph: patella 'high' if ligamentum patellae ruptured; patella 'low' with upper part tilted forward with quadriceps tear.

Treatment Operative repair of defect in the extensor mechanism. Immobilization for 8 weeks in plaster cylinder with knee in full extension.

FRACTURES AND DISLOCATIONS OF THE PATELLAE

Fractures

An avulsion or transverse fracture is caused by a violent contraction of quadriceps against resistance. A comminuted fracture is caused by direct violence, e.g. a blow from a bat or in an RTA.

Treatment This depends whether the extensor mechanism is intact and the degree of comminution. If the extensor mechanism is intact and there is no severe comminution, treatment in a plaster cylinder for 3–4 weeks will suffice. Transverse fractures with separation are held with a circumferential wire or a longitudinal screw. Mobilization is possible after 3 weeks in a plaster cylinder. If the extensor mechanism is ruptured, surgical repair with or without patellectomy is required. Severely comminuted fractures require patellectomy. A long-term complication is OA of the patellofemoral compartment.

Dislocation of the patella

This may be acute or recurrent and occurs laterally.

Acute or traumatic This results from a blow on the side of the knee. The patella is visibly displaced. The knee remains flexed until the patella is reduced by medial pressure. There is usually a tear in the medial capsule or avulsion of the medial side of the patella. May be associated with haemarthrosis. Treatment is by rest in a plaster cylinder followed by quadriceps exercises.

Recurrent Usually affects adolescent girls. Associated with flattening of lateral condyle, small high-riding patella, or genu valgum. Dislocation occurs spontaneously or with minor trauma. The knee locks in semiflexion. Spontaneous reduction usually occurs. After a single incident, intensive physiotherapy to strengthen vastus medialis. Surgery is indicated in recurrent cases.

FRACTURES OF THE TIBIAL SHAFT

These are common fractures occurring as a result of RTAs, sports injuries, and industrial accidents. They are often compound. Oblique and spiral fractures are commonly unstable when reduced. Up to 20% of cases develop non-union.

Treatment Numerous methods are available depending on fracture:

- Stable fractures; closed reduction under GA is suitable for a transverse fracture. The leg hangs over the end of the operating table, gravity maintaining position of the fragments. The ankle is dorsiflexed to a right angle and a full leg plaster applied with the knee in slight flexion. Positions should be checked with radiographs immediately after plastering, and at weekly intervals until stable.
- Unstable fractures; with spiral, oblique or comminuted fractures, a long leg plaster is insufficient. Closed injuries should be fixed with an intramedullary nail. Severe compound injuries should be fixed with an external fixator. Either method can be used for open fractures with minimal soft tissue damage.
- Open wounds; all compound wounds must be explored, irrigated and treated in conjunction with a plastic surgeon if bone is exposed at the base of the wound.

Complications Delayed union. Non-union. Infection. Stiffness of knee, ankle, foot. Ischaemia of muscles leading to claw toes.

Isolated fractures of the fibula

These are uncommon. They are usually associated with tibial fractures and with direct violence. Beware common peroneal nerve injury in fractures of neck of the fibula. Exclude ankle injury, e.g. diastasis (→ below). Treatment is by strapping or below-knee plaster until pain settles.

FRACTURES AROUND THE ANKLE

These are due to indirect forces transmitted from the foot (e.g. twisted ankle). The ligaments and malleoli may be injured in various combinations. Severe force may cause associated dislocation.

Classification

There are several classifications of ankle fractures. Most are based on the mechanism that is thought to have caused the injury. The classification given below is simplified and is hopefully adequate for the introductory medical student.

External rotation injuries (→ Fig. 17.7) When a patient 'goes over' with full weight on the ankle, the forced inversion of the

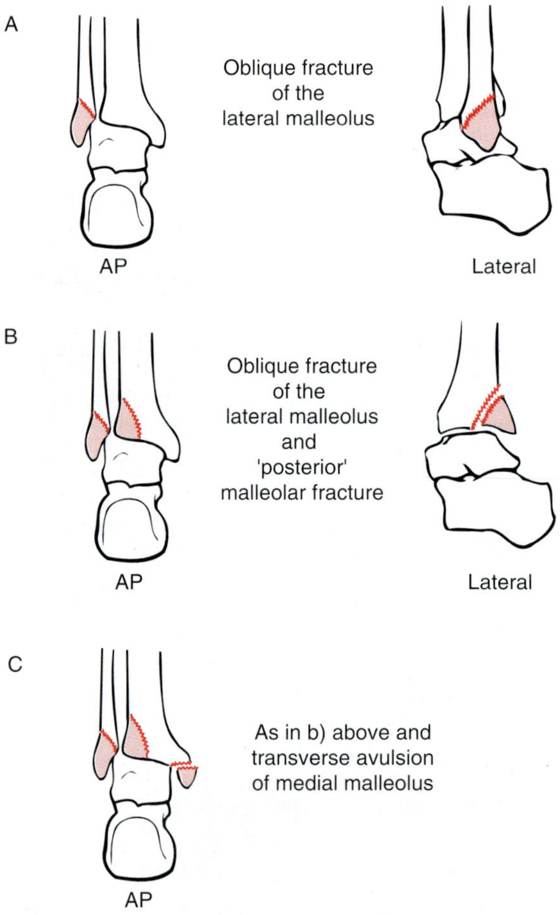

Fig. 17.7 External rotation injuries at the ankle. AP and lateral views.

foot is associated with external rotation of the talus. The talus attempting to rotate externally within the fixed ankle mortice causes both ligamentous and bony injury. As the talus rotates externally:

- The lateral malleolus is fractured, the line of the fracture running obliquely upwards and backwards, i.e. a uni-malleolar fracture which is stable.
- Further rotation stresses the posterior tibiofibular ligament, rupturing it or avulsing the 'posterior malleolus' (→ Fig. 17.8).
- If rotation continues, the medial malleolus may be pulled off transversely or the medial ligament ruptured. This is a bi-malleolar fracture, which is unstable.

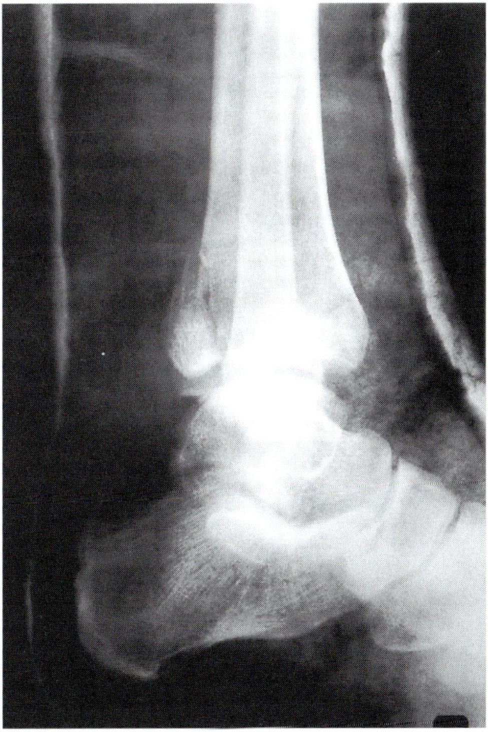

Fig. 17.8 A lateral radiograph of the ankle showing an oblique avulsion fracture of the 'posterior' malleolus.

In some external rotation injuries, disruption starts with the medial ligament, extends up the interosseous ligament and then causes a high fibular fracture (→ Fig. 17.9). Although the ankle is severely damaged (diastasis of the inferior tibiofibular joint), no fracture is seen on the initial ankle X-ray. A radiograph of the whole fibula is essential.

Adduction fractures (→ Fig. 17.10) The foot is fixed and the talus is driven medially, obliquely fracturing the medial malleolus and pulling off the tip of the lateral malleolus. Rupture of the lateral ligament may occur.

Abduction fractures (→ Fig. 17.10) The foot is fixed and the talus is driven laterally. Rupture of the medial ligament or avulsion of the tip of the medial malleolus with a transverse fracture of the fibula occurs, i.e. bi-malleolar.

Vertical compression fractures These are caused by a fall on the foot from a height. The talus is driven into the articular surface of the tibia, which is disrupted. This is a severe injury which is difficult to treat. Consider using a hinged external fixator from tibia to tarsal bones.

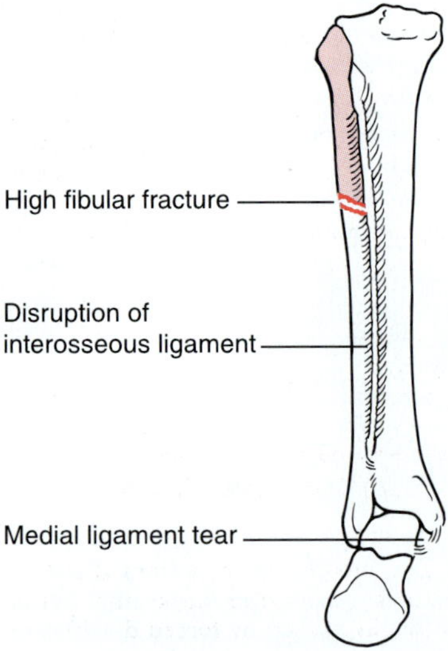

Fig. 17.9 Diastasis of the inferior tibiofibular joint with rupture of the interosseous membrane. There is an associated high fibular fracture.

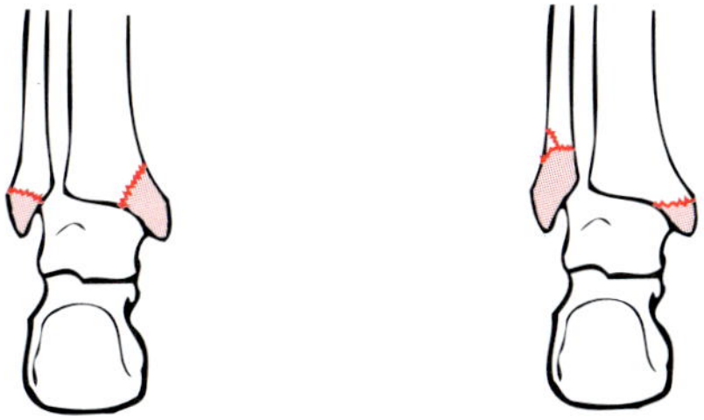

Fig. 17.10 Adduction and abduction injuries at the ankle. Rupture of the lateral ligament may also occur in adduction fractures. In abduction injuries rupture of the medial ligament may occur.

Investigations • AP and lateral films • Note site of fractures and talus shift or tilt • Stress films may be necessary.

Treatment This may be conservative or operative.

Uni-malleolar It is usually intrinsically stable and may be treated in plaster. 6 weeks' weight-bearing mobilization is required.

Bi-malleolar Reduced stable injuries can be treated in plaster extended above the knee for added stability. Unstable or displaced injuries require internal fixation, usually with plates and screws. Active ankle movements are encouraged but weight bearing is not permitted. When a good range of movement is achieved, a partial weight-bearing plaster cast is added for 6 weeks.

Tri-malleolar These fractures are always unstable and require internal fixation.

FRACTURES AND DISLOCATIONS IN THE FOOT

Os talus

This is rare. The blood supply is from distal to proximal and therefore fractures across the neck may result in avascular necrosis. It is usually caused by forced dorsiflexion. Undisplaced fractures are treated in plaster. The foot should be maintained in plantar flexion following closed reduction of displaced fractures. 8–12 weeks' immobilization is required. Avascular necrosis leads to OA. Displaced fractures require internal fixation after reduction.

Os calcis

This is caused by a fall from height on to the heel. It may be bilateral. Look for fractures elsewhere especially crush fractures of the spine. Conservative treatment is by bed rest and elevation of the legs to reduce swelling. Operative treatment is controversial; severe damage to the subtalar joint may be helped by open reduction, fixation and bone grafting. Ankle exercises are required. Partial weight bearing on crutches is permitted as pain allows. Healing takes up to 10 weeks. Complications include pain, stiffness at the subtalar joint, and local nerve and tendon entrapment.

METATARSAL FRACTURES

Avulsion fracture of the base of the 5th metatarsal is common and is caused by an inversion injury combined with forced plantar flexion, e.g. mis-stepping on a stair. The peroneus brevis tendon avulses the styloid process at the base of the 5th metatarsal. Treatment is in a below-knee walking plaster for 3–6 weeks. Fracture of the proximal 5th metatarsal is due to direct trauma and may require open reduction and fixation.

Shaft fractures

These occur with crushing injuries and are often multiple. Elevation of the foot followed by mobilization in a below-knee walking plaster for 6 weeks is required. If displacement is gross, manipulation or internal fixation may be required.

Stress fracture ('march' fracture)

This usually affects the second metatarsal neck and is caused by the stress of long hours of walking, e.g. new army recruits. It may not be apparent on an early radiograph but only show on a repeated radiograph when callus is forming. Treatment is a below-knee walking plaster for 6 weeks. In mild cases, rest only is required.

FRACTURES OF THE TOES

These are common injuries. Fracture occasionally interferes with circulation, and amputation is required. Otherwise splintage by strapping of the adjacent toe will suffice. Great toe fractures may require fixation.

INJURIES TO THE UPPER LIMB

FRACTURES AND DISLOCATIONS AROUND THE SHOULDER

Dislocation of the sternoclavicular joint

This is uncommon. Usually the medial end of the clavicle dislocates forward and the deformity is obvious. Posterior dislocation is rare and may lead to tracheal compression. Treatment is by bracing the shoulder in a 'figure of 8' bandage. Posterior dislocation requires open reduction to relieve tracheal compression.

Clavicular fracture

This is caused by falls on the outstretched hand or point of the shoulder. The bone usually breaks between the middle and outer third. Fractures of the outer end may be associated with fractures of the coracoid and damage to the coracoclavicular ligament.

Symptoms and signs Pain in shoulder region. Supports weight of arm with other hand. The proximal portion is drawn upwards by sternomastoid. The distal portion droops owing to the weight of the arm. Tenderness over the site.

Investigations • Radiograph.

Treatment Support the arm in a triangular sling. With displaced fractures a 'figure of 8' bandage may be appropriate. 3 weeks of support is usually sufficient. Rarely, displacement may be sufficient to warrant internal fixation.

Complications Rare. Occasionally injury to brachial plexus or axillary artery may occur.

Acromioclavicular joint

Subluxation Seen in rugby players who present with a lump over the joint. Treatment is by rest in a sling until symptoms subside. The lump over the joint often persists.

Dislocation Complete dislocation occurs only when the coracoclavicular ligament is disrupted. The clavicle is elevated and the point of the shoulder lowered. Tenderness and bruising occur. Radiographs show a gap between coracoid process and clavicle. Treatment is via a sling with strapping over the joint. Occasionally open reduction and repair of the ligament is advisable.

Scapular fracture

This is usually caused by direct violence. There may be extensive bruising. Treatment is by rest, analgesia, collar and cuff. Mobilize when pain allows.

Dislocation of the shoulder

The commonest form is anterior, and is caused by a fall on the outstretched hand. In the younger patient the capsule is strong and does not tear. The glenoid labrum and capsule are avulsed from the bone allowing recurrent dislocations to occur. In the older patient the capsule is torn and this heals after reduction. Recurrent dislocation is less common in the older patient.

Symptoms and signs Fall on outstretched hand. Pain. Patient supports arm, which is abducted. The normal contour of the shoulder is lost. Check for axillary nerve damage – anaesthesia over skin at insertion of deltoid.

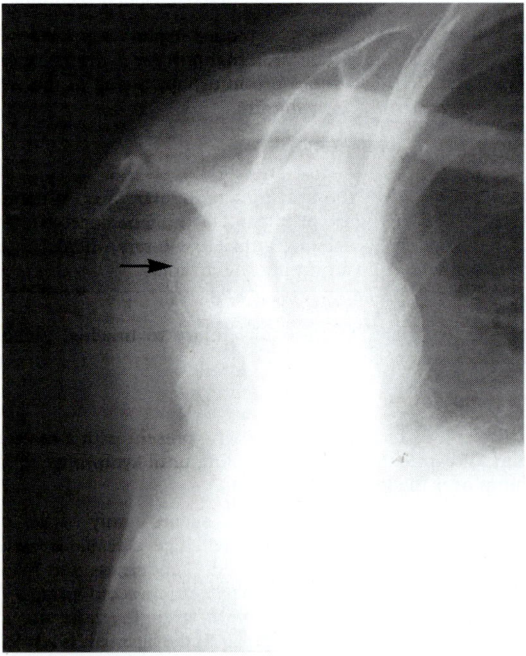

Fig. 17.11 Anterior dislocation of the shoulder joint. The humeral head lies below and medial to the glenoid (arrow).

Investigations • Radiograph (→ Fig. 17.11): humeral head not in contact with the glenoid; check for associated fractures of the neck of the humerus.

Treatment Reduction under GA or intravenous sedation. Two methods are available:

Kocher's method Flex the elbow to a right angle and apply slow gentle traction in the line of the humerus. Rotate the humerus externally using the forearm as a lever. Adduct the humerus across the trunk. Then internally rotate the humerus. Avoid this method in the elderly owing to risk of iatrogenic fracture.

Hippocratic method Place the stockinged foot in the axilla and pull downwards on the arm. Use the toes to slip the head back into position. Confirm the position with radiograph. Immobilize the arm in a sling for 3 weeks.

Complications Early complications include axillary nerve damage and associated fractures. Late complications include stiffness and recurrent dislocation. Complete rotator cuff tear in the elderly.

Recurrent dislocation

This usually follows damage to the glenoid labrum or humeral head at the time of original dislocation. Dislocation occurs on movement of the arm especially if raised and externally rotated. Radiograph may reveal a depression on the humeral head.

Treatment Operative: either the torn glenoid labrum is reattached to the bone (Bankart's operation) or the anterior capsule is pleated and reinforced, restricting external rotation (Putti–Platt operation). Results of surgery are good.

Posterior dislocation is rare. A lateral radiograph is essential for diagnosis.

FRACTURES OF THE HUMERUS

Proximal humerus (→ Fig. 17.12)

This is usually due to indirect violence, i.e. a fall on the shoulder, often in the elderly.

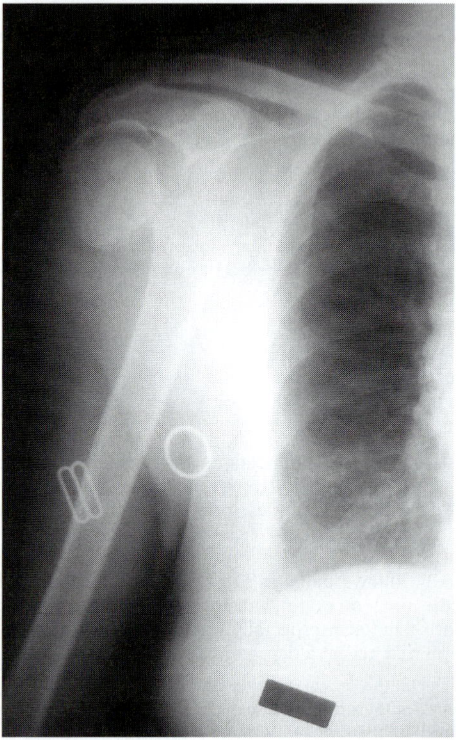

Fig. 17.12 A fracture of the neck of the humerus. This shows severe displacement. The axillary nerve is in danger with such a fracture.

Treatment Undisplaced fractures are treated with a collar and cuff (for gravitational traction) then physiotherapy. Significantly displaced avulsion of the tuberosities or anatomical neck fractures should be internally fixed with repair of the rotator cuff. Surgical neck fractures are usually treated in a collar and cuff for 3–6 weeks and then physiotherapy.

Complications Axillary nerve damage. Axillary vessel damage. Shoulder stiffness.

Shaft of the humerus

This is caused by a direct blow or a fall on the outstretched hand. The fracture is usually oblique and may be displaced. Check for radial nerve damage (wrist drop and anaesthesia in the first web space on the dorsal aspect).

Treatment The weight of the arm effects reduction. A 'U' slab is applied to the upper arm and the wrist supported with a collar and cuff. The 'U' slab extends over the shoulder and under the elbow. Occasionally open reduction and internal fixation may be required using a plate or an intramedullary nail. Internal fixation is approriate if the patient requires bed rest for other injuries.

Complications Radial nerve damage and non-union.

FRACTURES AND DISLOCATIONS AROUND THE ELBOW

Supracondylar fracture

This is chiefly a fracture of childhood but may occur in adults. There is a history of a fall on the outstretched hand followed by pain and swelling around the elbow. The lower fragment is usually displaced and rotated backwards. The brachial artery and median nerve are vulnerable to injury.

Treatment Attempted reduction under anaesthesia. Longitudinal traction is inserted on the forearm, and thumb pressure is used to position the distal fragment. Continue thumb pressure on distal humerus while the elbow is flexed to about 60°. Check radiograph for position. Check that the radial pulse does not disappear through overflexing the swollen elbow. Reduction is maintained by a collar and cuff. The elbow should not be flexed much above 90° particularly if swelling is severe. Admission is necessary to observe the circulation for 24 hours. If all is well the patient is discharged after 24 hours, the fracture being immobilized for 4–5 weeks after which active exercise is commenced.

Problems may occur after this type of treatment:

- The pulse may not return after manipulation but provided the hand remains pink with good capillary return there is no cause for alarm. Pallor, poor capillary return, excessive pain and inability to bring about full passive extension of the fingers are signs for alarm. Reduce the degree of flexion. If the pulse does not return, extend the arm vertically. If →

the circulation is not restored, the forearm needs surgical decompression with exploration of the brachial artery.

- If the fracture will not reduce or reduction cannot be held, internal fixation with K wires may be required.
- Late loss of reduction.

Complications This fracture is prone to several complications, particularly in children. Damage to brachial artery. Nerve injury (median). Stiffness. Mal-union. Epiphyseal damage with later deformity. Myositis ossificans. OA. Volkman's ischaemic contracture. Sudek's atrophy may occur in adults.

Lateral condyle/epicondyle

Lateral condylar fractures occurring in young children are injuries of the capitellar epiphysis. Displaced lateral condyles should be fixed to prevent valgus deformity and late ulnar neuritis due to traction. Lateral epicondylar avulsions are very rare and should be fixed if displaced.

Medial condyle/epicondyle

Medial condylar fractures are rare and should be fixed if displaced. Medial epicondylar fractures are more common and are associated with elbow dislocations (50%). They should be fixed if displaced or fragments need washing out of the joint.

Dislocation of the elbow

It is caused by a fall on the hand with the elbow partly flexed. Dislocation is almost always posterior. Occasionally there are fractures of adjacent bones. Median or ulnar nerve palsy may occur. Damage to the brachial artery is rare.

Treatment Reduction is usually easy. The elbow is held in slight flexion and then pressure is applied to the olecranon posteriorly until reduction occurs. The elbow is immobilized for 1–3 weeks in a collar and cuff, after which active exercises are encouraged.

Fracture-dislocation of the elbow is a more serious injury involving fractures of the humeral condyles, radial head or olecranon. Manipulative reduction and internal fixation may be necessary. A stiff elbow is the usual outcome. Vascular injury and myositis ossificans may also occur.

FRACTURES OF THE RADIUS AND ULNA

These are caused by either indirect violence from a fall on the outstretched hand with or without rotation, or direct violence which usually causes fracture of a single bone.

Fracture of the radial head

This varies from a fine vertical crack to severe comminution. There is localized tenderness over the radial head with minor injury. With comminution the elbow is painful and swollen with restriction of all movement. Minor cracks and undisplaced fractures may be rested in a collar and cuff sling for 2 weeks. Displaced large fragments may be internally fixed. Comminuted fractures may require excision of the radial head.

Fracture of the olecranon

This is caused by direct violence as an isolated injury, or as part of a fracture-dislocation of the elbow. Displaced fractures are internally fixed.

Fractures of the radial and ulnar shafts

These injuries are common and are often compound. They are usually caused by direct violence. An injury to the forearm usually affects the two bones, or one bone plus one radioulnar joint. A displaced fracture of the midshaft of either bone alone can occur if the radial head dislocates with an ulnar fracture (Monteggia's fracture) or the lower end of the ulna dislocates with a fracture of the radius (Galeazzi fracture). Radiographs of the forearm must therefore include both wrist and elbow joints. Occasionally direct violence fractures only one bone, e.g. the ulnar as when lifting up the flexed arm to ward off a blow. In children, fractures are of the greenstick type with angulation. In adults the fractures are transverse or oblique.

Treatment

Children Manipulative reduction is usually successful. Position is maintained in an above-elbow plaster cast from axilla to metacarpal heads with the elbow at a right angle.

Adults Accurate alignment is essential to allow pronation and supination. Open reduction and plating is usually undertaken followed by 4 weeks in plaster.

FRACTURES OF THE DISTAL RADIUS

Colles' fracture (→ Fig. 17.13)

This is a dorsally displaced fracture 2.5 cm from the wrist joint. It is common in elderly osteoporotic women following a low-energy fall. In young people this is a high-energy injury and is commonly intra-articular.

Symptoms and signs Fall on outstretched hand. Pain. Limitation of wrist movement. 'Dinner fork' deformity. Check for distal neurovascular deficit.

Investigations Radiograph in two planes (→ Fig. 17.14): distal fragment is displaced dorsally, radially (with pull off of the ulnar styloid) and supinated; check for intra-articular fracture lines and associated scaphoid fracture.

Treatment Undisplaced or greenstick fractures require immobilization in a below-elbow plaster for 3–4 weeks. Significant displacement requires manipulation under general or regional anaesthesia (Bier's block). The fracture is disimpacted by traction and increasing the deformity. The distal fragment is levered over the proximal, the wrist flexed, ulnar deviated and pronated. A dorsal plaster slab is applied to hold this position. A check radiograph is taken and the arm supported in a sling. A further radiograph is taken 1 week later to check reduction. Swelling has usually subsided by this time and the plaster is completed and the sling abandoned. The plaster is removed at 6 weeks and exercises commenced. Operative treatment is required for intra-articular fractures and failed reduction or failed plaster immobilization.

Complications Stiffness and oedema of the hand. Mal-union with angulation. This may be associated with pain from subluxation of the inferior radioulnar joint. Median nerve symptoms occur but usually subside spontaneously. Later rupture of the tendon of extensor pollicis longus may occur where it crosses the fracture. Sudek's atrophy.

Smith's fracture

This is a fracture of the lower end of the radius with forward angulation. It is the reverse of a Colles' fracture. Conservative treatment is manipulation using the reverse procedure for Colles' fracture. An above-elbow plaster is applied for 6 weeks with the wrist dorsiflexed and the forearm fully supinated. Operative treatment is often required owing to instability of the fracture in plaster.

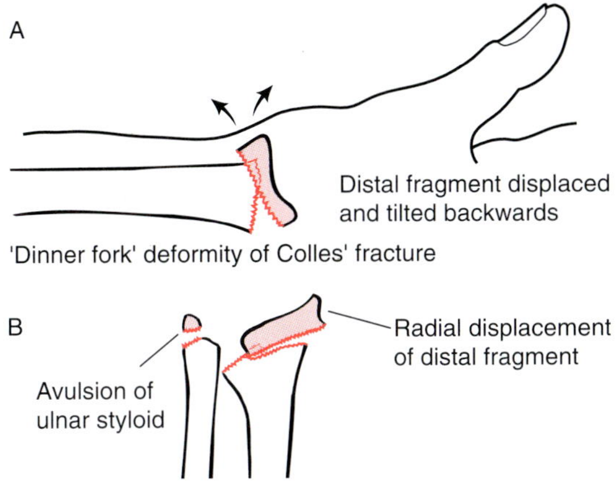

Fig. 17.13 A Colles' fracture. A. Lateral view. B. Anteroposterior view.

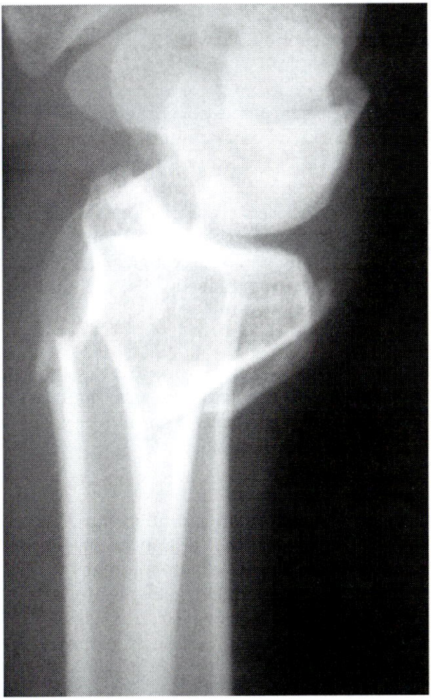

Fig. 17.14 A radiograph of the wrist (lateral view) showing a typical Colles' fracture. There is anterior angulation, dorsal displacement, and impaction.

Barton's fracture

This is a fracture-dislocation of the radiocarpal joints. It usually needs internal fixation.

Distal radial epiphyseal fractures

This occurs in children and is usually extra-articular. Treat as Colles' fracture but it heals faster (4 weeks).

FRACTURES AND DISLOCATION OF THE CARPAL BONES

Fracture of the scaphoid

Caused by a fall on the outstretched hand or a blow to the palm of the hand. The blood supply to the bone comes from distal to proximal, and hence there is a risk of avascular necrosis of the proximal fragment. The scaphoid spans both rows of carpal bones hence the high risk of non-union.

Symptoms and signs Fall on outstretched hand. Painful swollen wrist with tenderness in the anatomical snuff box and on AP compression of the scaphoid.

Investigations • Radiograph: scaphoid views.

Treatment If this fracture is suspected clinically but is not confirmed on radiograph, treat on clinical grounds as a fracture to scaphoid. Re-radiograph in 2 weeks when the fracture may show. A bone scan may be helpful. The wrist is immobilized in a plaster which extends from the elbow to the knuckles including the thumb as far as the interphalangeal joint. The plaster is worn for 6 weeks initially when radiological evidence of union should be apparent. Union may be delayed and a plaster may need to be worn for 6 months.

Complications Avascular necrosis of the proximal segment. Delayed union and non-union. If the latter is associated with symptoms, bone grafting and internal fixation should be undertaken. OA of the wrist is a long-term sequel.

Dislocation of the carpus

Commonly missed. Caused by a fall on an extended hand. If the radiograph looks unusual, especially the lateral view, obtain specialist advice. Anterior dislocation of the lunate is the commonest and may cause acute median nerve compression. Closed or open reduction is performed. Methods of immobilization are controversial but application of a plaster for 6–8 weeks may be required.

FRACTURES AND DISLOCATIONS OF THE METACARPALS AND PHALANGES

When assessing fractures of the metacarpals or phalanges, beware of rotational displacement. This may not be obvious until the fingers are flexed, when they cross over each other abnormally.

Fractures at the base of the thumb

Extra-articular fractures can usually be treated conservatively by manipulation and plaster casting. Intra-articular fractures of the thumb may produce late OA. Bennett's fracture is oblique and the small fragment is on the ulnar side of the base of the first metacarpal where the deep oblique ligament attaches. Open reduction and internal fixation with early mobilization is required to avoid stiffness and later OA.

Fractures of the metacarpal bones

These are caused by direct violence or by punching with a closed fist.

Treatment Undisplaced fractures are treated in a back slab or by strapping the injured finger to its neighbour. Displaced or multiple fractures require reduction and/or internal fixation. Active movements are encouraged.

Fractures and dislocations of the phalanges

These are often serious injuries and may be associated with tendon and nerve damage.

Treatment Dislocation can usually be reduced under local anaesthetic. Undisplaced fractures may be treated by strapping the injured finger to its neighbour. Active movements are encouraged. Unstable or displaced fractures may need open reduction and internal fixation with crossed Kirschner wires or miniscrews.

Fractures of the terminal phalanges

These are usually crush injuries and may be compound. There may be subungual haematoma which contributes to the pain. The latter can be drained by piercing the nail with a hot wire giving instant relief. Compound fractures are treated with wound toilet, leaving the wound open, tetanus toxoid and broad-spectrum antibiotics. Occasionally partial amputation of the finger is required.

Mallet finger

This injury is caused by 'stubbing' a finger when it is actively extended. Forced passive flexion leads to avulsion of the extensor tendon from the base of the terminal phalanx often with a flake of bone. Examination reveals a finger in which the distal phalanx is flexed and cannot be extended. Treatment is by immobilization of the distal interphalangeal joint in a 'mallet finger' splint which hyperextends the terminal interphalangeal joint while allowing flexion of the proximal interphalangeal joint. The splint is worn for 6 weeks. Occasionally healing does not occur but the disability is slight.

CONDITIONS OF JOINTS

ARTHRITIS

This is inflammation of a joint. The term is used to describe both inflammatory and degenerative disease.

Osteoarthritis (osteoarthrosis: OA)

This is a term applied to degenerative disease of a joint caused by wear and tear which affects the articular cartilage and subchondral bone. At first, the synovial membrane is normal but later thickening and fibrosis occurs. OA may be primary or secondary. In the former there is no underlying cause. It may arise as a result of senile changes and may affect more than one joint. Secondary OA occurs if there has been previous damage to the joint, e.g. congenital deformity, trauma, infection, avascular necrosis, gout, haemophilia.

Symptoms and signs Pain. Stiffness. Deformity. Pain increases in severity as the disease progresses. Sleep is often disturbed. Synovial thickening and bony enlargement of joint because of osteophytes. Effusions. Tenderness. Loss of movement. Crepitus. Fixed deformities. Disturbances of gait.

Investigations • Radiographs (→ Fig. 17.15): narrowing of joint space, subchondral bone sclerosis, subchondral cysts, osteophytes, evidence of other underlying pathology. Symptoms do not necessarily correlate with the severity of radiological changes.

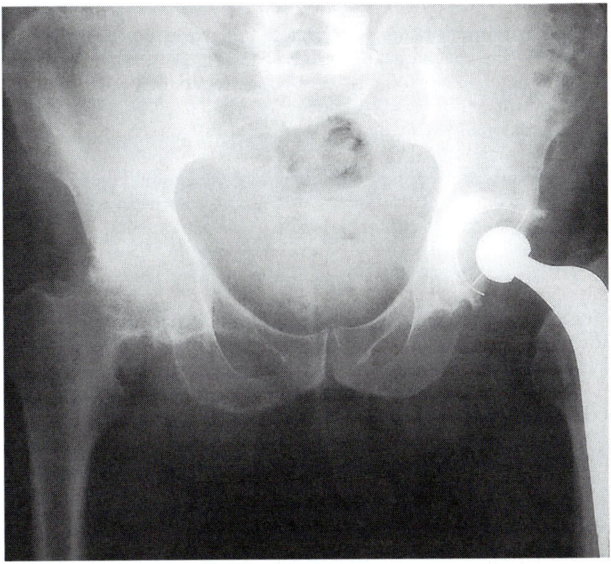

Fig. 17.15 There is osteoarthritis of the right hip joint. The joint space is diminished and there is sclerosis of the surrounding bone. On the left side, the patient has had an arthroplasty (hip replacement).

Treatment Principles of treatment involve pain relief, improvement of mobility and correction of deformity. Management may be conservative or surgical.

Conservative
- Analgesia: start with mild analgesia, e.g. paracetamol; NSAIDs are usually required eventually.
- Lose weight.
- Walking stick or shoe raise.
- Physiotherapy, i.e. heat treatment or short-wave diathermy.
- Changing occupation to a lighter job.

Surgical Disturbance of sleep, severe uncontrolled pain and gross lack of mobility are indications for surgery. The following procedures may be undertaken depending upon the level of symptoms and joint involved:

- Arthrodesis: surgical fusion of the joint, relieves pain, e.g. first MTP joint in hallux rigidus.

→

- Osteotomy: it is not known how this works but it probably alters the mechanics of weight bearing. Pain relief is often dramatic. The bone is usually sectioned below the joint, e.g. upper tibia for OA knee.
- Occasionally synovectomy and removal of osteophytes can give temporary relief.
- Excision arthroplasty: for small joints, e.g. small toes.
- Replacement arthroplasty (→ Fig. 17.15): most joints can be replaced by artificial joints, e.g. hip and knee.

Rheumatoid arthritis (RA)

The reader is referred to a textbook of medicine for the details of the symptoms and medical management of this disease. Only surgical aspects of management will be dealt with here. Surgery is undertaken to improve function not for cosmetic effect. Procedures include:

- Synovectomy gives good pain relief. The knees and finger joints are most suitable for this treatment.
- Repair of ruptured tendons.
- Joint fusion, e.g. painful wrist; atlantoaxial subluxation.
- Arthroplasty: the same prostheses and procedures are used as for OA. However, hand deformities are often most trouble in RA and various arthroplasties of the finger joints are indicated. Flexible silastic implants giving stability whilst allowing movement are the most popular. Infection can be a problem as the patients have often been on long-term steroids.

OTHER CONDITIONS OF JOINTS

Loose bodies

These may occur in any joint but the knee is by far the commonest site. Causes include osteochondritis dissecans (see below), detached osteophytes in OA, osteochondral fractures, torn menisci and synovial chondromatosis, where cartilaginous nodules form in the synovium and may become detached.

Symptoms and signs Pain and swelling. 'Locking' (an inability to fully extend the knee). Giving way. Occasionally the loose body may be palpable.

Investigations • Radiograph • Arthroscopy.

Treatment Open or arthroscopic removal.

Osteochondritis dissecans

In this an area of bone with its overlying articular cartilage becomes necrotic, separates and drops into the joint cavity as a loose body. It is associated with local trauma (50%).

Symptoms and signs Late childhood or young adults. Commonly affects the knee. Occasionally multiple joints. Knee – usually medial femoral condyle. Pain and swelling. Loose body may cause locking or giving way.

Investigations • Radiographs.

Treatment In the early stages before separation, rest in a plaster cast or bandage may allow healing. If separation is incomplete pinning may help revascularization. A loose body needs removal. Drilling the defect may help healing.

Neuropathic joints (Charcot's joints)

A joint which has lost pain and proprioception appreciation is subject to harmful stresses and strains. Destruction of the joint results. The patient usually presents with a painless, deformed joint. Causes include diabetic neuropathy, tabes dorsalis, syringomyelia and leprosy. Vibration sense, position sense and deep pain sensation are absent or reduced. Treatment is difficult. Arthrodesis and arthroplasty are usually unsuccessful. Supporting appliances may be the most appropriate treatment.

Haemophilia and related disorders

The main orthopaedic problems relate to acute haemarthroses and bleeding into muscles. They may occur spontaneously or as a result of injury which may be minor. Recurrent bleeding into the same joint results in degenerative changes, capsular fibrosis, contracture and deformity. The knee, elbow and ankle are the joints most frequently effected.

Symptoms and signs Pain, muscular spasm, swelling over joint. Local tenderness. Bruising. Long-standing cases show deformity of joint. Muscle wasting and synovial thickening. Patients presenting for the first time with a haemarthrosis need detailed haematological investigation.

Treatment Analgesia, splintage, factor VIII replacement. Large haemarthroses require aspiration under factor VIII cover. The chronically damaged joint is prone to repeated bleeds and a splint (a caliper in case of a knee joint) may be necessary for long-term protection. Synovectomy and soft tissue release for severe contractures.

ARTHROPLASTY

This is surgical refashioning of a joint, the aims being to relieve pain, restore mobility and provide stability. There are basically three types of arthroplasty:-

Excision The joint surfaces are excised. Fibrous tissue forms across the gap. Although considerable pain relief is gained there is residual instability. This method is usually regarded as a temporary measure following failure of a joint replacement where the prosthesis has to be removed and infection allowed to settle before proceeding with a 're-do' joint replacement.

Partial or hemiarthroplasty This is used where one surface of the joint is in good condition, e.g. a Thompson's prosthesis in fractured neck of femur where the acetabulum is normal. It is rarely suitable for OA.

Total (→ Fig. 17.15) Both articular surfaces are replaced, e.g. Charnley's prosthesis in hip replacement.

Design of joint replacements

- Metal on metal (stainless steel, chrome, cobalt, or titanium) or metal on plastic (high-density polyethylene). The material must be biologically inert.
- Strength must resist fatigue.
- Low friction.
- Firm bonding to bone, using a cement (polymethyl methacrylate) or ceramic materials or 'sintering' to stimulate osseo-integration to the prosthesis.
- Adequate range of movement.
- Stability against dislocation.

Practice of joint replacement

Indications Pain limiting activity despite adequate analgesia, and especially pain disturbing sleep.

Preoperative preparation DVT prophylaxis. Prophylactic antibiotics. Operative procedure. Ultraclean air with unidirectional laminar flow ventilation ('Charnley's tent'), body exhaust suits.

Strict aseptic technique. Inclusion of antibiotics in bone cement. Meticulous dissection, positioning of prosthesis, soft tissue reconstruction. Closed drainage to minimize haematoma.

Complications

Early As for any major operation, especially bleeding, DVT, PE. Neurovascular injury. Dislocation. Wound infection.

Intermediate Recurrent dislocation. Heterotopic calcification.

Late Septic or aseptic loosening (failure of the interface to bone). Implant wear or failure.

CONDITIONS OF MENISCI, LIGAMENTS, TENDONS, CAPSULES AND BURSAE

KNEE

Meniscus tears

This is a common knee injury. The medial is affected more often than the lateral. It occurs in patients whose occupation involves kneeling, crouching, or trauma, e.g. miners, footballers.

Symptoms and signs Often young male. Twists the knee. Usually knee is flexed and weight is on injured leg. Pain on side of knee where meniscus is torn. Knee may 'lock'. Knee swells. Settles with resting. Symptoms may then recur with 'recurrent locking'. At time of injury, tenderness, swelling, tender over meniscus, effusion. In the chronic phase – wasted quadriceps, effusion, tenderness over meniscus in joint line. McMurray's test is positive if the tear is posterior. Diagnosis is usually made on classical history and signs.

Investigations • Plain radiographs normal • Exclude other conditions, e.g. radio-opaque loose bodies • Arthrography • Arthroscopy.

Treatment

Acute phase Tears in the periphery of the meniscus can be repaired. Otherwise, minimal meniscal resection. Avoid total menisectomy because of the high risk of OA.

Chronic phase Menisectomy usually by arthroscopic technique followed by course of quadriceps exercises.

Ligamentous damage

Damage to the collateral ligaments and cruciate ligaments occurs frequently in sportsmen. Strains may be associated with an effusion into the joint and tenderness over the affected ligament. In contrast to complete tears the joint remains stable. Strains settle with rest and support followed by graded exercises.

Collateral ligaments

Medial An abduction strain on the tibia ruptures the medial ligament. Valgus straining with 10° of flexion will demonstrate opening of the joint. If a cruciate ligament is also damaged, the joint will open even in full extension. Radiographs under GA with joint stressed.

Lateral Rarely occurs in isolation. Instability is rarer because the biceps femoris tendon helps stabilize the lateral side of the knee.

Cruciate ligament tears

Anterior Usually caused by hyperextension or forward movement of the tibia on the femur with the knee flexed. There may be associated meniscal tears or damage to collateral ligaments. Examination reveals an effusion and a positive 'anterior draw sign' – the tibia can be pulled forwards on the femur with the knee flexed.

Posterior Usually torn by a force drawing the tibia backwards on the femur with the knee flexed. There is almost always other ligamentous injury. Examination reveals posterior 'set back', i.e. the tibia moves backwards on the femur when eliciting the 'posterior draw sign'.

Treatment of ligamentous injuries Isolated collateral ligament injuries are initially treated in plaster or a brace. Acute, multiple or complex injuries are best treated surgically. Chronic injuries with symptomatic instability benefit from surgery.

Bursae around the knee

Housemaid's knee (prepatellar bursitis) Rarely seen now that women do not scrub floors. Leaning forward on the knees brings the prepatellar bursa in contact with the floor. Treatment is by aspiration or excision.

Clergyman's knee (infrapatellar bursitis) Rarely seen now that clergymen infrequently pray on their knees. After prolonged periods of prayer the clergymen sat back on his heels bringing the infrapatellar bursa in contact with the floor. Treatment is by aspiration or excision.

Semimembranosus bursa It occurs between the tendon of semimembranosus and deeper structures. Cystic swelling on medial aspect of popliteal fossa. Usually occurs in children and young adults. Requires treatment by excision only if tense and painful. Often resolves spontaneously in children.

Baker's cyst This is included here for convenience but is not a bursa. It is a cystic lesion of the knee joint caused by chronic disease in the joint. It presents as a swelling in the popliteal fossa. The cyst usually communicates with the back of the joint through a small defect in the capsule. Surgery is required if the cyst becomes tense and painful. If there is any doubt about the diagnosis MRI should be carried out. The cyst may rupture and cause pain behind the knee and in the calf. It may be difficult to distinguish from a DVT (venography will confirm the diagnosis of DVT). A thrombosed popliteal aneurysm enters into the differential diagnosis of a painful Baker's cyst. Check the other limb (popliteal aneurysms may be bilateral) and the distal circulation.

ANKLE

Sprained ankle

The anterior fibres of the lateral ligament may be torn during an inversion injury. Pain, swelling and tenderness occur below and in front of the lateral malleolus. Treatment is by analgesia, strapping and, occasionally, a below-knee walking plaster.

Rupture of the Achilles tendon

This usually occurs during sport, e.g. tennis. The patient feels 'something give' and feels like 'being kicked in the back of the heel'. Examination usually reveals a gap in the tendon. The patient cannot stand on tiptoe. Conservative treatment is by plaster immobilization in full plantar flexion followed by progressive plasters up to the neutral position. Surgical repair may be necessary and is followed by a similar shorter period of immobilization in plaster.

Plantar fasciitis

This occurs in late middle age. The pain is under the heel. In the younger patient it may be associated with Reiter's disease. The pain is often worse on standing after a period of rest and improves somewhat with walking. Examination reveals tenderness at the attachment of the plantar fascia to the under surface of os calcis. A lateral radiograph may show an associated calcaneal spur. Treatment is by a soft heel pad, or local injection of steroid and local anaesthetic or both. The condition is self-limiting.

SHOULDER

A variety of conditions may occur in middle life at the shoulder girdle. They probably represent a spectrum of related conditions of low-grade inflammatory or degenerative aetiology. They include conditions variously known as frozen shoulder, rotator cuff syndrome, painful arc syndrome, subacromial bursitis, supraspinatus tendinitis, tendinitis of the long head of biceps, rupture of supraspinatus tendon or rupture of the long head of biceps.

Supraspinatus tendinitis

This may be due to inadequate blood supply with consequent inflammation and degeneration of the tendons. Progressive calcification of the tendon may develop and rupture may occur. A painful arc occurs when the tendon impinges on the acromion usually between 30 and 60°. Thereafter painless abduction of the arm is possible.

Subacromial bursitis

This may occur with partial rupture of the rotator cuff or spontaneously. The painful arc affects mid abduction between 45 and 120° when the greater tuberosity passes under the acromion.

Tendinitis of the long head of biceps

This occurs where the tendon passes through the bicipital groove. Pain occurs on flexion and abduction especially if the forearm is supinated.

Investigations • Radiographs to exclude arthritis of glenohumeral or acromioclavicular joints • Arthrogram • CT.

Treatment The treatment of the above inflammatory conditions in the acute phase is rest in a sling and analgesia. Injection of steroid and local anaesthetic into the tender spot may help. Exercises, both active and passive, when acute symptoms settle. Surgical decompression of demonstrable impingement if symptoms are persistent.

Frozen shoulder

As the consequence of the pain associated with the above conditions the patient tends to hold the shoulder still. Adhesions form which limit shoulder movement and the shoulder becomes stiffer until only scapular movement remains. This is known as frozen shoulder and is not a pathological entity but a response of the shoulder to the local painful condition.

Treatment Early stages require rest and injection of local anaesthetic and steroid until movement returns when physiotherapy is started. Spontaneous improvement is usual over 12–18 months. Advanced cases may need manipulation under anaesthesia to break down adhesions following physiotherapy.

Rupture of supraspinatus tendon

This usually occurs in a tendon that is already degenerate. It follows trivial trauma or normal everyday activity. There is a sudden pain in the shoulder and an inability to initiate abduction. If initial abduction can be started passively (e.g. by tilting the body to the side to initiate abduction by gravity) deltoid can continue abduction. Treatment is as for acute tendinitis. Surgical repair for large tears demonstrated by arthrography.

Rupture of the long head of biceps

This usually occurs in a previously diseased tendon. There is acute pain, tenderness and 'bunching up' of the muscle in the lower part of the upper arm when the elbow is flexed. There is little residual functional disability.

ELBOW

Tennis elbow

This is chronic inflammation or degeneration of the extensor muscles of the forearm at their insertion at the lateral epicondyle. It affects tennis players and anyone whose work involves extending and twisting the forearm. In some cases there is no obvious cause. There is pain on the outer side of the elbow radiating down the back of the forearm. It becomes worse on gripping. Tenderness is localized to the lateral epicondyle. Flexing and pronating the forearm while extending the elbow exacerbates the pain. Treatment is by rest and injection of local anaesthetic and hydrocortisone. Surgery is rarely indicated.

Golfer's elbow

This is similar to tennis elbow but affects the medial epicondyle. Pain occurs on hyperextending the fingers and wrist. Treatment is by rest and injection of local anaesthetic and steroid. If the latter treatment is given remember the close proximity of the ulnar nerve.

Student's elbow (olecranon bursitis)

This occurs owing to prolonged pressure over the olecranon bursa, e.g. a student studying long into the night and resting his head in his hand and his elbow on the table. For obvious reasons the condition is uncommon in present-day students. Examination reveals a swelling over the olecranon which may be acutely inflamed. In the acute phase, aspiration (occasionally pus is obtained) and antibiotics are required. In the chronic phase, straw-coloured fluid is aspirated. Surgical excision may be required.

WRIST

Tenosynovitis

This is inflammation of a tendon sheath. It is caused by the trauma of repetitive movements and affects the tendons of the fingers and thumb especially dorsally, where they cross the wrist within their synovial sheath. There is localized tenderness and crepitation on movement of digits. Treatment is by rest, local splinting and NSAIDs. A specific form affects the tendon sheaths of abductor pollicis longus and extensor pollicis brevis as they cross the radial styloid (De Quervain's tenosynovitis). Pain occurs at the site and is exacerbated by gripping and by extending the thumb. Forced flexion of the thumb with ulnar deviation of the wrist exacerbates the pain. Treatment in the acute phase involves splints and local injection of hydrocortisone. Chronic cases require surgical division of the tendon sheath.

HAND

Ganglion

A ganglion is a cystic swelling in relation to a joint or tendon sheath. It may represent cystic-myxomatous degeneration of fibrous tissue. It is common on the dorsum of the hand, and also occurs in relation to the wrist and ankle. It is a painless, cystic swelling that is fluctuant and transilluminates, and filled with a crystal clear gel (some authorities believe it is a protrusion of synovium through an opening in a joint or fibrous sheath and that the fluid is derived from synovial fluid). Treatment is by dispersion by a blow directly over it (from the family bible in bygone days), although this treatment is not recommended at the present time when aspiration, or complete surgical excision is recommended. The latter should be done under GA or brachial block using a tourniquet as they often extend down inside the underlying joints. It may recur.

Trigger finger

The fibrous flexor sheath thickens and the lumen narrows. The tendon sheath thickens because of local trauma in the narrowed sheath and a nodule develops on it. The condition occurs at the level of the metacarpal head or neck. As the nodule passes through the area of stenosis, a click or snap is felt and the digit 'triggers'. If the finger is fully flexed the patient may have to extend it passively. A nodule may be palpable at the site of thickening. Spontaneous resolution may occur. Surgical treatment is by longitudinal division of the sheath. Multiple 'triggering' digits should arouse the suspicion of RA.

Dupuytren's contracture

This is a condition of the palmar fascia involving nodules and contractures. Aetiology is unknown but it is associated with family history, alcoholism, liver disease and antiepileptic drugs. It may be associated with Peyronie's disease and retroperitoneal fibrosis.

Symptoms and signs Mainly elderly males but can occur in females. Nodular thickening of the palmar fascia. Contracture of the proximal interphalangeal joint and the metacarpophalangeal joint usually affecting the ring or little finger.

Treatment If the patient cannot place the hand flat on the table, surgery is required. This involves careful dissection of the palmar fascia, fasciotomy and local fasciectomy. Recurrence may occur. If the deformity is great and involves a single digit, amputation may be appropriate.

MISCELLANEOUS CONDITIONS OF THE LIMBS

UPPER LIMB

Ulnar neuritis

The ulnar nerve lies in a groove behind the medial epicondyle. Pressure or chronic friction may occur in the groove. Cubitus valgus (increased carrying angle) may stretch the nerve. Symptoms include pain in the forearm, paraesthesia in the medial one and half fingers and wasting of the small muscles of the hand supplied by the ulnar nerve. EMG studies confirm the diagnosis. Treatment is by decompression or by transposition of the ulnar nerve anterior to the medial epicondyle.

Carpal tunnel syndrome

In this condition the median nerve is compressed in the carpal tunnel. It may be associated with pregnancy, RA, myxoedema, OA, anterior dislocation of the lunate, and arteriovenous fistula at the wrist for dialysis. Middle-aged women are most affected.

Symptoms and signs Pain, paraesthesia, in the thumb, index and middle fingers. Worse in bed at night. Relieved by hanging arm out of bed. Clumsiness when carrying out fine movements. Wasting of thenar muscles and reduction of sensation in distribution of median nerve in hand occur in advanced cases. No objective findings in early cases. Pressure over the carpal tunnel may reproduce symptoms.

Investigations • Nerve conduction studies may help.

Differential diagnosis Thoracic inlet syndrome, cervical spondylosis, peripheral neuritis.

Treatment Mild cases may be treated by splintage at night. Carpal tunnel decompression by operative division of the flexor retinaculum. Cases presenting in pregnancy often settle spontaneously after delivery.

LOWER LIMB

Metatarsalgia

This is pain under the metatarsal heads. It is caused by a dropped transverse arch often in elderly obese ladies. It is tender over the second and third metatarsal heads with callosities. Treatment is with a weight-relieving insole. Morton's metatarsalgia is due to a plantar digital neuroma probably due to chronic trauma. It also affects middle-aged women. Usually it affects the cleft between the third and fourth toes. Treatment is weight-relieving insoles. If symptoms do not settle, exploration and excision of neuroma may be necessary. Other causes include: stress fracture, plantar warts, inflammatory conditions (e.g. RA), Freiberg's disease.

Hallux valgus

This is common in females. The first metatarsal deviates medially and the great toe laterally creating a bulge often covered with a 'bunion' due to a thickened overlying bursa. The great toe may overlap or under-ride the second toe. It may be a result of wearing unsuitable footwear, especially in adolescence. It is often familial. Metatarsalgia may coexist.

Treatment Mild cases require appropriate wide shoes. Surgery is necessary for gross deformity or associated arthritis. If there is no arthritis, realignment operations are appropriate, e.g. Mitchell's osteotomy (the osteotomy is through the neck of the metatarsal head and the head is displaced inwards and allowed to unite). Arthrodesis or resection arthroplasty is required if there is secondary OA (e.g. Keller's procedure – trimming of the prominent metatarsal head combined with removal of the base of the proximal phalanx. This operation is appropriate in the older patient).

Hallux rigidus

This is OA of the first metatarsophalangeal joint. It is a common condition which occurs in young adults, but the cause is unknown. There is pain on walking, especially 'pushing off', and a stiff, painful, enlarged joint. Radiographs show OA. Treatment in mild cases is by a metatarsal bar in the shoe. Severe cases require arthrodesis.

Hammer toes

This is a toe (usually the second) with a fixed flexion deformity of the proximal interphalangeal joint and compensatory hyperextension of the adjacent joints. Painful overlying corns occur. Treatment is by arthrodesis or excision of the proximal interphalangeal joints.

Mallet toe

This is a toe with flexion deformity of the distal interphalangeal joint with a corn at the tip of the toe or over the joint. Distal interphalangeal joint fusion is indicated.

INFECTION OF BONES AND JOINTS

ACUTE INFECTIONS OF BONES AND JOINTS

Acute osteomyelitis

This is a disease of growing bones or immunosuppressed or diabetic adults. It is usually due to *Staphylococcus aureus*, and rarely due to streptococci, pneumococci, haemophilus or salmonella. The infection usually starts at the vascular metaphysis of a long bone or centre of a short bone. Common sites include the lower end of the femur, upper end of the tibia, humerus, radius, ulna and vertebral bodies. Suppuration occurs and pus under tension causes bone necrosis. Pus breaks out under the periosteum, strips it up, and penetrates through, forming a sinus. Alternatively the pus can decompress into the joint causing septic arthritis. Necrotic bone is called a 'sequestrum'. New subperiosteal bone forms around the dead bone forming a shell (involucrum).

Symptoms and signs Young patient. Recent history of infection (e.g. respiratory) or trauma. Pain in limb. Aggravated by movement. Swelling and redness of affected area – usually localized to metaphyseal area. Loss of function. Malaise. Pyrexia. Tenderness and head over site of infection. Oedema. Pus with fluctuation is a late sign. Sympathetic effusion in nearby joint.

Investigations • WCC↑ • ESR↑ • Blood cultures • Radiographs: negative in early stages • Later, areas of osteoporosis with subperiosteal new bone and later sequestration is seen • Technetium bone scan • Indium-labelled WCC scan • CT scan • Sinogram.

Treatment After obtaining blood cultures start antibiotics, e.g. fusidic acid and flucloxacillin i.v. Splint the limb to relieve pain. If pus has already formed, drainage is necessary. Prolonged antibiotic therapy up to 6 weeks may be necessary. Resolving temperature and falling ESR are good guides to recovery.

Acute pyogenic arthritis

This is a blood-borne infection especially in infants. Staphylococci, streptococci and gonococci may be causative organisms. It may arise following osteomyelitis where the metaphysis is intracapsular, e.g. hip joint. It is a complication of RA in patients on steroids. Occasionally it follows penetrating injuries of joints.

Symptoms and signs Hot, tender, painful, swollen joint. All movements are painful and there is surrounding muscle spasm. High fever. Rigors.

Investigations • WCC↑ • ESR↑ • Blood culture • USS • Joint aspiration with Gram film • Culture and sensitivity • Radiographs are of little value in early stages; later, subperiosteal new bone with periarticular porosis.

Differential diagnosis Osteomyelitis with sympathetic effusion. RA. Reiter's disease. Gout. Rheumatic fever.

Treatment Aspiration and washout of joint. Antibiotic. Fusidic acid and flucloxacillin initially and then according to culture. Splintage. Analgesia. Surgical drainage may be necessary.

CHRONIC INFECTIONS OF BONES AND JOINTS

CHRONIC OSTEOMYELITIS

This may follow acute osteomyelitis but is more common following surgery for a compound fracture, especially when foreign material is implanted. It may be chronic from the outset, e.g. tuberculosis.

Secondary to acute osteomyelitis

In this condition the bone becomes sclerotic and thickened. Sequestra are present and involucrum and sinuses may be present.

Symptoms and signs Flare-ups with pain, swelling, discharging sinus and abscess formation. Spontaneous recovery may occur.

Investigations • Radiographs: show thickening of bone and cavity formation, sequestra (denser than normal bone) may be present • ESR↑ • WCC↑ • Culture and sensitivity. Drainage if discharge present.

Treatment Treat acute episodes with appropriate antibiotic. Surgery is indicated if discharge is marked, sequestra or large cavities are present, or attacks of pain and pyrexia are frequent. Open the cavity, allow the wound to granulate, excise sequestra. Rarely, amputation may be necessary.

Complications Amyloid. Pathological fracture. Squamous carcinoma in a sinus track.

Chronic osteomyelitis may occur secondary to trauma or secondary to insertion of a joint replacement or internal fixation device. Chronic osteomyelitis secondary to trauma is treated as above but fracture stabilization needs an external fixation device. If an internal fixation device or joint replacement is associated with chronic osteomyelitis it must be removed.

Chronic osteomyelitis due to specific chronic infections

This may arise as a result of tuberculosis, syphilis (tertiary) or mycotic infections. Tuberculosis is the most common.

Tuberculosis of bones and joints

This occurs worldwide especially in Third World countries. In Europe it is more common in the immigrant population and in the elderly. It is blood-borne usually. The primary site is usually in the lung. Destruction of bone and articular cartilage occurs. The synovial membrane is studded with tubercles which extend under the articular cartilage, destroying it. Abscess formation occurs especially in spinal tuberculosis. This may discharge into the psoas sheath and present under the inguinal ligament of the groin as a psoas abscess. Joints are often destroyed and undergo fibrosis or bony ankylosis.

Symptoms and signs History of TB contact. Infection of bone alone unusual. Usually involves both bone and joint. Malaise, weight loss, night sweats. Local pain, stiffness or limping. Local tenderness, soft tissue swelling, joint effusion. Local muscle atrophy. Discharge of cold abscess with sinus formation. Backache with TB of spine (Pott's disease). Wasting of back muscles, spasm, movement restricted. Localized kyphosis or 'gibbus' due to vertebral collapse. Paraplegia may occur.

Investigations • WCC↑ with lymphocytosis • ESR↑ • Mantoux test • Joint aspiration with Ziehl–Neelsen staining and culture

• Biopsy: needle or open • Sputum and urine culture • Radiographs show: osteoporosis around joint; erosion of joint surfaces; destruction of bone and intervertebral discs; soft tissue shadows, e.g. psoas abscess • CXR: initial pulmonary infection.

Treatment Antituberculous drugs. Rest. Splintage. Traction, e.g. TB hip. Surgery – drainage of abscess, excision of affected bone with grafting, synovectomy, arthrodesis of diseased joints. Spinal tuberculosis is treated initially by immobilization in a spinal support until stability achieved, usually by bony fusion of the vertebral bodies. Drainage of cold abscesses and removal of necrotic bone may be necessary, with surgical fusion of adjacent vertebrae.

BONE TUMOURS

These may be benign or malignant. Secondary tumours are much more common than primary. Secondaries occur from the lung, breast, prostate, thyroid and kidney. Primary malignant tumours are rare but they have a bad prognosis and affect patients in a younger age group. The management of suspected primary bone tumours is a specialist multidisciplinary task.

Investigations Diagnosis of primary bone tumours is very difficult. Radiographs show an overlapping spectrum of changes. Various imaging techniques can be used to determine the extent of the lesion. Pulmonary and cerebral metastases should be sought.

Biopsy Careful surgery reduces dissemination of the tumour and may allow limb-conserving surgery. Histology may be very difficult to interpret.

Treatment Some combination of surgery (curettage and bone grafting, wide local excision, amputation), and for malignant tumours radiotherapy or chemotherapy. The margin for resection is determined by staging the involvement of adjacent muscles and joints.

BENIGN TUMOURS

Osteoma ('ivory' osteoma)

This is a growth from the surface of bone. It is common on the surface of the vault of the skull. A smooth, non-tender mound, it rarely causes symptoms. If symptomatic it can be cured by excision.

Osteoid osteoma

It usually occurs in long bones in young males. There is severe continuous boring pain usually worse at night and relieved by aspirin. It is probably not a true neoplasm. Radiographs show dense sclerosis surrounding a central small lucent zone (osteoid). Treatment is by excision which gives dramatic relief of pain.

Chondroma

A cartilaginous tumour, common in the phalanges and metacarpals. An enchondroma is a chondroma growing in the centre of a bone. An ecchondroma is a chondroma growing on the surface of a bone. Osteochondroma is a cartilage-capped bony outgrowth (commonest bone tumour, malignant potential, especially if >2 cm or multiple). Treatment is indicated only when the swelling is large, when excision should be undertaken. Occasionally multiple enchondromatosis occurs in the long bones (Ollier's disease).

Fibroma and fibrous dysplasia

This is a spectrum of conditions with failure or partial failure of ossification replaced by fibrous tissue. These are usually asymptomatic and often regress at puberty or after a fracture.

Bone cysts

These are fluid- or blood-filled cavities. They vary from multiloculated cysts containing clear fluid in children and adolescents to large aneurysmal bone cysts which may cause 'bulging out' of one side of a bone. Pathological fractures are common. Treatment is by excision and bone grafting.

MALIGNANT TUMOURS

PRIMARY

Osteosarcoma (osteogenic sarcoma)

This is the most common primary tumour of bone. It occurs under the age of 30 years and is more common in males. It occurs in long bones. In older patients it is usually associated with Paget's disease: in the young it commonly affects the lower end of the femur or upper end of the tibia. It usually affects the metaphysis. Spread is via the bloodstream to the lungs.

Symptoms and signs Bone pain. Swelling. Limp. Cough due to lung metastases. Tumour grows rapidly. Hot, tender swelling on examination.

Investigations • Radiograph (→ Fig. 17.16): bone destruction, grows out of cortex elevating periosteum with deposition of subperiosteal bone (Codman's triangle), radiating spicules of bone

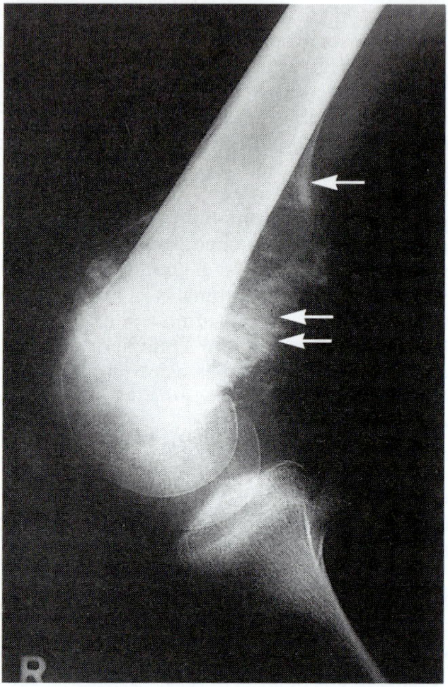

Fig. 17.16 Osteogenic sarcoma of the lower end of the femur showing 'Codman's triangle' (top arrow) and 'sunray spicules' (bottom two arrows).

('sunray' spicules), soft tissue invasion • ESR↑ • Alkaline phosphatase↑ • CT scan: shows invasion of the tumour, lung secondaries • Biopsy.

> ***Treatment*** Classically, amputation as soon as diagnosis is made. Recently, wide local excision with joint replacement and chemotherapy. If multiple pulmonary metastases at time of presentation, treatment is by chemotherapy alone. Solitary pulmonary metastases may be resected.

Prognosis 15–20% 5-year survival.

Osteoclastoma (giant cell tumour)

This occurs in young adults, at the ends of long bones. It has a low malignant potential but is locally recurrent. Metastases are uncommon, occur late and are to the lungs.

Symptoms and signs Pain. Swelling. Pathological fractures.

Investigations • Radiograph: multilocular cystic lesion expanding the cortex • Biopsy.

Treatment Excision. Joint replacement may be necessary. Recurrence is common if curettage and bone grafting is the only treatment undertaken.

Ewing's tumour

It is highly malignant. It arises from the marrow; it is not confined to the ends of long bones and may occur in any bone. It affects children and young adults and spreads rapidly via the bloodstream to lungs, liver and other bones.

Symptoms and signs Pain. Tenderness. Swelling. Pyrexia.

Investigations • WCC↑ • Radiographs: bone destruction, intense periosteal reaction, soft tissue swelling, 'onion-skin' layers of new bone around lesion • Biopsy.

Treatment Radiotherapy. Chemotherapy. Surgery when excision is easy. Amputation for very large lesions or fractures.

Prognosis Poor. The 5-year survival rate is approximately 20%.

Chondrosarcoma

This is a slow-growing tumour arising from chondroblasts. It occurs between 30 and 50 years and may arise de novo or in a pre-existing osteochondroma. It occurs in long bones, pelvis and ribs. Radiographs reveal a diffuse swelling with spicules of calcification. Metastases occur to the lungs. Treatment is by wide excision or amputation. 50% of patients survive 5 years.

Fibrosarcoma

This is more common in soft tissues (malignant fibrous histiocytoma) and much less aggressive in bone.

Myeloma

The commonest primary bone malignancy, it arises from marrow plasma cells. It is rare before 50 years. There is very early dissemination with widespread marrow replacement (multiple myelomatosis).

Symptoms and signs Anaemia. Malaise. Bone pain (backache). Pathological fracture.

Investigations • ESR↑ • Anaemia • Hypercalcaemia • Increased gamma globulins • Urinary Bence Jones protein • Bone marrow aspirate • Radiographs: multiple punched-out lesions.

Treatment Chemotherapy with radiotherapy for localized pain or surgery for compression symptoms.

SECONDARY

Secondary deposits occur in bone from the lung, thyroid, breast, prostate and kidney.

Symptoms and signs Bone pain. May be past history of primary tumour or primary may not be apparent. Pathological fracture. Full clinical examination of likely primary sites.

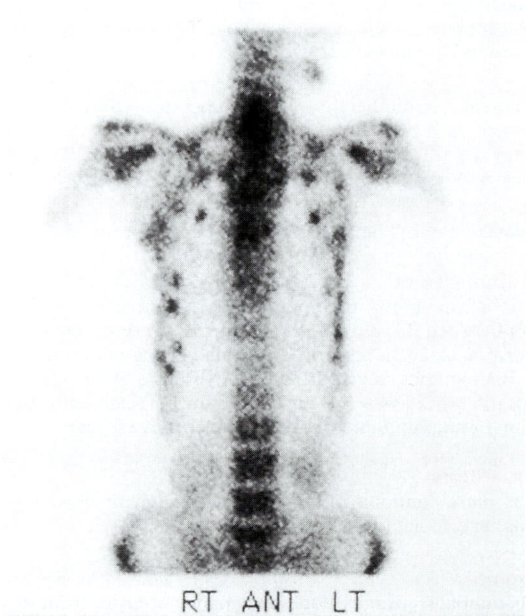

Fig. 17.17 A bone scan showing secondary deposits (hot spots) in the bony skeleton, especially in the ribs.

Investigations • Radiograph individual bone: osteolytic or osteosclerotic (prostate) lesions • Bone scan (→ Fig. 17.17) • Alkaline phosphatase↑ • PSA↑.

Treatment
- Severe bone pain at one site may be treated by local radiotherapy or systemic irradiation (thyroid with radio-iodine).
- Pathological fractures are treated by internal fixation and radiotherapy.
- Hormonal manipulation. Breast responds to oophorectomy. Prostate responds to orchidectomy.

BACKACHE

This is an extremely common complaint accounting for about 20% of orthopaedic referrals. Most cases are either traumatic or degenerative but other causes are numerous (→ Table 17.1 shows a list of causes). The more common causes will be described in this section.

Table 17.1
Causes of backache

Congenital	Kyphoscoliosis Spina bifida Spondylolisthesis
Acquired	
Traumatic	Vertebral fractures Ligamentous injury Joint strain Muscle tears
Infective	Osteomyelitis – acute and chronic, TB
Inflammatory	Ankylosing spondylitis Discitis Rheumatology disorders
Neoplastic	Primary tumours (rare) Metastases (common)
Degenerative	Osteoarthritis Intervertebral disc lesions

Table 17.1
Causes of backache (*Contd*)

Metabolic	Osteoporosis Osteomalacia
Endocrine	Cushing's disease (osteoporosis)
Idiopathic	Paget's disease Scheuermann's disease
Psychogenic	Psychosomatic backache is common
Visceral	Penetrating peptic ulcer Carcinoma of the pancreas Carcinoma of the rectum
Vascular	Aortic aneurysm Dissecting aneurysm
Renal	Carcinoma of the kidney Renal calculus Inflammatory disease
Gynaecological	Uterine tumours Pelvic inflammatory disease Endometriosis

Osteoarthritis of the spine

In this condition disc degeneration causes narrowing of the space between vertebral bodies. The posterior intervertebral joints may become osteoarthritic. Osteophytes form and may encroach on nerve roots.

Symptoms and signs Back pain radiating to buttock or thigh but not beyond. Usually cyclical in nature associated with overuse or episodes of abnormal movement.

Investigations • Radiographs: disc space narrowing, osteophyte formation.

Treatment Simple analgesia. NSAIDs. Physiotherapy, heat, exercises, manipulation. Spinal support. General advice re: posture, weight loss, lifting, etc. In severe cases decompression and surgical fusion may be required.

Prolapsed intervertebral disc

This is a common cause of low back pain and sciatica. There is often a history of pain or mild injury, e.g. while lifting. Backache and radicular pain occur. The prolapse can occur through the annulus fibrosus, or through the 'end' plate into a vertebral body. In the latter case, acute pain occurs and eventually a translucent area is seen on radiograph, adjacent to the disc in the vertebral body, i.e. a Schmorl's node. Most disc prolapses are backwards or lateral and cause nerve root compression. A central directly posterior prolapse may cause pressure on the spinal cord causing cauda equina syndrome (see below).

Symptoms and signs

Back pain Worse on movement, coughing, straining. May radiate to buttock and thigh without nerve root entrapment. Associated spasm and loss of lordosis. Restricted movements.

Nerve root compression Most commonly L5 or S1. Dermatomal distribution of pain and anaesthesia. Segmental weakness (L5 – toe extensors, S1 – foot evertors). Sciatic stretch test (restricted passive straight leg raising due to leg pain). Depressed reflexes, e.g. L3/4 – depressed knee jerk, L5/S1 – depressed ankle jerk.

Cauda equina syndrome Compression of sacral outflow, saddle paraesthesia. Reduced anal sphincter tone. Reduced bladder coordination, painless retention and overflow. Loss of anal reflex. Bilateral leg symptoms.

Investigations • Radiograph: often of little help, mild scoliosis, loss of lumbar lordosis, may be loss of disc spacing in chronic cases • CT • MRI (→ Fig. 17.18) • Myelography is undertaken prior to surgery or if there is doubt about the level of the disc herniation.

Treatment

Conservative Reassurance. Analgesia. Physiotherapy. Avoid prolonged bed rest. Mobilization in a corset.

Surgical An absolute indication for urgent surgery is bladder paralysis. Muscle weakness is also an indication for urgent surgical assessment. Other indications include failed conservative management, repeated attacks. Operative treatment includes:

- Surgical removal of the disc (the disc material is removed following laminectomy).
- Chemonucleolysis – the disc is dissolved with chymopapain. It is administered by direct injection into the disc under radiographic control.

Spondylolisthesis

In this condition one vertebra slips forward relative to the one below, usually L5 on S1 or less commonly L4 on L5. It is due to a breach in ossification between the lamina posteriorly and the

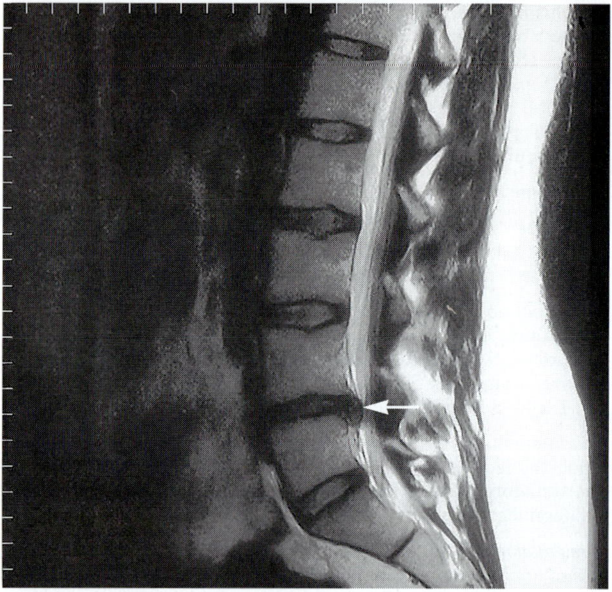

Fig. 17.18 MRI showing a prolapsed intervertebral disc (arrow).

body and pedicles anteriorly. It is usually congenital although, rarely, a fracture may be responsible.

Symptoms and signs Chronic backache, worse on standing. May present in late childhood or early adult life. Sciatica. Neurological symptoms in lower limbs. 'Step' palpable in the line of the spinous processes with marked skin creases below the ribs.

Investigations • Radiographs: oblique views show defect in pars interarticularis ('Scottie dog' decapitation sign).

Treatment Mild slips require exercise to improve muscle tone and a lumbosacral corset may suffice. With severe slips, decompression and spinal fusion are indicated.

Scheuermann's disease (adolescent kyphosis)

The ring epiphyses of the vertebral bodies are affected by osteochondritis. The vertebral bodies grow abnormally and become wedge-shaped. The condition occurs between 12 and 18 years.

Symptoms and signs Mild backache or no pain at all. A gradual curve or kyphosis develops.

Investigations • Radiographs: wedging of vertebrae and irregularity of vertebral end-plates.

Treatment Other than postural exercises, treatment is rarely necessary. Occasionally bracing or spinal fusion may be necessary.

Ankylosing spondylitis

This affects young adults, males more commonly than females. It usually starts in the sacroiliac joints and extends to involve the whole spine. Ossification occurs in the ligaments of the spine and intervertebral discs and the spine is converted to a solid column of bone with an increasing kyphosis (bamboo spine). There is an association with HLA-B27.

Symptoms and signs Young adult males. First sign is often reduced chest expansion. Low back pain, stiffness in the lumbar region. Most marked on rising in the morning and improving with activity initially. Eventually deformity occurs with flexion in the spine and hips and the patient may have difficulty raising the head to look forwards. Iritis and plantar fasciitis may occur.

Investigations • ESR↑ • Radiographs: special views of sacroiliac joints, irregularity, sclerosis, fusion. Later changes of ossification in spinal ligaments and discs (bamboo spine) (→ Fig. 17.19).

Treatment The progress of the disease is rarely influenced. Analgesics. Physiotherapy. Joint replacements may be necessary to deal with deformities. Osteotomy of the spine may be required.

Complications In the past this condition was treated with radiotherapy. Leukaemia may develop as a complication of this. Excessive use of analgesia in the past may cause CRF.

Cervical spondylosis

This is a degenerative condition of the cervical spine with narrowing of the intervertebral discs and osteophyte formation of the adjacent vertebral bodies. OA develops in the synovial intervertebral joints. The condition is common in the middle-aged and elderly. It may cause pressure on the nerve roots or the cord itself.

Symptoms and signs Painful, tender, cervical spine with reduced neck movement. Pain may radiate over the occiput and

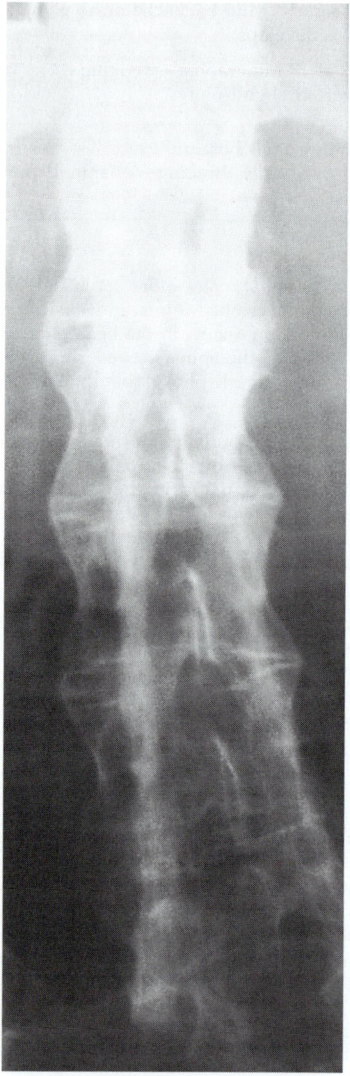

Fig. 17.19 Ankylosing spondylitis. The vertebral bodies are fused with early 'bambooing' of the spine. There is ossification of the interspinous ligaments.

to the shoulders. When nerve roots are involved pain radiates into the arm and hand. Stiff neck, limited movement of neck. Diminished reflexes in the arm, dermatomal sensory loss, signs of lower motor neuron weakness. Rarely bladder involvement from cord compression. Rarely spasticity of legs.

Investigations • AP and lateral radiographs of cervical spine (→ Fig. 17.20): narrowing of disc space, lipping of vertebrae, osteophytes, sclerosis of posterolateral joints with encroachment on foramina • If neurological symptoms, myelography or MRI.

Differential diagnosis Thoracic inlet syndrome, shoulder disorders, carpal tunnel syndrome, peripheral neuropathy, spinal cord tumour, syringomyelia.

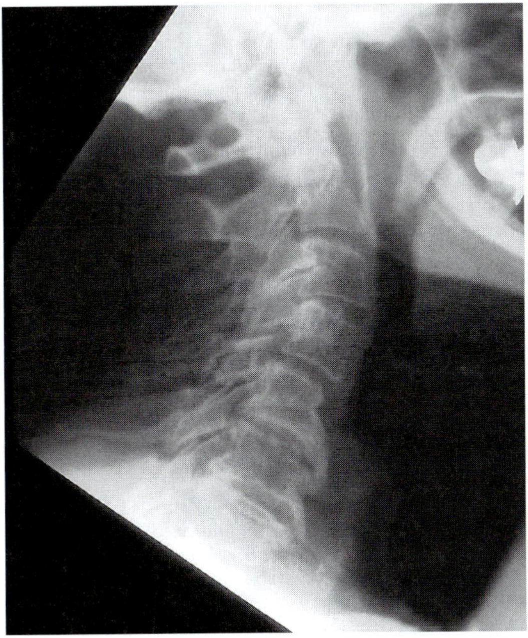

Fig. 17.20 A lateral radiograph of the cervical spine showing cervical spondylosis. There is gross anterior lipping of C5, 6 and 7. There is marked narrowing of the disc spaces.

Treatment Reassurance and symptomatic treatment in mild cases. NSAIDs, collar, short-wave diathermy. Gentle traction. The need for surgery is rare but may be required to decompress the nerve roots or cord.

Cervical disc prolapse

This should be distinguished from cervical spondylosis. It usually occurs in a young adult.

Symptoms and signs

Lateral cervical protrusion Acute neck pain often with severe pain radiating into the arm or hand with paraesthesia and weakness. Restricted neck movement, spasm in neck muscles, paraesthesia in dermatomal pattern in arm and hand. Weakness of muscle supplied by affected nerve root. Diminished reflexes.

Midline protrusion If massive, may cause no root pain but may produce a spastic quadriplegia by interfering with the anterior and lateral columns of the spinal cord. There may also be bladder symptoms. Milder degrees of midline protrusion may cause a spastic gait with reduced fine movements in the hand and associated bladder involvement.

Investigations • AP and lateral radiographs of cervical spine • MRI is the investigation of choice • Myelography if MRI not available.

Treatment In mild cases, analgesia, collar, heat treatment. Traction may be required. Acute onset of neurological signs or progressive appearance of neurological signs is an indication of surgery. Surgery involves removal of the disc material by an anterior approach with or without intervertebral fusion.

METABOLIC BONE DISEASE

Osteomalacia and rickets

Vitamin D deficiency causes the failure of osteoid to ossify. Rickets is the childhood form of osteomalacia. In children classical deformities occur, i.e. bowing of the femur and tibia, large head, chest deformity with thickening of the costochondral junctions (rickety rosary), enlarged epiphyses. In adults bone pain and pathological fractures occur (especially in the elderly with associated osteoporosis). Treatment is with vitamin D and calcium. Orthopaedic correction may be required for severe deformities in children.

Osteoporosis

This is a reduction in bone mass per unit volume. The causes are multifactorial. It is common in postmenopausal women. Pathological fractures are common (hip, wedge fractures of vertebrae, Colles' fracture). Radiograph show osteopenia, i.e. loss of bone density and cortical thickening, when 30–40% of bone mass has been lost. Treatment is difficult but should correct any underlying cause. Calcium and vitamin D should be given if the diet is deficient. HRT helps prevent postmenopausal osteoporosis at the expense of a small risk of endometrial carcinoma.

Hyperparathyroidism (→ Ch. 11)

Pathological fractures may occur.

Paget's disease of bone

This is a difficult disease to categorize but is included here for convenience. The aetiology is unknown. Disorderly bone resorption and replacement leads to softening, increased vascularity, painful enlargement and bowing of bones. It occurs in middle to old age and is more common in males. The skull, vertebrae, pelvis and long bones are affected. Some cases are symptomless, being

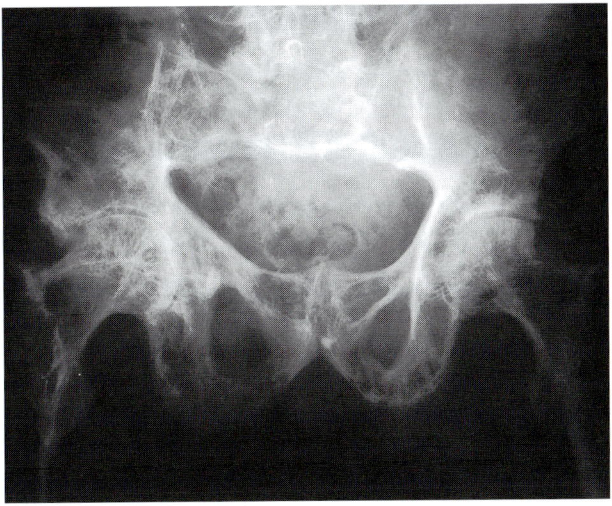

Fig. 17.21 Paget's disease of bone. The pelvic bones are thickened and patchily sclerotic.

picked up on routine radiograph (→ Fig. 17.21). Complications include compressive symptoms due to skull enlargement (e.g. blindness, deafness, cranial nerve entrapment), paraplegia, pathological fractures, high-output cardiac failure due to vascularity of bone. Osteogenic sarcoma may develop after many years. In mild cases no treatment is required. In severe cases calcitonin and diphosphonates may help.

PAEDIATRIC ORTHOPAEDICS

SCOLIOSIS

This is a lateral curvature of the spine. Untreated the condition may progress to obvious embarrassing deformities, embarrassment of respiratory function and neurological lesions. Scoliosis may be postural or structural. Postural scoliosis is usually mild, disappears on recumbency and is seen only in children. It may be due to a short lower limb, hip deformity, or spasm of the paravertebral muscles, e.g. associated with a prolapsed intervertebral disc. In structural scoliosis, in addition to the lateral curve, the vertebral bodies are also rotated. In the thoracic region this leads to rib asymmetry with flatness on the concave side and a hump on the convex side which produces the hunchback deformity initially best seen on flexion. Structural scoliosis may be:

- congenital – often associated with vertebral anomalies
- infantile
- paralytic – associated with trunk muscle paralysis
- adolescent idiopathic scoliosis (this is met most commonly; should be picked up early and referred for appropriate assessment).

The management of the latter type of scoliosis is described below.

Adolescent idiopathic scoliosis

This is more common in girls aged 10 onwards. It is usually convexed to the right and thoracic curves are most common.

Symptoms and signs Usually noticed by parents. One shoulder higher than other. Development of rib hump. More obvious on flexion.

Investigations • Radiograph in two planes: used to measure the degree of deformity and to assess progress.

Treatment Many cases progress. If the scoliosis is minor and not progressing it can be watched. Curves >30–40° or progressive curves require bracing using a polythene jacket. More severe curves at presentation and those which progress rapidly require surgery. Internal fixation is carried out using various implants to hold the correction until fusion occurs.

CONDITIONS OF THE HIP

Congenital dislocation (CDH)

The incidence is 1.5 : 1000 live births and girls are affected more than boys. There are hereditary factors – an increased risk if one parent has CDH. There is an association with breech delivery.

Symptoms and signs Routine examination in the neonate. The hips and knees are flexed to a right angle and the thighs are then abducted. There is jerk or 'clunk' as the head slips into the joint over the acetabulum (positive Ortolani's test). When reassessed at 3 weeks after the initial test only 1 : 10 of hips will remain unstable. If the diagnosis is missed at routine testing, the child may present in later life with a limp or a typical waddling Trendelenburg's gait (if the condition is bilateral).

Investigations • Radiographs are not very helpful and difficult to interpret in young infants as the epiphyses for the femoral heads are not yet present. Positioning the limb in 45° abduction shows a break in continuity of a line drawn around the margins of the obturator foramen and carried down onto the femoral neck (Shenton's line) • USS is the investigation of choice.

Treatment Ideally, all cases should be diagnosed at birth and treatment started immediately. In early infancy, all that is required is to hold the hip(s) in abduction with a malleable splint or harness for 3 months or less. The hip is held in the 'frog' position. Check radiographs should be carried out to assess acetabular development. If the condition is diagnosed between 6 and 18 months it is necessary to reduce the hip and maintain reduction until the acetabulum develops enough to hold the femoral head. This may be achieved by traction, a hip spica plaster, or open reduction. In older children, acetabuloplasty or osteotomies may be required to correct the deformity.

Prognosis The earlier the treatment the better the result. Delayed diagnosis especially beyond 18 months makes it difficult to achieve a good result. OA may develop in later life.

Irritable hip

This usually occurs under the age of 10 years and is more common in boys. The aetiology is unknown and the condition is self-limiting, the diagnosis being one of exclusion of other conditions.

Symptoms and signs Pain in hip. Limp. Occasionally mild constitutional upset. Mild spasm and restriction of movement.

Investigations • Radiographs are normal • ESR • FBC to exclude sepsis.

> *Treatment* Bed rest. Occasionally traction. Usually settles within 2 weeks.

Differential diagnosis It is important to distinguish the condition from Perthes' disease, TB and septic arthritis. The patient must be carefully followed up with physical examination and radiographs to exclude other conditions, e.g. developing Perthes'.

Perthes' disease

This is an osteochondritis which affects the capital femoral epiphysis. It is bilateral in 10%, is commoner in boys and usually occurs between 3 and 12 years, being maximum around 7–8 years. The aetiology is unknown although ischaemia may be the cause, resulting in avascular necrosis of the femoral head.

Symptoms and signs Pain in hip. Limp. Otherwise well. May present as groin pain or pain may be referred to knee. Decreased range of movements at joint.

Investigations • Hip radiographs: early changes include increased joint space and flattening of the epiphyses; later changes include increased density of the epiphyses which is followed by fragmentation of bone. If weight bearing continues the femoral head collapses and reduction in the neck-shaft angle occurs.

> *Treatment* Controversial. Depends upon the degree of damage to the epiphyses. In milder cases restriction of weight bearing is necessary during the active phase until the symptoms settle (2–3 weeks). This may be achieved by a short period of traction or immobilization in a weight-relieving caliper. In severe cases with most of the epiphysis affected, bed rest with the hip abducted to maintain it in the acetabulum may be required. This may be achieved by an abduction frame or plaster. This is continued until reconstitution of the femoral head occurs. Surgery with osteotomy may be required.

Prognosis Younger children with partial involvement of the epiphyses do well. Complete involvement in older children may result in later development of OA.

Slipped upper femoral epiphyses

This occurs from ages of 10 to 18 years and boys are more affected than girls. The child may be overweight and may have delayed sexual development in some cases. The capital femoral epiphyses slips downwards and backwards. 25% are bilateral of which 15–30% occur simultaneously.

Symptoms and signs Pain in hip. Limp. Pain may be referred to knee. Leg lies in external rotation and passive internal rotation is diminished.

Investigations • Radiographs: AP and lateral views; both hips should be radiographed. A line drawn through the centre of the femoral neck should pass through the centre of the head on both AP and lateral radiographs. If not, displacement has occurred.

Treatment If the patient presents acutely, the head is fixed in situ with pins or a screw to prevent further slipping. Reduction is rarely performed as it increases the risk of avascular necrosis. In the chronic case, pinning should be carried out if feasible, i.e. if the slip is not too great to allow this. Osteotomies may be necessary either as a primary or secondary procedure. Prophylactic fixation of the other side is controversial.

Complications Avascular necrosis of the femoral head and osteoarthritis may occur.

CLUB FOOT (TALIPES EQUINOVARUS)

The aetiology of this is unknown but there may be a neurological defect in some cases, and in others intrauterine factors, e.g. pressure or position may be involved. It is more common in boys and may be bilateral. There are three elements of the deformity:

- equinus – the hind foot is drawn up with a tight Achilles tendon
- varus – the sole faces inwards
- adduction of the forefoot – the inner border of the forefoot is concave.

Symptoms and signs The deformity is as described above. Usually picked up at routine postnatal examination. Exclude associated CDH and spina bifida.

Treatment Commenced at birth. Manipulation – usually slightly overcorrected. Held in position with strapping, plaster cast or malleable splint. Manipulation is repeated as necessary until the deformity is fully corrected. If correction is not obtained by 3 months, surgery is undertaken. Posteromedial soft tissue release is carried out. The Achilles tendon and posterior capsule of the ankle joint are released, the varus deformity corrected, and the tibialis posterior tendon may require lengthening. Splintage in either a plaster or a Denis Browne's splint is required postoperatively, usually until 1 year old.

Prognosis Usually good but relapses may occur. Follow-up for several years is required. Further surgery may be required if relapse occurs.

OSTEOCHONDRITIDES

A group of conditions in which developing epiphyseal areas, in children and adolescents, are affected. The underlying pathology may be avascular necrosis but trauma and stress injuries have been implicated. Several epiphyses may be involved and there are a number of eponyms in common usage to describe the various conditions: vertebral epiphyseal plates (Scheuermann's disease); femoral capital epiphyses (Perthes' disease); tibial tuberosity (Osgood–Schlatter disease); carpal lunate (Kienböch's disease), os calcis (Sever's disease); tarsal navicular (Köhler's disease); metatarsal heads (Freiberg's disease – usually second metatarsal).

Symptoms and signs Local pain and muscle spasm.

Investigations • Radiographs: dense and fragmented bone. Progress of the disease is followed by radiograph.

Treatment These conditions are usually self-limiting. Treatment of the various conditions involves rest, splinting or excision of bone fragments. The three most common of the conditions are Scheuermann's disease, Perthes' disease and Osgood–Schlatter disease. The former two conditions are described elsewhere in the chapter. The latter is described below.

Osteochondritis of the tibial tubercle (Osgood–Schlatter disease)

This is a common condition affecting adolescent boys in which the epiphyses of the tibial tubercle are involved.

Symptoms and signs Boys 10–14 years. Often related to physical activity, e.g. football. Pain and swelling accurately localized to the tibial tubercle. Examination reveals a tender, swelling. Knee joint is normal.

Investigations • Radiographs: fragmentation of the tubercle.

Treatment Restriction of physical activity. In severe cases, rest in a plaster cylinder or rarely surgery to remove fragments of bone may be necessary. Most cases settle spontaneously but it may take up to 2 years.

18

Neurosurgery

HEAD INJURIES

In the UK, head injuries account for annual attendance rates at A&E departments of almost one million people. Head injuries account for 9 deaths per 100 000 population and in young males account for 15–20% of all deaths. 20% of all patients attending A&E departments with head injuries are admitted, and over 25% of these have alcohol-related head injuries. More than 50% of all patients admitted with head injuries are discharged within 24 hours. Head injuries, therefore, cause a considerable workload and bed occupancy. It is therefore necessary to have a protocol to decide which patients need admission and which patients need further investigation.

It is recommended that all patients are monitored using the Glasgow Coma Scale after initial resuscitation (→ Table 3.1, p. 42).

Criteria for CT scan and consultation with a neurosurgical unit

The presence of one or more of the following:

- confusion, or other neurological disturbances persisting for more than 2 hours even if there is no skull fracture
- coma continuing after resuscitation
- suspected open injury of the vault or the base of the skull
- depressed fracture of the skull
- neurological deterioration despite adequate resuscitation
- penetrating injuries
- fractured skull in combination with either confusion or other depression of the level of consciousness or focal neurological signs or fits.

Criteria for hospital admission after recent head injury

The presence of one or more of the following:

- confusion or any other depression of the level of consciousness at the time of examination
- skull fracture
- neurological signs or headache or vomiting
- difficulty in assessing the patient, e.g. alcohol, the young, epilepsy
- other medical conditions, e.g. haemophilia
- the patient's social conditions or lack of responsible adult/relative.

- Post-traumatic amnesia with *full* recovery is not an indication for admission.
- Patients sent home should be given written instructions about possible complications and appropriate action.
- If a patient has been knocked out, hospital admission is not mandatory. If the patient is fully orientated, has no skull fracture, and no neurological deficit, the chances of an intracranial haematoma are small (<1 : 500 000).

Criteria for skull radiography after recent head injury

CT scan, when available, is the preferred option. A skull radiograph can be helpful if no other form of imaging is available but clinical judgement is necessary. The presence of one or more of the following indicates a need for skull radiograph in patients with a history of recent head injury and who are clinically stable:

- loss of consciousness or amnesia at any time
- neurological symptoms or signs (a CT scan is preferable)
- CSF or blood from the nose or ear
- suspected penetrating injury or scalp bruising or swelling
- alcohol intoxication
- difficulty in assessing the patient (e.g. the young, epilepsy).

Simple scalp laceration is not a criterion for skull radiography.

TYPES OF BRAIN INJURY

Primary

This is the damage caused as an immediate result of trauma. It results in contusions, lacerations or diffuse brain damage. Treatment cannot reverse primary brain injury.

Secondary

This develops as a result of complications. Secondary brain injury results in intracranial bleeding, cerebral hypoxia, cerebral oedema and infection. The prevention, recognition and treatment of these secondary complications is the mainstay of treatment of the patient with head injuries.

ASSESSMENT OF HEAD INJURY

Emergency

- Establish an airway.
- Ensure adequate breathing.
- Maintain the circulation
- Make a thorough but rapid examination of the patient.
- Evaluate the CNS with GCS (→ Table 3.1, p. 42).
- Splint long bone fractures.
- Assume cervical spine injury until proved otherwise.

Evaluate CNS injury

Assess the level of consciousness as this is the most significant factor after head injury. Use GCS (→ Table 3.1, p. 42) and check pupillary reactions. Pupillary changes may indicate brain swelling or compression. Pressure on a cerebral hemisphere causes the third nerve on that side to be stretched over the edge of the tentorium. The resultant paralysis of the nerve allows unopposed action of the dilator pupillae under the control of the sympathetic nervous system and the pupils dilate. There is also loss of light reaction of the pupil on the affected side. If compression continues, the contralateral third nerve is compressed and the opposite pupil also dilates and is fixed to light. Bilateral fixed dilated pupils in a patient with a head injury are a grave prognostic sign and recovery is rare. Pupillary changes are always late signs ('undertaker signs'), and are always preceded by an alteration in conscious level.

Pulse, respiration and blood pressure As further compression occurs, the pulse slows, the respirations become slow/irregular and eventually of the Cheyne–Stokes type. The BP rises. These are signs of midbrain compression and, properly managed, are avoidable in those with salvageable head injuries.

CNS examination

This may be difficult in the unconscious patient. Observe the pattern of limb movement in response to painful stimuli. Progressive unilateral weakness or focal epilepsy may be helpful localizing signs. Obtain a history from witnesses to the event, e.g. speed of impact, height of fall, state of crash helmet.

Check for CSF rhinorrhoea, or otorrhoea

Check for these signs. Periorbital bruising and retromastoid bruising imply basal skull fracture.

Scalp lacerations or depressed fractures

Check for these using a gloved finger.

Assess amnesia

Post-traumatic amnesia (loss from time of the injury) gives an assessment of the severity of the injury. Retrograde amnesia correlates poorly with the severity of the injury. Amnesia of several days or several weeks carries a poor prognosis with respect to return of mental function. Patients seen initially may appear fully conscious and oriented. Do not make allowances when assessing. They are often amnesic of events in A&E when asked at a later date.

CT AND MRI BRAIN SCANNING

Computerized tomography and magnetic resonance imaging provide very rapid and highly accurate detail of the brain. CT also provides excellent bone detail and should be considered instead of a skull X-ray if a significant brain injury is suspected. Resuscitation must always precede any form of imaging, however sophisticated. MRI is not at present necessary for management of acute head injury but may provide important prognostic data. A cervical spine X-ray is mandatory for all head injuries and must include C7/T1

SKULL FRACTURES

> A skull fracture is an indication for hospital admission. Patients with skull fractures are more likely to suffer secondary brain damage. Skull fractures are classified as closed, i.e. the skin over the underlying fracture is intact, or open (compound) where the skin overlying the fracture is broken, or the fracture connects with an air sinus or the external auditory canal.

They may be further classified as follows:

Linear, stellate or comminuted non-depressed These fractures are serious if they cross major vascular channels, e.g. the groove for the middle meningeal artery.

Depressed fracture A portion of the vault of the skull is depressed inwards. Surgery may be required to elevate the fracture.

Compound comminuted fractures with damage to the underlying brain These are treated by removing all bony fragments, debridement and closure. Failure to remove all bony fragments may lead to development of cerebral abscess. They are associated with epilepsy.

Fractures of the base of the skull They involve the anterior or middle cranial fossa. Those affecting the anterior fossa may cause nasal bleeding, periorbital haematoma, subconjunctival haemorrhage, CSF rhinorrhoea and cranial nerve injuries (I–V). Middle cranial fossa fractures involving the petrous temporal bone may cause bleeding from the ear, CSF otorrhoea, bruising over the ear over the mastoid and cranial nerve injuries (VII and VIII).

Summary The emphasis in the management of head injuries is on damage to the underlying structures rather than on the skull fracture *per se*. CT scanning is the investigation of choice for patients with severe head injuries, and no patient with a significant head injury should be admitted to a hospital A&E department that does not have immediate 24-hour access to CT scanning.

Management of CSF leakage It may be difficult to distinguish bleeding from blood mixed with CSF. Place a drop of the blood-stained discharge on a clean white gauze. If CSF is present there will be a spreading yellowish ring around a central stain of blood (halo sign). CSF leakage implies that the dura and arachnoid are torn and there is therefore a pathway allowing infection to spread to the meninges and brain. Antibiotics should be given. The head of the bed should be elevated 30°. The patient should be advised not to blow the nose. In many cases the leakage settles spontaneously but all CSF leaks should be referred for a neurosurgical opinion.

INTRACRANIAL BLEEDING

This may be extradural, subdural (acute or chronic) and intracerebral. Subarachnoid haemorrhage commonly follows trauma.

EXTRADURAL

This results from bleeding between the bone and the dura. It is most likely to occur when a fracture occurs in the temporal region crossing the middle meningeal artery. It may occasionally occur without a fracture. Usually low-speed injury.

Symptoms and signs History of head injury (may be relatively minor). Temporary concussion. Recovery ('lucid interval'), then headache, decreased conscious level, coma. There may be no lucid period or the patient may have the signs when admitted unconscious. Falling pulse rate. Rising BP. Reduced and irregular respiration. Dilated ipsilateral pupil. Contralateral hemiparesis or focal fits. May be boggy swelling overlying the site of the fracture as extradural blood may track through the fracture and into the subcutaneous tissues.

Investigations • CT scan. This should *always* be done immediately before surgery is contemplated.

Treatment This is a true emergency and requires neurosurgical assistance. If none is immediately available, make a burr hole over the suspected site of clot. Enlarge the hole with bone-nibbling forceps. Gently evacuate the clot. Clip or diathermy the bleeding vessel.

SUBDURAL

Acute

This results from tearing of small bridging veins which bleed into the subdural space and is usually associated with a lacerated brain resulting from high-speed injuries. The haematoma spreads over a large area. The patient usually has marked brain injury at the outset and is comatose but the condition deteriorates further.

Symptoms and signs Severe head injury. May be rapid deterioration. Signs of raised ICP. Localizing signs. Pupillary inequality.

Investigations • CT scan.

Treatment Craniotomy. Evacuation of clot. Recovery depends on degree of underlying brain damage.

Chronic

Usually in the elderly. Brain shrinkage makes the bridging veins between cortex and venous sinuses vulnerable. May have only been trivial and forgotten head injury. It may occur weeks or months after the injury, presenting with neurological signs, headache or coma, confusion or personality change. A brain tumour may be suspected in the differential diagnosis. There may be fluctuating level of consciousness.

Investigations • CT scan.

Treatment Evacuation of clot via burr holes and short course of dexamethasone. Reaccumulation may occur.

Intracerebral

This occurs as a result of primary brain injury but may expand causing secondary brain damage. It may extend into the ventricles. A discrete haematoma may require craniotomy if the patient's condition deteriorates.

Complications

Meningitis Organisms enter via compound skull fractures. Prophylactic antibiotics should be used for all compound fractures. Current prophylaxis includes cefuroxime given for a minimum of 1 week. It is not necessary for the drug to cross the blood–brain barrier if given for prophylaxis but it is necessary for it to cross the blood–brain barrier if given for specific treatment of meningitis.

Cerebral hypoxia This is a major and preventable cause of secondary brain injury. Respiratory failure after head injury may be peripheral or central. Peripheral causes include upper airway obstruction, e.g. tongue, vomit; chest injuries; pneumothorax; pneumonitis; shock lung. Central causes include primary brainstem injury or depressant drugs, e.g. alcohol. Hypertension may also contribute.

MANAGEMENT OF HEAD INJURIES

Minor

The most important question is: does the patient need a skull radiograph and to be admitted (see indications for skull radiography and admission)? The patient should be monitored for 24 hours. The majority of complications will occur during this time. If no problems occur after 24 hours, the patient can be discharged into the care of a responsible adult. Patients should be given an information sheet detailing symptoms and signs for which they should be on the look-out with instructions to return to the hospital should any of these symptoms occur. They should also be referred to a head injury clinic for management of any post-concussional symptoms.

Observations during admission The primary observations are the GCS (→ Table 3.1, p. 42). In addition pulse, BP, respiratory rate and pupillary size and reaction are monitored. These are carried out by the nursing staff on the ward, the frequency depending on the severity of the symptoms. Hourly observations are usually the norm. Signs of deterioration include falling coma score, falling pulse rate, raised BP, reduced or irregular respirations, dilatation of the pupils, loss of light reflex and asymmetrical pupils. An alteration of conscious level occurs before signs of brainstem compression.

Major

Does the patient need a CT scan and a neurosurgical referral (see indication earlier in the chapter)? If the patient deteriorates rapidly and an extradural is suspected, burr holes may be required, but if appropriately diagnosed it is usually preferable to transfer the patient immediately to a neurosurgical unit. In many patients with head injury, no surgical intervention is warranted. These patients may be in coma with diffuse cerebral injury and oedema and may require ventilation. Other injuries may be present. Intensive care will be required. The following may be required in management:

- Monitoring of vital signs and neurological status.
- Assisted ventilation.
- i.v. fluids and nasogastric aspiration.
- Avoidance of fluid overload.
- Maintain electrolyte balance, avoid hyponatraemia which exacerbates cerebral oedema.
- Control raised ICP, e.g. i.v. mannitol (osmotic effect reduces cerebral oedema): frusemide; controlled hyperventilation reduces $P\text{CO}_2$ and causes cerebral vasoconstriction, reduces cerebral oedema and therefore reduces raised ICP; dexamethasone is not used in head injuries to control cerebral oedema.

Other complications of head injury

Epilepsy Post-traumatic epilepsy may occur. It occurs in 0.5% of children with head injuries. In adults the frequency is similar and is associated with prolonged post-traumatic amnesia, depressed fractures and intracerebral haematoma. It is associated with cortical damage and subsequent scarring. Long-term anti-convulsive therapy is usually required. Prophylactic anti-convulsants are given to patients in high-risk categories.

Post-concussion syndrome Headache, dizziness, fatigue and poor memory are common after head injury. Loss of ability to concentrate and a labile emotional state are often sequelae. Management includes reassurance and symptomatic treatment. Often strong reassurance is necessary to explain that the condition is usually self-limiting within a few weeks or months. In most patients, symptoms cease within 12-months. Imipramine may be helpful. Strong codeine-based analgesics should be avoided.

Brain death Regrettably, some patients do not recover from head injury and are dependent on life-support systems. The brainstem death criteria were drawn up to allow a way of determining which patients had sustained irreversible brain damage so that they were not kept on life-support systems to no avail and to the distress of relatives and the nursing staff. The diagnosis of brain death depends on the demonstration of permanent and irreversible destruction of brainstem function.

There are prerequisites for the diagnosis of brainstem death:

- The patient must not be medicated with any CNS depressant drugs or neuromuscular blocking agents.

- The core temperature must be above 35°C.
- There should be no metabolic disturbance.
- The cause of the brain damage must be known.

The following tests reflecting brainstem reflexes must then be carried out by two doctors, on two occasions. Both doctors must have been registered for at least 5 years and be of consultant or senior registrar grade. They must be completely independent of any organ transplant team.

- Fixed pupils not reacting to light. Absent corneal reflexes.
- Absent vestibulo-occular reflexes. No eye movements should occur after injection of 20 ml iced water into each external auditory meatus. Clear access to the tympanic membrane is essential.
- No motor response within the cranial nerve distribution can be elicited by adequate stimulation of any somatic area.
- No gag reflex or response to bronchial stimulation with a catheter.
- No respiratory effort after discontinuation of ventilation and allowing the $P\text{aCO}_2$ to rise above 6.7 kPa. 100% O_2 is administered by tracheal catheter to maintain oxygenation.

There is no set time period recommended between the two sets of tests but 6–24 hours is usual. Once two sets of brainstem death criteria are satisfied, the decision to discontinue ventilation is made. The official time of death is that of the timing of the second set of tests. The possibility of a patient becoming an organ donor should be discussed sensitively with the next of kin. Many relatives gain some consolation out of the death of their loved ones, knowing that their organs are giving life to others.

MANAGEMENT OF RAISED INTRACRANIAL PRESSURE (ICP)

Causes Head injury, meningoencephalitis, haemorrhage (extradural, subdural, subarachnoid, intracerebral), tumour, infection, hydrocephalus.

Symptoms and signs Headache, drowsiness, vomiting, fits, irritability, listlessness, slowing pulse, rising BP. Irregular respiration. As the pressure increases the cerebral hemisphere is pushed through the tentorial hiatus alongside the brainstem. The third nerve is compressed against the edge of the tentorium and the brainstem is compressed by the herniating cerebral hemisphere. The following symptoms and signs: deepening coma, irregular slow breathing progressing to Cheyne–Stoke respiration and apnoea. Pressure on the third nerve causes ipsilateral and then bilateral pupillary dilatation. Eventually the patient exhibits the decerebrate posture.

A sixth nerve palsy may be an early false localizing sign. The long intracranial course of this nerve makes it susceptible to stretching.

Investigations • CT scan • Cerebral angiography.

> ⚠ Lumbar puncture should *not* be carried out in the presence of raised ICP. If the spinal CSF pressure is reduced by removing CSF, the high ICP may force the brainstem and cerebellar tonsils through the foramen magnum (coning) with fatal results.

Treatment

- Monitor conscious level with GCS (→ Table 3.1, p. 42).
- Ensure adequate oxygenation.
- Avoid fluid overload.
- Nurse with head elevated at 15–20° to promote cerebral venous drainage.
- Hyperventilate to maintain $P\text{a}CO_2$ at around 3.5 kPa which causes cerebral vasoconstriction and lowers ICP.
- Hyperosmolar agents, e.g. mannitol – osmotic diuretic which reduces oedema in the relatively normal parts of the brain.
- Dexamethasone is very valuable in some forms of cerebral oedema, e.g. that associated with cerebral tumours, but not head injury.
- ICP monitoring may be helpful in some patients.
- Neurosurgical intervention may be required. This must be carried out before signs of midbrain compression become established.

CEREBRAL TUMOURS

These may be broadly classified as glial and non-glial depending on the cell of origin (→ Table 18.1).

Symptoms and signs

- General, e.g. confusion, dementia, and epilepsy.
- Raised ICP, e.g. drowsiness, headache, vomiting.
- Focal signs.
- Epilepsy.

Symptoms vary depending upon the site of tumour. A full neurological examination should be carried out. Papilloedema

Table 18.1
Classification of cerebral tumours

Primary	
Glial (gliomas)	Astrocytoma Medulloblastoma Ependymomas Oligodendrogliomas
Non-glial	Meningiomas Acoustic neuroma Pituitary tumours
Secondary	Lung Breast Kidney Melanoma

is uncommon (about 15%). Symptoms occur alone or in combination.

Investigations • MRI • CT scan • Angiography • CXR to exclude primary • Burr hole • Biopsy.

Treatment

Medical Dexamethasone 4 mg q.d.s. to reduce cerebral oedema. Avoid overhydration. Consider a diuretic, e.g. frusemide 20 mg b.d.

Surgical The aim of treatment should be excision with a view to a cure. This is not always possible. If the tumour cannot be completely excised, subtotal removal may be required to decompress the surrounding brain. Postoperative radiotherapy or chemotherapy may give good results after 'debulking' the tumour.

Radiotherapy For inoperable tumours radiotherapy may give good palliation.

Chemotherapy This is rarely used except for pineal tumours.

Shunting Ventriculoperitoneal diversion of CSF is required if the tumour blocks CSF flow causing hydrocephalus.

TYPES OF CEREBRAL TUMOUR

Astrocytoma

The peak incidence of astrocytoma is in early middle age. They vary in malignancy and some are slow growing. All are infiltrative. Most malignant astrocytomas are radioresistant and survival overall is usually less than 5 years. Surgical cure is usually impossible as they extend into deep structures. In children, the tumour is often well differentiated and cystic, and occurs in the cerebellum. This type is histologically benign and may often be completely excised with potential cure.

Glioblastoma multiforme

This is the most malignant brain tumour It is rapidly growing and usually occurs between 40 and 60 years. It is rarely removable surgically and is radioresistant. Most patients are dead within a year of diagnosis.

Medulloblastoma

This is the commonest glioma of childhood. It occurs in the first decade of life arising in the roof of the fourth ventricle and infiltrates into the cerebellum. It may cause obstructive hydrocephalus. Spread is by the CSF and it may seed on the spinal cord. Radical removal is followed by radiotherapy. Chemotherapy may be required. Cure rates of 25% have been reported.

Ependymomas

Those arising from the choroid plexus of the ventricles may be totally removable. Those arising from the ventricular walls are difficult to remove. The more malignant forms may seed via the subarachnoid space. Craniospinal irradiation is required and gives good results.

Oligodendrogliomas

These occur in the cerebral hemispheres and are slow growing. Treatment is by tumour debulking and radiotherapy. Most patients are dead within 5 years of diagnosis. Relatively few survive 10 years or more.

Meningiomas

Meningiomas arise from arachnoid cells. They usually occur in females in the 40–60 age group. They compress the cerebral cortex early in their growth and therefore fits may be an early sign. They may rarely cause osteoblastic change in the overlying bone giving rise to exostosis producing a palpable lump over the vault of the skull. Common sites include parasagittal, along the falx; sphenoid – lesser wing; and olfactory groove. They are usually slow growing and do not invade brain tissue but compress it. Small tumours are usually curable by surgical excision. Even with subtotal excision for large tumours the prognosis is good. They may respond to hormonal therapy.

Acoustic neuroma

This arises from Schwann cells of the nerve sheath of the VIIIth cranial nerve at the internal auditory meatus. As the tumour grows it expands the internal auditory canal, extends into the cerebellopontine angle compressing the pons, cerebellum, and adjacent cranial nerves. It may be a feature of von Recklinghausen's disease.

Symptoms and signs An acoustic neuroma should always be considered in a patient with unilateral sensorineural deafness, especially with tinnitus. Occurs in those aged 30–60. Facial weakness with unilateral taste loss is a later manifestation. The corneal reflexes are lost relatively early when the trigeminal nerve is stretched by the tumour. Dysphagia, hoarseness and dysarthria may arise owing to involvement of nerves IX, X, XII. Ultimately cerebellar signs and features of raised ICP may occur, but these are now a rare occurrence.

Investigations • CT • MRI.

Treatment Surgical excision. Most can be completely removed with cure. Early diagnosis ensures preservation of facial nerve function and occasionally hearing. Stereotactic radiosurgery may be used.

PITUITARY TUMOURS

These cause symptoms due to their endocrine capacity or due to their effects on the optic chiasma.

Secretory tumours (e.g. prolactinoma) Many tumours contain a mixture of secretory cells. Presentation is influenced by the hormonal production and size of the tumour. These tumours are usually small.

Non-secretory tumour Null cell adenomas – usually grow to a larger size and present because of local effects.

Symptoms and signs These depend on whether the symptoms are due to the endocrine capacity or local pressure effects. Bitemporal hemianopia results from compression of the optic chiasma. Compression of secretory cells by non-secretory tumours may result in hypopituitarism. Symptoms include reduced libido, infertility, amenorrhoea, myxoedema, depression, loss of sex characteristics and hypoadrenalism. In children, growth arrest may occur. Hormonally active tumours may result in the following:

- Overproduction of growth hormone: before fusion of the epiphyses this will cause gigantism; in adult life, acromegaly results.
- Hyperprolactinaemia: this is characterized by amenorrhoea, infertility, galactorrhoea and impotence.
- Cushing's disease (→ Ch. 11).

Investigations • MRI • CT is contraindicated if MRI available because of radiation of optic chiasma • Visual field assessment • Hormonal analysis • Skull radiograph is never the primary investigation but a pituitary tumour may be discovered incidentally on a skull radiograph (expansion of sella turcica).

Treatment Surgery or radiotherapy. Tumour removal may be carried out by the transnasal route. Some pituitary tumours are radiosensitive and radiotherapy may be used as an adjunct to surgery or rarely as primary therapy in those with large tumours or in poor general health. Radiotherapy may be administered by external beam or stereotactic radiosurgery. Hormonally responsive tumours, e.g. prolactinoma, acromegaly, can be treated with hormonal antagonists.

Craniopharyngioma

This a cystic benign tumour arising in a remnant of Rathke's pouch. It may present in childhood or adult life. Symptoms are those of hypopituitarism due to compression, visual defects or raised ICP. The treatment of choice is radical excision but this may be difficult because of their size.

INTRACRANIAL VASCULAR LESIONS

These include:

- Aneurysms of the circle of Willis at the base of the brain. Most of these are acquired, the remainder being congenital.
- Angiomas which may occur in any part of the CNS. AV malformations may be associated with these.

Aneurysms

The majority are acquired as a consequence of cerebrovascular disease. Most patients are smokers. Mycotic aneurysms are very rare. Some are associated with polycystic kidney disease, Ehlers-Danlos syndrome, coarctation of the aorta and Type III collagen deficiency.

Symptoms and signs The classic history is one of sudden severe headache with nausea, vomiting, collapse and often coma.

Death may occur within minutes in major bleeds. With less serious bleeding there may be photophobia, and neck stiffness. Isolated cranial nerve palsy may occur, e.g. third nerve.

Investigations • CT scan (may miss small bleeds) • LP (only if the diagnosis is in doubt and the patient is conscious without focal neurological signs): if positive, carry out urgent cerebral angiography only when the patient is fit and if surgery is contemplated. The latter is usually indicated when the patient makes a good recovery from the initial bleed.

Treatment Early consultation with a neurosurgeon. If the patient is conscious with little neurological deficit, angiography is undertaken with a view to surgery. Surgery involves an intracranial approach to the aneurysm with clipping of the neck of the aneurysm with a non-magnetic metal clip. Occasionally, angiography fails to show an aneurysm, possibly indicating that thrombosis has taken place in the aneurysm. Such cases may be treated conservatively and often do well.

Prognosis 25% of patients die without regaining consciousness. 5% bleed again within 3 weeks of the initial haemorrhage and in rebleeding, the mortality is high. After 6 weeks the chances of a rebleed are about 10% per annum. Surgery is the treatment of choice but intravascular coiling may replace surgery in future for the majority of aneurysms.

HYDROCEPHALUS

This may be divided into two types:

Non-communicating or obstructive In this type the CSF cannot escape from the brain through the duct system and ventricular dilatation alone occurs. The duct system may be blocked by congenital stenosis, e.g. Arnold–Chiari malformation (downward herniation of the fourth ventricle and cerebellar tonsils), infection or tumour.

Communicating The ventricles communicate with a subarachnoid space and the CSF can escape within the brain but absorption via the arachnoid villae is prevented. This may result from meningitis, intraventricular haemorrhage in premature infants or malignant deposits on the meninges.

Clinically, hydrocephalus may be divided into two groups, congenital and acquired.

Congenital

The commonest causes are stenosis of the aqueduct of Sylvius, stenosis of the foramina of Magendie and Lushka, and Arnold–Chiari malformation.

Symptoms and signs Developmental delay. Abnormal skull enlargement. Frontal bossing. Prominent scalp veins. 'Setting sun' sign (eyeballs displace downwards). 'Crackpot' sign on percussion of skull. Diffuse transillumination of the skull only if the hydrocephalus is very gross. Bulging fontanelles which fail to close at the appropriate time. Later there may be epilepsy and profound mental impairment. Associated congenital deformities may occur, especially spina bifida.

Investigations • USS if fontanelles open • CT/MRI: ventricular dilatation and may confirm cause.

Treatment In some infants natural arrest of the condition occurs. A shunting procedure is usually required to direct the CSF to an absorptive area. In obstructive hydrocephalus the CSF is shunted from the ventricles into the peritoneal cavity. The shunt incorporates a unidirectional valve set at a specific opening pressure.

Acquired

This usually presents with signs of raised ICP unless it occurs before the age of 3 when the skull may expand as in congenital hydrocephalus. Causes include meningitis, trauma, intrauterine infection, e.g. rubella, syphilis, CMV and cerebral tumours.

Investigations • USS if fontanelles open • CT • CSF (ventricular tap) to exclude infection.

Treatment In obstructive hydrocephalus the obstructing tumour or abscess may be removed. Infections, e.g. TB and meningitis, are treated. Ventriculoperitoneal shunting may be required.

SPINAL TUMOURS

Spinal tumours are classified in Table 18.2.

Symptoms and signs Pain especially nocturnal. Radiation in dermatomal patterns. Progressive symptoms. Symptoms and signs of cord compression. Sensory changes below lower level of involvement. Motor weakness with spasticity. Bowel or bladder sphincter impairment. Cord compression causes spasticity with increased reflexes and extensor plantar response together with

Table 18.2
Classification of spinal tumours

Extradural	Secondary spinal deposits are most common Primary bone tumours, e.g. osteoblastoma and myeloma
Intradural-extramedullary	Meningioma Neurofibroma
Intramedullary	Rare and include astrocytomas and ependymomas

retention of urine with overflow and constipation. Cauda equina lesions cause a lower motor neuron lesion with flaccidity, diminished reflexes and paralysis of the anal and bladder sphincters with incontinence.

Differential diagnosis Intervertebral disc lesions especially central disc protrusions. Cord infarction (e.g. vasculitis due to polyarteritis nodosa, syphilis). Syringomyelia. Motor neuron disease. Osteoporosis. Fractures. Extradural abscess. Haematoma. Myelitis. Subacute combined degeneration.

Investigations • MRI scan is initial investigation. • Spinal radiographs: erosion, vertebral collapse, enlarged intervertebral foramina, calcification in tumour (meningioma) • CT myelography if MRI not available.

Treatment

Primary tumours Laminectomy. Surgical intervention is aimed at obtaining tissue diagnosis, removal of tumour and cord decompression. Microsurgery has improved results. Meningiomas and neurofibromas may be completely excised as may ependymomas.

Metastatic lesions Radiotherapy and chemotherapy may be helpful in palliation. The prognosis is poor. Surgical biopsy and decompression with stabilization may be required.

SPECIFIC NEURALGIAS

Trigeminal neuralgia

This is a severe lancinating pain in the distribution of usually the lower branches of the trigeminal nerve. Exacerbations and remissions may occur. Aetiology is thought to be due to vascular compression of the trigeminal sensory nerve route at the pons.

Symptoms and signs Severe lancinating pains. Shooting or burning. Exacerbation and remissions. ‘Trigger’ zones occur on the face, mouth or tongue and patients avoid ‘trigger’ stimuli, e.g. afraid of eating or shaving.

Investigations • MRI scan for microvascular compression and to exclude tumour.

Treatment Initially medical with carbamazepine. Surgery should be considered in all patients. If fit, microvascular decompression. If patient frail, thermocoagulation of ganglion or phenol injection is very helpful. Stereotactic radiosurgery may also be helpful.

Glossopharyngeal neuralgia

This is a pain of similar character to trigeminal neuralgia and is felt deep in the neck at the angle of the jaw and the region of the tonsillar fossa. Diagnosis is confirmed by applying local anaesthetic to the tonsillar fossa, which relieves the pain. Aetiology is thought to be due to vascular compression of the nerve. Surgical treatment involves partial section of the IXth nerve.

Postherpetic neuralgia

Severe burning pain may persist in the involved segment long after the infection of herpes zoster has settled. Medical treatment should be tried initially. Amitriptyline or carbamazepine may help. TENS may be tried. In severe forms, dorsal route entry zone destruction or dorsal ganglionectomy may be required.

NEUROSURGICAL PROCEDURES FOR PAIN RELIEF

Destructive operations of the nervous system for the treatment of pain should only be used when other simpler measures have been used and failed. These should be undertaken in specialist neurosurgical centres. They are mainly used for relieving the pain of malignant disease.

Cordotomy

The spinal cord tracts which transmit pain to the brain are the anterolateral spinothalamic tracts. If these are divided, the appreciation of pain and temperature is lost on the contralateral side of the body. The procedure can be carried out via a laminectomy but also percutaneously under radiographic control. In the latter procedure the patient is awake and a radiofrequency current is passed through a needle placed percutaneously in the spinothalamic tract.

Trigeminal thermocoagulation

This is used in the treatment of trigeminal neuralgia in patients who have not responded to medical treatment. Percutaneous radiofrequency rhizotomy of the trigeminal nerve is carried out by introducing a needle into the foramen ovale under radiographic control. 75% of patients get relief at the expense of an area of anaesthesia on the face.

Neurovascular decompression

The aetiology of trigeminal neuralgia is thought to be due to distortion of the nerve by blood vessels. Decompression may be carried out through a small retromastoid craniectomy. No neural tissue is destroyed and therefore there is no anaesthesia. The vessels are separated from the nerve and muscle or silicone sponge interposed. Results are excellent.

Dorsal root entry zone destruction

This may be used for treatment of pain resulting from nerve injury. Suitable conditions include phantom limb pain, post-herpetic neuralgia, and brachial plexus avulsion. Results have been encouraging.

Sacral neurectomy

This may be used for the pain of pelvic cancer. Open laminectomy is carried out. If the sections are limited to the nerve roots below S3, sphincter function is spared.

19 Plastic surgery

This chapter will cover some of the more common conditions which present to the plastic surgeon. It will also cover some plastic surgical procedures with which medical students should be familiar. Although the treatment of burns is more properly covered under the heading of major trauma, it will be included here since subsequent management after resuscitation is normally undertaken by the Plastic and Burns Unit. Work typically undertaken by a plastic surgeon includes: trauma to the hands and face and acute burn care (30%); skin, and head and neck malignancy (30%); congenital deformities and late effect of injury (30%); with less than 10% of the work involving cosmetic surgery, e.g. rhinoplasty, prominent ear correction and other facial aesthetic surgery. The procedure of breast reduction is usually performed for functional reasons, i.e. intertrigo, backache or shoulder ache.

CLEFT LIP AND PALATE

Cleft lip occurs in 1 : 750 live births. Cleft palate occurs in 1 : 2000 live births. In half the affected children cleft lip and cleft palate occur together. Cleft lip may be complete or incomplete and it may occur unilaterally (70%) or bilaterally (25%) or, rarely, in the midline. A unilateral cleft lip usually occurs on the left. Clefts of the palate may be unilateral and usually affect the soft palate and posterior third of the hard palate. They may be complete, incomplete or submucous. Bilateral clefts usually affect the soft and hard palate.

Symptoms and signs Cleft lip is obvious at birth. Cleft palate is discovered on routine inspection soon after birth or may be discovered when difficulties occur with feeding. Beware missing a submucous cleft in which the palate initially appears intact. Late presentation may occur with speech and hearing difficulties.

Treatment The problem and its treatment must be explained to the parents. Feeding may be a problem. Sucking may be difficult making breast-feeding and bottle-feeding a problem. Swallowing is normal. Feeds may be delivered to the back of the tongue via a spoon or pipette. Feeding in the upright position prevents regurgitation.

Operation on cleft lip should be undertaken at 10 weeks, although some surgeons are now carrying out neonatal lip repair. The aims of surgery are to achieve an intact lip, alveolus and palate and to permit normal speech and dentition. Operation on cleft palate should be undertaken before the child learns to speak. This should be around 9–12 months. The aims of treatment of cleft palate are:

→

- to close the cleft thus separating nasal and oral cavities
- to ensure adequate length of the soft palate allowing separation of the nasopharynx and oropharynx on phonation.

Various relaxing or plastic procedures may be necessary to achieve this.

Prognosis Surgery for cleft lip and cleft palate is confined to some 10 centres nationally. A good cosmetic result is normally achieved in closing cleft lip. With cleft palate satisfactory speech is achieved in about 80% of cases. 20% may require a pharyngoplasty. All children need speech therapy. Occasionally secondary procedures may be required such as secondary alveolar bone grafting at 9–11 years and corrective rhinoplasty around the age of 16 years. A Cleft Lip and Palate Association is available for advice and support.

PROVIDING SKIN COVER

FREE GRAFT

A graft is removed completely from one part of the body and grafted onto another site on the body. It is separated from its blood supply and therefore depends on being placed on a healthy vascular bed for its revascularization. (For indication for skin grafting → Table 19.1.)

Split-skin graft (partial thickness or Thiersch)

This consists of the epidermis and upper capillary dermis. The graft is cut with a special knife which controls the skin thickness (dermatome). This may be carried out with either a freehand knife or a power dermatome. A thin split-skin graft is approximately 0.25 mm thick. The usual donor sites include arms, thigh and buttocks. The donor site heals quickly. The site can be reused as

Table 19.1
Indications for skin grafting

Traumatic skin loss, e.g. burns
Pressure sores (sometimes require flaps)
Extensive ulcers
Following wide excision of skin tumours
Skin flap donor defects
Covering large granulating areas

a donor site in 7–10 days. Infection can significantly slow healing and cause loss of deeper structures.

The main use for split-skin grafts is in the treatment of burns, and to close defects after removal of skin tumours. Advantages include rapid vascularization with rapid healing of the donor site. Disadvantages include postgraft contracture, lack of resistance to trauma, and absence of normal skin properties, e.g. suppleness, hair growth. Factors affecting 'take' of the graft include a poorly vascularized bed, haematoma, seroma, infection and movement. A bolus or 'tie over' stent pressure dressing can be applied to prevent movement and keep all parts of the graft in contact with the bed.

Skin grafts may be meshed. This has two advantages:

- greater coverage may be obtained
- seroma or haematoma may escape through the interstices.

The graft is passed through a 'mesher' which creates multiple holes so that the graft looks like a string vest. Wide meshing allows large areas to be covered and clearly this is an advantage in major burns. A disadvantage is that the final result also resembles a string vest because the interstices heal by epithelialization alone as they contain no dermal elements. Partial thickness grafts if kept moist can be stored at 4°C for 3–4 weeks.

Full thickness graft (Wolfe graft)

This consists of the epidermis and dermis and therefore includes all skin elements, e.g. hair follicles, sweat glands. Only areas of thin skin can be used as donor sites. Main uses are for facial areas and hands. Usual donor sites include supraclavicular, postauricular, submammary, antecubital and inguinal areas. The donor area requires closure and if this cannot be closed primarily a split-skin graft may be required.

Advantages include the fact that full thickness grafts include all skin elements, are more supple, withstand trauma and undergo the least contraction. Disadvantages include limited donor sites, failure of take (less than with split skin) and problems closing donor sites. Successful 'take' depends on the same factors as split-skin grafting. A 'tie over' stent dressing should be used. Prior to all skin grafting, wound swabs should be taken for culture and sensitivity to check for Group A β-haemolytic streptococcus.

PEDICLE FLAPS

These are composed of skin and subcutaneous tissue created on one part of the body and transferred to another. The thickness of the flap renders survival impossible if transferred like a graft. Survival depends on a vascular attachment to the body through-

Table 19.2
Indications for pedicle flaps

Wound closure in areas of poor vascularity, e.g. over ribs after extended mastectomy
Areas of bone where padding is needed, e.g. over sacrum or ischial tuberorsity
Facial reconstructive surgery

out the transfer procedure. Pedicle attachment is required until a new blood supply develops from the recipient site. This usually takes 2–3 weeks, following which the flap is detached from the donor site. General indications for pedicle flaps include: relatively avascular areas, e.g. exposed bone or joint surfaces, the chest wall after extensive procedures for breast carcinoma, irradiated areas and extensive sacral pressure areas with exposed bone. (For indications for pedicle flaps → Table 19.2.)

Types of pedicle flaps

Skin flaps

Random flaps A skin flap raised on a random blood supply, i.e. no specific artery or vein is included in the flap, which depends on subdermal vessels for its blood supply. Examples include simple advancement flaps, V–Y advancement flaps, Z-plasty, rotation flaps, transposition flaps.

Axial flaps These have a known vascular supply based on a named artery and vein. Flaps of greater length may be obtained, the flap being up to four times the length of the base of attachment. Examples include forehead flaps based on the superficial temporal artery, deltopectoral flaps based on perforating branches of the internal mammary artery and the radial forearm flap.

Myocutaneous flaps These consist of skin, subcutaneous tissue and underlying muscle. They are axial flaps, having a named supply. They are used to cover large defects or bare bone. Examples include latissimus dorsi flaps for breast reconstruction after mastectomy and pectoralis major flaps for head and neck reconstruction.

Fasciocutaneous flaps These consist of skin, subcutaneous tissue and fascia. They are less bulky than myocutaneous flaps and leave less functional disability at the donor site. The lack of bulk is advantageous in some situations, e.g. grafting on the back of the hand. They may also be random, e.g. on the lower limb.

Free flaps The blood supply to the flap is completely divided and the flap transferred to another area of the body where revascularization is effected by microvascular anastomosis. Free flaps may be axial, muscle, myocutaneous or fasciocutaneous. Advantages include single-stage reconstruction, a wide choice of donor sites allowing a better cosmetic result, better tailoring to fit the defect without the constraint of a pedicle and a good success rate (up to 95%). Disadvantages include long operating time and the need for specialized equipment.

Care of the donor site

This heals by epithelialization from the remaining epithelial structures, i.e. hair follicles, sebaceous glands and sweat glands. The thinner the graft the more rapid the healing. Traditional management of the donor site involves application of paraffin gauze, cotton wool and a crepe bandage for 10 days. Many patients find the donor site more painful than the recipient site and the pain may be treated by the application of local anaesthetic gel. More modern dressings promote rapid healing with less pain. These include alginate dressings and synthetic semipermeable membranes.

Survival of skin grafts

Survival depends on the graft being placed on a healthy vascular bed to allow ingrowth of a new vascular supply into the graft. Factors leading to failure include:

- Loss of contact of graft:
  - tension on graft
  - fluid beneath the graft, e.g. serum, blood, pus
  - movement between graft and bed.
- Infected wounds. Grafts will not take on an infected bed. The most common infective agent is Group A ß-haemolytic streptococcus.
- Grafting on to an unsuitable base, e.g. bone, cartilage, tendon: at these sites a flap procedure is required.

BURNS

A burn is a coagulative destruction of the surface layers of the body. Burns may be caused by heat, ultraviolet light, irradiation, electricity, chemicals and friction. In the UK there are about 750 deaths annually from burns, there being approximately 150 000 injuries each year. Domestic burns and scalds, especially in children and the elderly, are a common cause of attendance at A&E units.

CLASSIFICATION

Partial thickness

Some epidermal elements are spared, allowing spontaneous healing without the need for skin grafting.

Superficial This involves the superficial epidermis only. The underlying germinal layer is intact. Blistering occurs with superficial partial thickness burns. There is minimal tissue damage, the only clinical finding is erythema. Healing takes place in a few days.

Deep These extend beyond the germinal layer and the only epithelial elements remaining may be sweat glands and hair follicles. Blistering occurs and slough formation may occur. New skin forms from remaining areas of epidermis and from sweat glands and hair follicles. Healing occurs in 2–3 weeks and some scarring is inevitable especially if infection supervenes.

Full thickness

All layers of the skin are destroyed. If left, the wound would heal by contraction of fibrous tissue and centripetal growth of the peripheral epithelium. In all but the smallest full thickness burns, skin grafting is required to prevent dense scarring, contractures, and deformity.

MANAGEMENT OF BURNS

First aid

1. Quench the burning process. Dousing with cold water has both a quenching and analgesic affect. Beware copious cold water irrigation in the young scalded infant as this may induce hypothermia.
2. If scalding, remove clothes.
3. If a chemical burn, flush with neutral solution if available. Hosing down with cold water may be appropriate.
4. Remove from smoke. Ensure clear airway.
5. Cover the burn in a clean sheet soaked in cold water.
6. Get the patient to hospital.

Assessment of the patient

1. Assess the airway.
2. Make sure the patient is breathing adequately.
3. Ensure an adequate circulation.
4. Obtain a history: source of burning, e.g. fire or scald; duration of contact; contact with any toxic gases.
5. Estimate the site, degree and severity of the burns. Use the 'rule of nines' (→ Fig 19.1). Alternatively the palm and finger surface of the patient's hand may be used as representing 1%

Fig. 19.1 The 'rule of 9s'. A guide to estimating the percentage area of a burn.

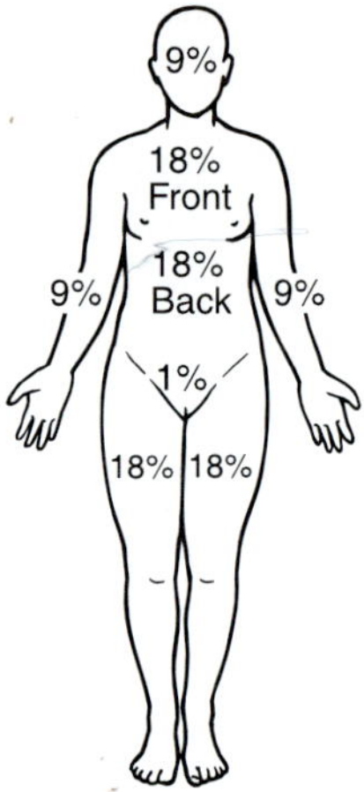

of the body surface area. It may be difficult to determine the depth of a burn clinically. Frequently there are areas of partial and full thickness burns. Partial thickness burns may show erythema. Pain is characteristic with normal pin-prick sensation. Full thickness burns are charred, or may be white, grey or leathery. They are usually dry. The surface is pain-free and pin-prick sensation is absent. However, final differentiation between partial and full thickness burns may be dependent on the degree of healing that occurs with time.

Treatment of burns

Patients with burns involving 15% or more of the body surface (10% in children) require hospitalization. Other indications for hospitalization include burns involving the face, hands, eyes, genitalia, and perineum; electrical burns; smoke inhalation or inhalation of other toxic fumes.

Local

Open The burn is exposed. Limbs should be elevated to reduce oedema. The open method is used for the face, limbs, or where only the front or back of the trunk is involved.

Closed The burn is cleansed, covered with silver sulphadiazine cream, Vaseline gauze and cotton wool. The dressings are changed if they become soaked with plasma. Burns on the hands and fingers are treated with silver sulphadiazine cream and are enclosed in a plastic bag. This allows for encouragement of hand movements.

→

By 10–14 days, whichever method is used, slough will separate from partial thickness burns leaving an epithelium. This does not occur with full thickness burns, the slough remaining adherent. Removal of the slough reveals granulation tissue which requires grafting. In some types of burns there is a need for immediate skin grafting. This is particularly the case if the eyelids are involved, where grafting is carried out in order to prevent ectropion and the risk of corneal ulceration. Scarring at certain other sites may cause considerable deformity or disability and these sites include the hands, joint flexures and the face. Circumferential burns of the extremities or the trunk may require escharotomy to prevent venous obstruction beneath the constricting eschar. Escharotomy of the chest may relieve constriction which may restrict ventilation.

Whilst traditionally skin grafting of burns occurred after 14–21 days when raw areas remained, in recent years early (within a few days of injury) excision of deep dermal or full thickness burns has become more popular. If successful it reduces the chances of invasive infection and limits catabolism and heat and water loss. In large burns the limitation is the availability of autogenous skin. In these situations homograft skin or synthetic skin substitutes may be used temporarily, later to be replaced by autograft skin.

General

Pain relief Frequent small doses of intravenous morphine should be given.

Fluid balance Oligaemic shock occurs from plasma loss. Anaemia occurs owing to destruction of red cells. Intravenous fluids should be given if the burn is greater than 15% (10% in the child). Fluid replacement may be given according to the Muir and Barclay formula:

$$\frac{\text{Weight (kg)} \times \text{\% burn}}{2} = \text{ml of fluid per 'ration'}.$$

The fluid in each 'ration' is given as follows: 3 rations in the first 12 hours, 2 rations in the next 12 hours and 1 ration for the third 12-hour period. For example, if a 70-kg patients sustained a 40% burn, then the fluid given in each ration is (70 × 40)/2, i.e. 1400 ml. This volume is given for each of three 4-hour periods, i.e. 4200 ml in the first 12 hours, 2800 ml in the next 12 hours and 1400 ml for the third 12-hour period. Fluid replacement is usually with 4.5% albumin or colloid, e.g. Haemaccel. The patient should be catheterized. Vital signs and urine output should be monitored hourly. The Muir and Barclay formula is only a rough guide to the likely

→

fluid needs, and the actual fluid volume given should be related to the clinical response of the patient.

An alternative resuscitation regimen of crystalloid (as Ringer lactate) developed at Parkland Hospital (Dallas, Texas) uses 4 ml/kg/% burns/24 hours. The actual amount given is dependent upon clinical response and urine output. Volumes of 5–6 ml/kg/% burns/24 hours have been found to be necessary if inhalation injury coexists with the cutaneous burn.

Airway Obstruction may be immediate or delayed. There may be burning around the mouth, nose, face and hair. Circumferential burns of the trunk may later interfere with breathing. Inhalation injuries may require humidified oxygen, antibiotics, steroids, intubation and ventilation. Tracheostomy should be avoided as it increases the chance of lung infection.

Anaemia This may result from direct destruction of red cells in the burning process. In extensive full thickness burns, blood may be given as part of a fluid 'ration'. Later, anaemia may occur from toxic depression of bone marrow especially if infection supervenes.

Infection Regular swabs should be taken. Prophylactic antibiotics are not usually indicated. The usual causes of sepsis are staphylococci, streptococci, and pseudomonas. Antibiotics should be given on the basis of culture and sensitivity.

Stress ulcers (Curling's ulcer) Prophylactic sucralfate or H_2 receptor antagonists should be given.

Renal failure This may occur and be due to delayed resuscitation, or myoglobinuria from muscle destruction. Ensure adequate CVP. Treat with mannitol, frusemide, dopamine. Haemodialysis may be required.

Nutrition Oral feeding via a nasogastric tube is preferred.

HAND INJURIES

The hand is a sophisticated mechanism from both motor and sensory considerations. Its importance is reflected in the size of its representation in the cerebral cortex. All hand injuries and infections should be referred to a specialist hand surgeon, usually a plastic or orthopaedic surgeon. Often joint management between both is necessary. Expert care is necessary from the outset to preserve or restore function. Careful history and examination are essential. Compensation claims or medicolegal problems may arise later. Accurate notes are essential.

PRINCIPLES OF MANAGEMENT

At place of injury

- Stop any bleeding by direct pressure. Never apply a tourniquet.
- Apply a clean, dry dressing.
- Do not bandage tightly.
- Save any avulsed or severed digit in a clean container. Cool with ice if possible (a bag of frozen peas will suffice). Place the digit on ice but do not cover in ice, in case the part gets frozen.

At hospital

History

- Age, occupation, dominant hand, any pre-existing anomaly or injury.
- The exact details of the injury – how it occurred, when it occurred, where it occurred. Risk of contamination.
- Treatment given at the site of accident.
- Tetanus prophylaxis status and allergies.
- Any drug history or past medical history.

Examination

- Skin loss and viability.
- Contamination.
- Swelling.
- Infection.
- Deformity – fractures, ligamentous injuries, flexor and extensor tendon injuries.
- Nerve integrity.
- Vessel integrity.
- Other injuries.

Transfer Any avulsed or severed digit should be transferred to a sterile plastic bag and placed on crushed ice.

Prophylaxis against infection Use tetanus prophylaxis; antibiotic.

Surgery

Immediate surgical management Irrigation of wound. Debridement. Repair – nerves, tendons, vessels, bones, reimplantation of digits. Wound closure and drainage – never close incision under tension. Drain to avoid oedema, haematoma, and infection. Appropriate dressings and splintage – dynamic splints may counteract deformity and assist weakened movements. Splint in the position of function. Elevation to prevent oedema. Physiotherapy – active exercises. *Never* force passive movements.

Delayed primary repair The injury is explored, cleaned and damaged structures identified at the time of injury. The skin is sutured and the hand splinted and elevated. The repair procedures are then carried out in a specialist centre as an elective procedure within 3 weeks of initial surgery. This procedure is used where there is initial gross contamination, or specialist skills are not immediately available. Every effort should be made to arrange immediate referral to a specialist centre.

Reconstructive surgery This may be required because of:

- extensive injury
- lack of opportunity for early exploration because of late diagnosis or late referral to a specialist centre.

The hand is splinted in the position of optimal function and mobilized by active or assisted active movement. When scarring has healed and the tissues are supple, reconstruction is carried out.

Rehabilitation This should start as soon as possible. A painful, stiff hand should be avoided. Appropriate early treatment is wasted unless early physiotherapy and occupational therapy are instituted. Career counselling may be appropriate.

HAND INFECTIONS

The incidence and severity of hand infections have decreased in the past two decades owing to earlier presentation and more appropriate treatment with antibiotics. The gross infections of the palmar spaces seen in the pre-antibiotic era are rare today. However, they should be recognized and treated appropriately to avoid long-term or permanent disability to the hand. Care should be taken with hand infections in patients with already compromising conditions, e.g. steroids, immunosuppressive therapy, diabetes, rheumatoid arthritis and other collagen diseases, and patients with poor peripheral circulation, e.g. Raynaud's phenomenon.

Paronychia (whitlow)

In this condition pus accumulates between the cuticle (eponychium) and the nail matrix. The pus tracks round the nail margin or under the nail. The causative organism is usually *Staph. aureus*. In chronic cases, candida may be responsible. In the acute case, spontaneous rupture may occur. If it is treated early, antibiotics and rest may suffice. Often surgical drainage is required. Incision is through the nail fold. Removal of the base of the nail may be necessary if pus is trapped beneath it. Chronic paronychia requires swabs and scrapings. If fungus is located, long-term oral antifungal agents may be used or the nail may be avulsed followed by application of a topical antifungal agent as the nail regrows.

Pulp space infection (felon)

The origin of the infection is usually a minor penetrating injury. Pressure builds up in the pulp space with oedema and suppuration, and the terminal branches of the digital vessel may thrombose owing to pressure from the pus. Necrosis and osteomyelitis of the terminal phalanx may result. Treatment is by surgical drainage via a longitudinal incision over the point of maximum tenderness. Antistaphylococcal antibiotics should be given.

Suppurative tenosynovitis

This is most common in the flexors of the fingers. Organisms reach the tendon sheath either from a direct puncture wound, or by extension from an undrained pulp space infection. An exudate which becomes purulent forms in the sheath and, if untreated, may discharge and infect the palmar spaces.

Symptoms and signs Following minor injury there is rapid onset of pain and swelling. The finger is held semiflexed and attempts at extension cause severe pain. Eventually a red, hot exquisitely tender finger results.

Treatment In early stages, i.v. antistaphylococcal antibiotics, rest and elevation may suffice. If there is no improvement in 24 hours or pus is present at presentation, the tendon sheath should be opened proximally and distally and a fine catheter passed down the sheath and irrigation with antibiotic solution carried out. Rest, elevation and systemic antibiotics should be given. Active exercises should be undertaken as pain subsides.

Deep palmar space infection

This is rare and may arise as a result of penetrating trauma, infection of a callosity, or as a complication of suppurative tenosynovitis. The infection occurs in the space deep to the flexor tendons but superficial to the interossei. The deep palmar space is divided into two by a septum attached to the third metacarpal. The space medial to the septum is the midpalmar space, the space lateral is the thenar space.

Symptoms and signs Oedema of the dorsum of the hand. The skin is looser here and the swelling initially forms on the dorsum of the hand although the infection is on the palm. Ballooning of the palm or thenar eminence. Acute throbbing pain. Fingers held flexed. Attempts at extension painful. Pain on pressure over affected space. Fever. Malaise.

Treatment Incision and drainage. The midpalmar space is drained by an incision in the web space between the fourth and fifth or third and fourth metacarpal heads. The thenar space is opened by an incision posteriorly in the web space between the thumb and index finger. Rest. Elevation. Anti-staphylococcal antibiotics.

Bites

Human or animal bites to the hand are serious. Most human 'bites' are the result of teeth and knuckles coming into contact in a fight. They frequently become infected, always with oral commensals, predominately anaerobic bacteria. Dog bites are common, and usually cause more extensive injury than human bites.

Symptoms and signs Obvious with dog bites. Check for teeth marks on the hand particularly the knuckle area after fights. Remember love bites may occur in strange places. Oedema, cellulitis, and frank suppuration may be apparent with delayed presentation.

Treatment Antibiotic and tetanus prophylaxis. Explore all wounds where the skin is breached. Remove foreign bodies or tooth fragments. Take swabs for bacteriology. With extensive dog bites excise any ragged areas of skin. Avoid primary closure. Elevate the hand postoperatively. If nerves or tendons are damaged, delayed repair is more appropriate.

COSMETIC SURGERY

In assessing a patient for cosmetic surgery the surgeon must assess the effect that the 'abnormality' is having on the patient and whether or not surgery will be truly beneficial. In many cases the patient wants a surgical improvement on nature or control of the natural ageing process. The patient must understand that whilst surgery may alter the appearance it rarely alters the person. In some cases a formal psychological assessment may be appropriate prior to surgery. The decision to operate on bat ears in a child who is the subject of taunts at school is easy, while to alter the facial appearance of a young woman simply because she does not like the way she looks is more difficult.

The following are some indications for cosmetic surgery.

RECONSTRUCTIVE BREAST SURGERY

Augmentation mammaplasty

Indications Small breasts (developmental or involutional after pregnancies); breast asymmetry with hypoplasia of one breast.

Treatment By silicone implant with textured silicone envelopes containing silicone gel. Implants may be placed in the plane between the breast and the underlying pectoralis major muscle or under pectoralis major via a submammary approach. Prophylactic antibiotics are usually given to prevent infection.

Complications Infection. Haematoma. Development of a firm capsule around the prosthesis may lead to distortion of the breast and discomfort. The latter complication is rare with the present textured prostheses. Silicone gel may leak out of the implant. There is no evidence that silicone prostheses increase the incidence of carcinoma.

Reduction mammaplasty

Indications Abnormally large breasts may cause backache, neck ache, intertrigo. Interfere with active sports. Taunts and sexual harassment.

Treatment Several techniques are available. All involve removal of breast tissue with transposition of the nipple and areolar to a higher level. Care must be taken to preserve the blood supply to the nipple. In very large breasts a free nipple graft may be required. Excised breast tissue should be examined to exclude an occult carcinoma. Surgical results are good and the satisfaction rate among patients is high.

Complications Haematoma, infection, nipple or flap necrosis.

Reconstruction following mastectomy

This may be carried out at the same time as mastectomy or several months later. If the soft tissue is adequate and pectoralis major has been preserved, the breast can be reconstructed with a silicone implant. A tissue expander may be necessary to form a space to insert a prosthesis later. If there has been extensive surgery and pectoralis major has been removed, reconstruction with vascularized tissue is required. A latissimus dorsi myocutaneous flap is most commonly used but myocutaneous flaps based on the rectus muscle (TRAM) may be used although they have a higher complication rate. Reconstruction of the nipple and areola may be carried out at a later stage.

Gynaecomastia

Treatment is by excision of breast tissue to restore the normal breast contour, preserving the nipple. A circumareolar incision is used when possible.

OTHER TYPES OF SUGERY

Rhinoplasty

This is correction of congenital or acquired nasal defects. It may be carried out for cosmetic or functional reasons (breathing difficulties). Controlled nasal bone fracture is combined with excision of varying amounts of bone and cartilage. Usually the operation is carried out totally through intranasal incisions. Complications are uncommon, the chief one being bleeding.

Bat ears

A child with bat ears is usually taunted at school. The operation should be carried out at about 7 years as the ear cartilage is actively growing up to this time.

Blepharoplasty

This is used to treat 'baggy' eyelids and involves removal of excess eyelid skin and fat through upper and/or lower lid skin crease incisions. The commonest complication is haematoma formation, although removal of too much skin from the lower eyelid may result in ectropion (out-turned lower eyelid) with a watery eye that is difficult to correct.

Face lift

This is used to treat the 'ageing face'. The skin of the face and neck is undermined following preauricular and postauricular incisions. Excess skin is excised at hair-bearing areas thus hiding the suture line. The skin of the face and neck are tightened smoothing out wrinkles and giving a more youthful appearance. Complications include haematoma, skin necrosis, infection and damage to branches of the facial nerve. The large majority of these operations are carried out in the private sector.

Apronectomy (abdominal dermolipectomy)

This is excision of excess abdominal skin and fat. It is indicated in the grossly obese and in women who have had repeated pregnancies where there are redundant skin folds and a lax anterior abdominal wall. For some minor or moderate degrees of tissue laxity a limited transverse lower abdominal excision may be sufficient (combined with umbilical transposition). When the operation is carried out after gastric partitioning operations or after massive weight loss a 'fleur de lys' excision pattern is used leaving a very obvious inverted T shaped scar. Apronectomy is not a substitute for the patient dieting.

Liposuction

This is carried out for the removal of localized deposits of fat, e.g. hips, thighs, buttocks. It is not indicated for generalized obesity and is therefore not a weight-reduction procedure. Cannulae are inserted through remote stab incisions and the subcutaneous fat removed through a series of tunnels using high-vacuum suction. Complications are rare, the chief problem being uneven removal of fat. Temporary numbness and bruising may occur. Occasionally when large amounts of fat are removed significant fluid replacement is required to prevent hypovolaemia.

Collagen injections

These are used for correcting localized irregularities of body contours usually on the face. The effect lasts up to 6 months. Repeated injections are required.

TISSUE EXPANSION

The principle involves localized stretching of the skin using an inflatable silicone implant which is surgically implanted underneath normal skin adjacent to the tissue that is to be excised. Over the ensuing weeks the implant is inflated through a remote valve by injecting normal saline. Once sufficient skin expansion has been produced, the silicone expander is removed, the lesion excised and the defect is repaired with the excess skin produced by the expander. Basically, a skin flap has been created at an adjacent site to the defect, which allows repair of the defect. The time required to inflate the balloon in order to produce more skin may take anywhere from 4 weeks to 6 months and depends on the site, amount of skin required and the age of the patient. The patient has to attend hospital at least twice weekly to have the expander further inflated. Complications include haematoma, infection and an erosion of the device through the skin. There are very few areas in which tissue expanders cannot be used. For example, they may be used:

- to replace hair-bearing scalp where there has been extensive hair loss from trauma, adjacent hair-bearing skin being expanded to replace the defect
- to allow expansion of skin following mastectomy prior to insertion of a permanent prosthesis
- in tattoo removal
- in facial reconstruction.

20
Paediatric surgery

This chapter will cover some of the paediatric surgical emergencies which arise in the newborn and also the more common paediatric surgical problems presenting at outpatient departments and common paediatric surgical emergencies.

ALIMENTARY TRACT EMERGENCIES IN THE NEWBORN

Oesophageal atresia

The commonest type is a blind-ended, upper oesophagus associated with a tracheo-oesophageal fistula involving the lower oesophagus (→ Fig. 20.1). Oesophageal atresia may occur alone or with a tracheo-oesophageal fistula. The incidence is approximately 1 : 3000 births. There may be coexisting anomalies of the heart, kidneys and intestines.

Symptoms and signs Association with maternal polyhydramnios. Dribbling of saliva, inability to swallow feeds, production of frothy mucus, choking, cyanotic attacks, aspiration pneumonia.

Investigations • Pass an orogastric tube – it will arrest at the obstruction • CXR including neck to see the position of tube at obstruction: cardiac anomalies, aspiration pneumonia • AXR: gas in stomach and intestine will indicate the presence of a tracheo-oesophageal fistula.

Treatment Rehydration. Treat any chest infection. Keep upper oesophageal pouch empty by continuous aspiration. Urgent surgical ligation of tracheo-oesophageal fistula and correction of atresia by primary end-to-end anastomosis of the oesophagus.

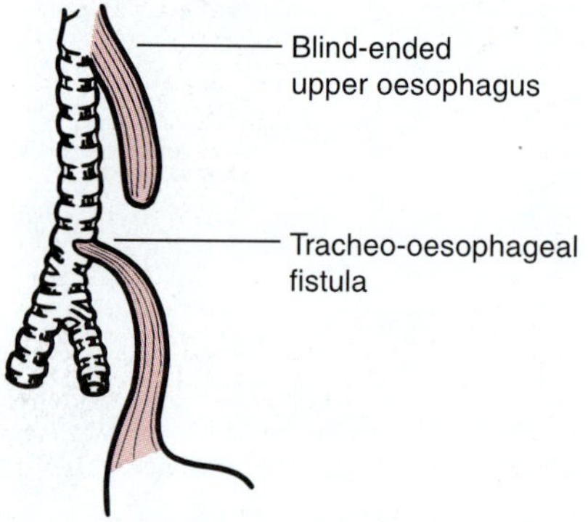

Fig. 20.1 The commonest form of oesophageal atresia.

Prognosis There is a 90% survival in regional paediatric surgical centres in the UK.

Duodenal atresia

This occurs in 1 : 6000 births. The common bile duct may open proximal or distal to an atresia. There is an association with Down's syndrome and congenital heart disease.

Symptoms and signs Associated with maternal polyhydramnios. Vomiting in first few hours of life usually bile-stained.

Investigations • Antenatal diagnosis is possible with USS • AXR shows 'double bubble' sign, i.e. gas bubble and fluid level on each side of upper abdomen owing to gas in stomach and proximal duodenum (→ Fig. 20.2).

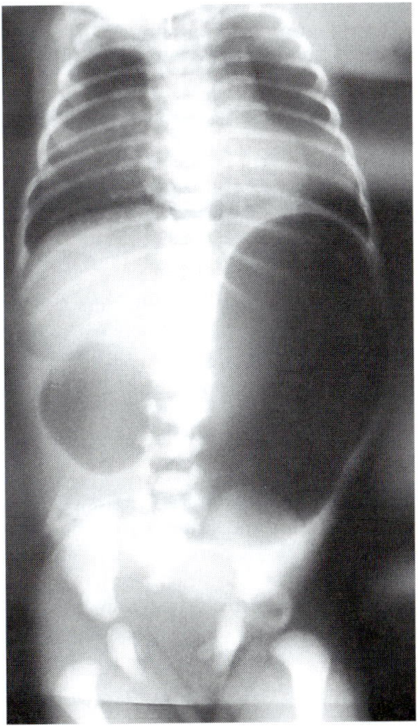

Fig. 20.2 Duodenal atresia. AXR with 'double bubble' gas sign and no gas pattern beyond the duodenum.

Treatment Rehydration. Urgent surgery. Duodenoduodenostomy, i.e. a side-to-side anastomosis between proximal and distal duodenal segments.

Prognosis Mortality depends on associated abnormalities and is high with Down's syndrome and cardiac anomalies.

Small bowel atresia

The incidence is 1 : 20 000 births in the UK. It is somewhat more common in other parts of the world. It may occur at any level and may be multiple.

Signs and symptoms Bilious vomiting. Abdominal distension. Visible peristalsis.

Investigations • AXR: distended bowel with fluid levels.

Treatment Rehydration. Urgent surgery. Resection of areas of atresia or stenosis with end-to-end anastomosis.

Malrotation (volvulus neonatorum)

In the first trimester, the midgut herniates outside the abdominal cavity but returns at the end of the third month, rotating as it does so. Several rotational abnormalities may result. Obstruction may consequently result from a variety of causes from peritoneal bands to volvulus of the midgut. Failure of normal rotation invariably occurs in patients with exomphalos and diaphragmatic hernia.

Symptoms and signs Bile-stained vomiting and abdominal distension. The symptoms are similar initially to duodenal atresia. However, volvulus will lead to venous and subsequently arterial obstruction, gut infarction and consequent potential short bowel syndrome.

Investigations • USS to identify mesenteric vein/artery relations – the position of the vein and artery in relation to one another changes with rotation • Contrast meal: abnormally placed duodenojejunal junction • Contrast enema: may show abnormally placed caecum but the latter may also be normal in position.

Treatment Emergency laparotomy. Untwist the volvulus. Tease out mesenteric base to prevent recurrence. Excise any gangrenous bowel.

Meconium ileus

This occurs in 15% of patients with cystic fibrosis. Meconium becomes inspissated in the terminal ileum with soft meconium above associated with distended proximal small bowel.

Symptoms and signs Infant born with distended abdomen. Bilious vomiting. Meconium is not passed and the rectum is empty.

Investigations • AXR: dilated loops of bowel • Gastrograffin enema will show an empty colon and may relieve the obstruction by refluxing into the terminal ileum and 'loosening' the meconium • Prenatal diagnosis may be made with USS.

Treatment 50% may have associated atresia, perforation, or volvulus and then laparotomy is required. The terminal ileum is opened and the inspissated meconium washed out. A temporary ileostomy may be required.

Complications Meconium peritonitis. May occur in utero or postnatally. The chemical peritonitis resulting is treated by peritoneal lavage and repair of the perforation. The mortality rate is 10%.

Anorectal abnormalities

These occur with an incidence of 1 : 5000 births. Management depends on accurate definition of the abnormality.

Symptoms and signs Infant fails to pass meconium. Rectal inspection reveals imperforate anus or other abnormality. There may be associated abnormalities of the GU system.

Investigations • Tape a metal marker over the anus (or if absent, anal dimple) • Place infant in knee–elbow position for 2 minutes and take a lateral shoot-through pelvic radiograph • Assess the distance between the gas shadow and metal marker.

Treatment Low lesions can be treated by a simple anoplasty. Higher lesions should be managed with a sigmoid loop colostomy allowing further evaluation prior to a more complicated reconstructive procedure.

Necrotizing enterocolitis

This is an ischaemic disorder of the intestine of the newborn. The aetiology of the disease is unknown but bacterial infection, hypoxia and umbilical artery cannulation have been implicated. It is more common in premature infants and 'epidemics' have occurred on neonatal intensive therapy units suggesting an infective aetiology.

Symptoms and signs Diarrhoea, blood, mucus per rectum. Abdominal distension and bilious vomiting.

Investigations • AXR shows distension of bowel with fluid levels • Later, a diagnostic radiological sign is intramural gas indicative of bowel wall necrosis • Free gas confirms intestinal perforation.

Treatment This is initially non-operative unless perforation occurs. Resuscitation includes i.v. fluids and NG suction together with intravenous broad-spectrum antibiotics. Laparotomy is required if there is evidence of perforation or failure of patient to improve on medical treatment. Gangrenous bowel is excised with a temporary ileostomy or colostomy.

Prognosis The mortality rate is high in severe cases. Stricture may develop in healing bowel and present later.

Diaphragmatic hernia

This occurs with an incidence of 1 : 4000 births. A hernia may occur through the foramen of Bochdalek, i.e. a defect in the pleuroperitoneal canal; through the foramen of Morgagni, between the xiphoid and costal margin; through a deficiency in the central tendon; or through a congenitally large oesophageal hiatus. Herniae through the foramen of Bochdalek are most common. Normal development of the ipsilateral lung is impaired and that of the contralateral lung may also be impaired.

Symptoms and signs May be diagnosed by prenatal USS. Presents with respiratory distress at birth. Apex beat displaced. Bowel sounds in chest. Scaphoid abdomen if the hernia is large and most of the bowel is in the chest.

Investigations • CXR • AXR: mediastinal shift, abdominal viscera in thorax; lack of intestinal gas pattern in abdomen (→ Fig. 20.3).

Treatment Urgent respiratory assistance and maintenance of circulation. When ventilation is adequate and the patient is haemodynamically stable, closure of the defect is undertaken. May require prosthetic patch.

Prognosis Mortality is high especially with large defects and is due to consequences of pulmonary hypoplasia.

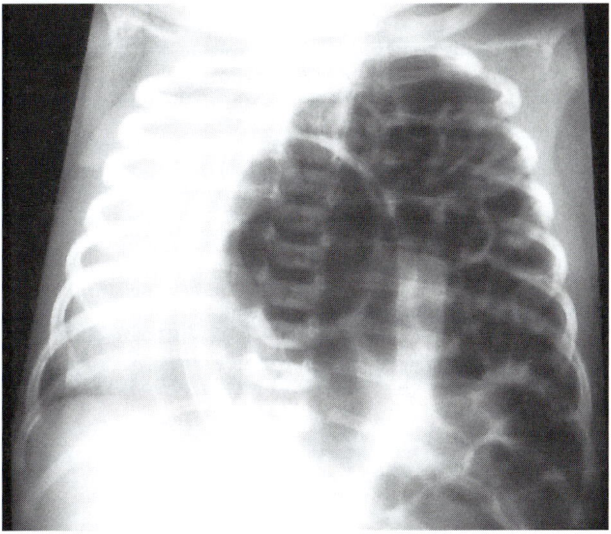

Fig. 20.3 CXR of a neonate with a left diaphragmatic hernia. Note the hypoplastic lungs, mediastinal shift to the right, and gas in abdominal viscera in the left chest.

Hirschsprung's disease

This occurs in 1 : 5000 births. There is a defect in the parasympathetic ganglia in the submucosal and myenteric plexus of the bowel wall. The aganglionic segment is present for a varying distance upwards from the anus and always involves the rectum. Rarely it affects the whole colon and even more rarely the small bowel. The peristaltic waves stop at the affected segment and the proximal bowel becomes dilated and hypertrophied. The aganglionic segment remains contracted. It is more common in males than females.

Symptoms and signs Delayed passage of meconium in the newborn period. However, presentation may be delayed, especially with short segment involvement, when it presents in infants and older children with constipation and abdominal distension. Digital rectal examination may demonstrate an empty rectum which feels 'tight' on the examining finger.

Investigations • AXR: dilated loops of bowel with fluid levels • Barium enema will demonstrate the level of obstruction • Rectal biopsy shows absence of ganglion cells.

Treatment

1. If the baby is healthy, and only rectosigmoid Hirschsprung's is suspected, it may be managed by regular rectal washouts to clear the bowel and early operation at 4–6 weeks, avoiding a colostomy if possible.
2. If the baby is ill and if a longer segment Hirschsprung's is suspected, then management is as follows:
   a. Initial defunctioning colostomy (normal innervation of the segment of bowel used for the colostomy should be confirmed by frozen section).
   b. Resection of the affected segment between 3 and 6 months of age and pull-through of the ganglionic bowel to the rectum.
   c. The defunctioning colostomy is closed 3–4 weeks later.

ABDOMINAL WALL DEFECTS

These occur with an incidence of 1 : 6000 births. There are two types, exomphalos and gastroschisis. Aetiology is unknown.

Gastroschisis

In this condition there is a defect in the abdominal wall immediately adjacent to the umbilicus but the abdominal wall itself is completely formed. Coils of gut have no protective covering and are thick, oedematous and matted together. The diagnosis is obvious at birth.

Treatment Primary closure of the defect may be possible after decompressing the gut and returning it to the peritoneal cavity. However, it may be necessary to cover the defect temporarily with a silastic sheet. Staged repair requires daily reduction of bowel into the peritoneal cavity, after which the defect may be repaired. It may be weeks or months before normal GI motility is restored and long-term TPN may be required.

Exomphalos

In this condition the opening is at the umbilicus. The umbilical cord coverings continue into a sac which covers the visceral protrusion. Chromosomal abnormalities, heart defects and also genitourinary malformations frequently occur, e.g. ectopia vesica and cloacal abnormalities. The condition is obvious at birth.

Treatment This is by either primary closure or staged repair with larger defects using a silastic sheet.

ALIMENTARY TRACT PROBLEMS IN OLDER INFANTS AND CHILDREN

Congenital hypertrophic pyloric stenosis

The aetiology of this condition is unknown. Progressive hypertrophy of the circular muscle of the pylorus occurs. The condition affects boys more than girls, being four times more common in boys, and occurs with an incidence of 1 in 4000 births. The first-born male child is most commonly affected. There is a familial tendency especially on the maternal side.

Symptoms and signs The infant thrives for the first 3–4 weeks of life and then presents with projectile vomiting after feeds. The vomit is rarely bile-stained. The infant is usually hungry and eager for further food after vomiting. Wasting is rare nowadays but weight loss and dehydration are presenting features.

Diagnosis This is clinical. A test feed is carried out. The abdomen is inspected for visible peristalsis passing from left to right across the epigastrium. Palpation is carried out during feeding for the classical 'lump' which is felt deep to the right rectus muscle in the RUQ. The 'lump' has the size and shape of an olive. Never sit facing the infant during this examination. You may experience the full impact of the projectile vomit.

Treatment Ramstedt's operation (pyloromyotomy). This is an elective operation and should be carried out only after correction of any dehydration and metabolic alkalosis. The stomach is emptied via an NG tube and saline lavage. The pylorus is exposed through an upper, right transverse abdominal incision. It is then incised longitudinally along its anterosuperior border. The incision is deepened by blunt dissection until the mucosa pouts out.

Complications Postoperative recovery is rapid. There should be no mortality. Morbidity relates to accidental mucosal perforation which if unrecognized at the time of surgery will lead to peritonitis.

Intussusception

This is the invagination of a portion of intestine into its lumen. It is commoner in children than adults. The peak incidence is between 6 and 9 months, although it may occur any time between 3 months and 2 years and occasionally in those younger and older than this age range. Most cases are ileocolic but ileo-ileal and ileo-ileocolic may occur. In most cases, the aetiology is unknown but hypertrophied Peyer's patches, polyps, Meckel's

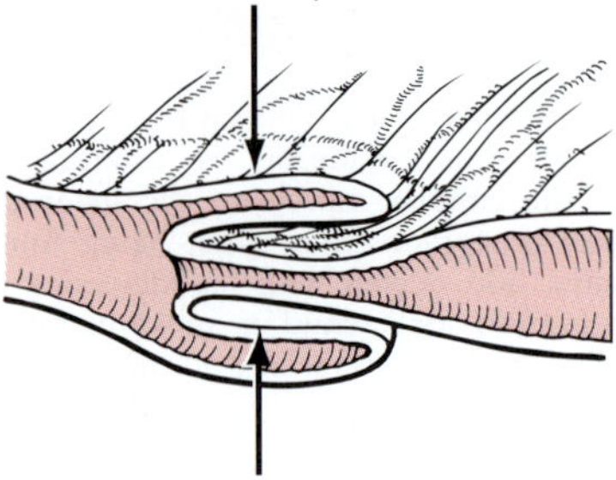

Fig. 20.4 An intussusception.

diverticulum or intramural haematomas (Henoch-Schönlein purpura) may be contributory. An intussusception is composed of three parts:

- the entering inner tube
- the returning or middle tube
- the sheath or outer tube.

The outer tube is called the intussuscipiens: the inner and middle tubes are called the intussusceptum (→ Fig. 20.4).

Symptoms and signs An otherwise healthy child presents with colicky abdominal pain and vomiting. The child often screams, draws up its knees to its chest, and goes pale with an attack of colic. In between bouts of pain the child appears normal. A first stool passed after onset of the pain may be normal but 30% of subsequent stools contain blood and mucus, the so-called 'redcurrant jelly stool'. Palpation of the abdomen reveals a palpable sausage-shaped mass in the line of the colon. An empty RIF may be apparent on palpation as the swelling moves into the upper abdomen with peristalsis. PR examination may reveal blood or mucus. Occasionally the apex of the intussusception may be palpable per rectum.

Investigations • AXR may show typical gas distribution and may show small bowel obstruction • USS or contrast enema (→ Fig. 20.5) • Adequate resuscitation with i.v. fluids.

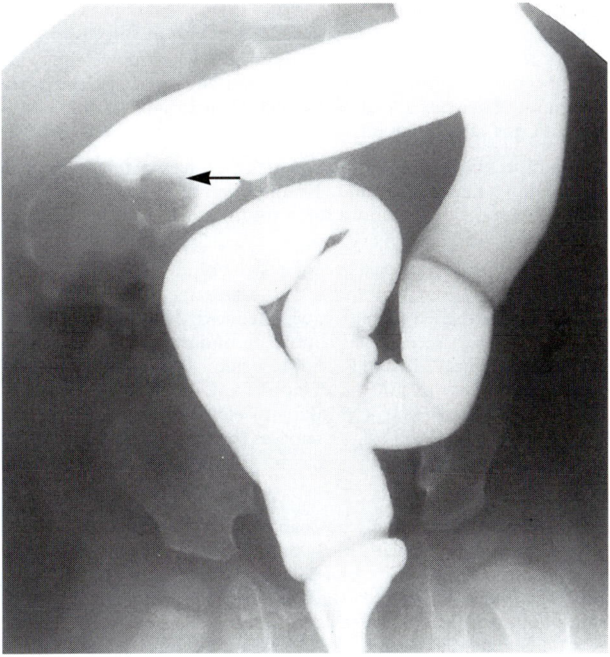

Fig. 20.5 Barium enema showing the typical appearance of an ileocolic intussusception. The ileum (arrow) has progressed as far as the proximal transverse colon.

Treatment At an early stage the intussusception may be reduced by the hydrostatic pressure of a contrast enema. Operation is required in patients with peritonitis, radiological signs of perforation, or failure of hydrostatic reduction. At operation, the intussusceptum is reduced by gentle retrograde reduction, squeezing the apex out of its containing bowel. Traction should not be applied to the proximal bowel. If the bowel cannot be reduced or is gangrenous, resection is required.

Prognosis Recurrence occurs in 1–2%. Mortality is very low if treatment occurs in the first 24 hours but increases if resection is required.

Obstructed inguinal hernia

This is a common cause of surgical admission in boys under the age of 2 years. It may also occur in girls when bowel or ovary may become irreducible. It is associated with a patent processus vaginalis. There is a high incidence in premature babies. The condition is often bilateral.

Symptoms and signs Mother usually notices a tense lump in the groin of her crying child. Examination reveals an irreducible lump which may extend into the scrotum.

Treatment If the lump is not red or tender, analgesia and sedation may be given and a gentle attempt made to reduce the hernia when the child is well sedated. If the hernia does not reduce, surgical repair should be undertaken. If infarcted bowel is found this must be resected. If the hernia does reduce, surgery should be delayed for 24–48 hours to allow oedema to resolve. It is prudent to electively repair inguinal herniae in young children as soon as they are discovered.

Acute appendicitis

This is dealt with more fully in Chapter 14. Certain points, however, are relevant to appendicitis in children. The condition is rare under the age of 6 months. The stool is liquid and the appendiceal lumen relatively wide. Therefore, acute obstructive appendicitis is rare. It does, however, occur and may present with diarrhoea and vomiting and consequently be mistaken for gastroenteritis. Careful and repeated examination is therefore essential.

Mesenteric adenitis

This is enlargement of mesenteric lymph nodes caused by an adenovirus infection. *Yersinia enterocolitica* has also been implicated. It affects young children and adolescents. Usually there is a preceding history of URTI, with sore throat and cervical lymphadenitis. Essentially, mesenteric adenitis is inflammation of Peyer's patches with secondary mesenteric lymphadenitis. The fever is usually higher than that of appendicitis, usually 38–39°C. The abdominal pain is more diffuse and examination reveals shifting tenderness rather than sharply localized tenderness in the RIF. Headache and mild photophobia may occur. These never occur in appendicitis. The WCC is usually raised but there is a relative lymphocytosis rather than neutrophil leukocytosis as seen in acute appendicitis. Treatment is symptomatic. If there is doubt over the diagnosis, appendicectomy is advisable.

Constipation

This is a common problem in children. The child is usually afebrile and relatively well despite the abdominal pain.

Urinary tract infections (UTIs)

There is abdominal pain and high pyrexia associated with dysuria, frequency and cloudy urine. Right pyelonephritis or cystitis may be mistaken for appendicitis. An FBC reveals neutrophil leukocytosis. An MSU and microscopy reveal cells and organisms. Beware the presence of cells alone. Pelvic appendicitis may irritate the bladder, producing frequency and pyuria but organisms will be absent on microscopy. Beware the presence of organisms *alone* as it may be due to contamination from the foreskin or vulva. Treatment of UTI is with appropriate antibiotics. Further investigation is with USS.

Lower lobar pneumonia

In this condition pain may be referred via the thoracic nerves to the lower abdomen. Right lower lobar pneumonia may refer pain to the RIF and be mistaken for acute appendicitis. It is important to observe the breathing pattern and auscultate the chest. Anteroposterior and lateral CXR will confirm diagnosis.

Testicular torsion

This may radiate to the iliac fossa. The child may be embarrassed to draw attention to scrotal symptoms. Always examine the scrotum in a child with abdominal pain.

Crohn's disease

Acute regional ileitis may occur in children.

Gynaecological problems

Remember pregnancy may occur in very young girls in this permissive society! Onset of periods may be associated with acute lower abdominal pain. Torsion of ovarian cyst or ovarian dermoid may occur.

INFANT WITH JAUNDICE

Neonates often develop physiological jaundice starting about 2 days after birth and lasting up to 2 weeks. Persistent jaundice beyond the first 3 weeks of life requires investigation. The two most common surgical causes are biliary atresia and choledochal cysts.

Biliary atresia

This occurs with an incidence of 1 : 25 000 live births. The aetiology is unknown. It appears to develop after birth.

Symptoms and signs It presents from 4 weeks to 4 months. Usually healthy child with jaundice. Jaundice may be intermittent. Pale stools. Dark urine. Later hepatosplenomegaly, ascites. Without treatment, death from liver failure occurs within 2 years.

Investigations • LFTs • USS: dilated ducts, absent gall bladder • Liver biopsy: bile duct proliferation with hepatocellular necrosis • Isotope scan demonstrates absence of bile drainage • Diagnostic laparotomy with operative cholangiography – if a normal duct system is demonstrated, hepatitis should be suspected as a diagnosis • α_1-antitrypsin deficiency and cystic fibrosis must also be excluded.

Treatment If an extrahepatic duct can be found a Roux loop of jejunum is anastomosed to it – this is called correctable biliary atresia. If an extrahepatic duct cannot be found (incorrectable biliary atresia), a hepatoportal enterostomy (Kasai procedure) is carried out. A patent duct is exposed in the porta hepatis and a Roux loop anastomosed to it. Intrahepatic biliary atresia (total absence of intrahepatic ducts) requires liver transplantation.

Prognosis Good with correctable form. Incorrectable extrahepatic and intrahepatic forms have a poor prognosis but this may be improved with a more widespread use of liver transplantation.

Choledochal cyst

Cystic dilatation of the bile ducts is usually extrahepatic involving the common bile duct. The aetiology is unknown.

Symptoms and signs It occurs between 3 months and adult life. More common in females. Pain, jaundice, abdominal mass.

Investigations • LFTs • USS • ERCP.

Treatment Excision of CBD with Roux choledochojejunostomy. Severe forms with involvement of the intrahepatic ducts require liver transplantation. Residual CBD can develop malignancy.

ABDOMINAL MASSES IN CHILDHOOD

An abdominal mass is an uncommon reason for surgical referral in children. (For causes → Table 20.1.)

Table 20.1
Abdominal masses in childhood

Gastrointestinal system	Pylorus (congenital pyloric stenosis) Crohn's disease Constipation (faecal masses) Intussusception
Hepato-pancreatico-biliary system	
Liver	Biliary atresia Portal hypertension Metastases Hepatitis Hepatoblastoma
Bile duct	Choledochal cyst
Pancreas	Pseudocyst (traumatic)
Genitourinary system	Hydronephrosis Nephroblastoma (Wilms') Bladder (urethral valves) Ovarian tumour or cyst
Other	Neuroblastoma Splenomegaly Retroperitoneal sarcoma Teratoma

Symptoms and signs In addition to the mass, failure to thrive, nausea, vomiting, weight loss, abdominal pain, constipation, diarrhoea. Anaemia. Jaundice. Uraemia. UTI symptoms. Spontaneous bruising.

Investigations • Hb • FBC • ESR • U&Es • LFTs • Urinalysis: 24-hour urine (VMA in neuroblastoma) • α-fetoprotein (tumour marker for teratoma and hepatoblastoma) • AXR • CXR (metastases) • USS: solid-v-cystic lesions • CT scan: solid-v-cystic spread • Bone scan, bone marrow aspirate • Biopsy.

Treatment This is of the underlying cause.

ABDOMINAL MALIGNANCIES IN CHILDHOOD

The commonest are neuroblastoma and nephroblastoma (Wilms' tumour). Neuroblastoma is the commonest extracerebral malignant solid tumour in children. Wilms' tumour accounts for about 10% of all the childhood tumours.

Abdominal neuroblastoma

This is a highly malignant tumour arising from the neural crest. The commonest site is the adrenal gland. It occurs in children under the age of 5. 70% occur under 1 year. Metastases occur early.

Symptoms and signs Abdominal mass. Failure to thrive. Anorexia, nausea, vomiting, diarrhoea. Metastases occur to liver, orbit, skull, long bones, spinal canal. Fever. Abdominal mass has a hard irregular surface and tendency to cross midline.

Investigations • AXR: calcification • USS: solid lesion • CT with contrast: size, site and metastases, and demonstrates displaced kidney • 24-hour urine VMA and HVA grossly elevated.

Treatment Localized tumours are excised. Unresectable primary and metastases require combination chemotherapy. Irradiation may be necessary. In neonates, tumour regression may be permanent. The older the child the worse the prognosis.

Nephroblastoma (Wilms' tumour)

This is an embryonic tumour of the kidney. The majority occur in the first 3 years of life. Less than 5% are bilateral. Metastases occur to the liver, lungs and regional nodes.

Signs and symptoms Abdominal mass. Pain. Haematuria. Weight loss. Pyrexia. May be associated with abnormalities of the GU tract. Aniridia.

Investigations • IVU: space-occupying lesion • USS: solid tumour • CT (→ Fig. 20.6): size, site, metastases.

Treatment Surgical excision. Chemotherapy with or without radiotherapy depending on the stage. 80–90% chance of cure. If the condition is bilateral dialysis will be required unless partial nephrectomy is possible. If there is no evidence of recurrence after 2 years renal transplantation is indicated.

RECTAL BLEEDING IN CHILDREN

This is not an uncommon problem. Causes include fissure-in-ano, rectal polyps, rectal prolapse, Meckel's diverticulum, intussusception and blood dyscrasia.

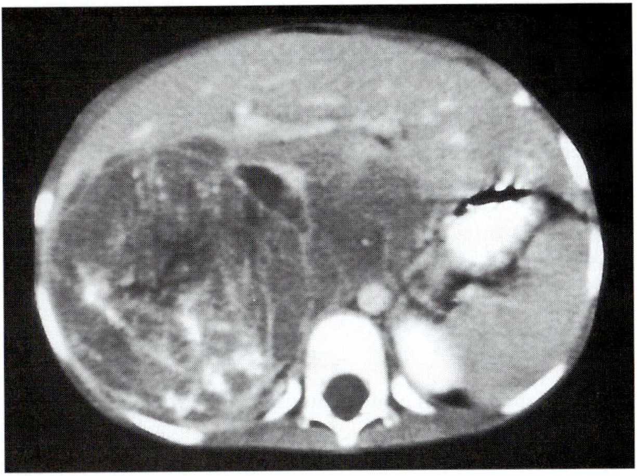

Fig. 20.6 An abdominal CT scan of a child with an abdominal mass. There is an extensive nephroblastoma (Wilms' tumour) of the right kidney.

Fissure-in-ano

Constipation causes a split in the mucosa of the anal canal. It is usually painful on defaecation. A vicious circle occurs with worsening constipation owing to fear of defaecation. There is blood on the stool and toilet paper. The fissure is often in the midline, usually posteriorly. Treatment involves explanation of the condition to the parent. Lactulose helps to relieve constipation, and LA is applied locally before and after defaecation. Most cases settle on this regimen. Persistent fissures require exclusion of Crohn's disease and TB.

Polyps

In addition to bleeding they may prolapse on their stalk if they are low enough in the rectum. Occasionally they may twist and auto-amputate and are passed PR. Occasionally they may precipitate intussusception. Treatment is by excision. If they are in the rectum, this may be done under GA using a proctoscope, the stalk being cut with diathermy. Higher polyps can be snared at colonoscopy.

Rectal prolapse

This usually occurs around 2 years. Most cases settle spontaneously. Straining at stool precipitates the condition initially which may then occur every time the child defaecates.

There may be an underlying abnormality, e.g. spina bifida, previous anoplasty for imperforate anus or cystic fibrosis. Prolapse may involve the mucosa only or may involve the full thickness of the rectum.

Symptoms and signs Usually prolapse occurs with defaecation and returns spontaneously. The prolapsed mucosa may ulcerate and bleed.

Treatment May settle spontaneously with toilet training and laxatives to relieve constipation. Persistent mucosal prolapse may be treated by submucosal injection of phenol in almond oil. Rarely rectopexy may be required.

Meckel's diverticulum

This is a remnant of the vitellointestinal duct which was attached to the umbilicus and is found on the antimesenteric border of the terminal ileum about 60 cm from the ileocaecal valve in an adult and proportionately nearer in a child. Rarely this may bleed if it contains gastric mucosa which produces acid and ulcerates the adjacent small bowel mucosa. This may cause either bright red or dark red bleeding depending upon the degree of haemorrhage. Abdominal pain is usually absent. The presence of gastric mucosa in a Meckel's diverticulum may be demonstrated by a technetium scan. Treatment is by excision.

Intussusception

In this condition, rectal bleeding may occur and is classically the appearance of a redcurrant jelly stool associated with attacks of abdominal pain. (For treatment of this condition → p. 479.)

General investigation of child with rectal bleeding

Full history and examination. Often the cause is obvious and no further investigation is required • Hb • FBC • Clotting screen • Examination under anaesthesia including PR, proctoscopy, sigmoidoscopy and colonoscopy under GA • Barium enema • Technetium scan.

Treatment This is of the underlying condition as indicated above.

CHRONIC AND RECURRENT ABDOMINAL PAIN

This is a common problem in children of school age and many are referred to general surgery clinics. In many cases the pain has a non-organic basis. Organic causes include chronic constipation, Crohn's disease, UTIs, hydronephrosis, peptic ulceration and, rarely, gallstones (may be associated with haemolytic anaemia). If the child has had previous abdominal surgery, adhesions may be responsible. It is the author's opinion that chronic and recurrent abdominal pain in children should initially be referred to a paediatrician and subsequently referred to a surgeon if necessary. The reader is referred to a textbook of paediatrics for further discussion of this topic.

NECK LUMPS IN CHILDREN

The general management of lumps in the neck is dealt with in Chapter 8. However, lumps in the neck are common in children, the most common cause being due to reactive lymphadenitis secondary to tonsillitis. The other causes of lumps in the neck in children are shown in Table 20.2.

Table 20.2
Lumps in the neck in childhood

Anterior triangle	Lymph nodes: • primary infection, e.g. atypical mycobacterium, TB, toxoplasmosis • secondary infection, e.g. lymphadenitis • primary tumours, e.g. Hodgkin's, leukaemia • secondary tumour – rare Thyroglossal cyst Dermoid cyst Goitre Submandibular gland Branchial arch remnant
Posterior triangle	Lymph nodes Cystic hygroma (lymphangioma) Sternomastoid tumour Parotid swelling

Symptoms and signs Child may otherwise be well. Malaise. Pyrexia. Lethargy. Weight loss. Bruising. Bleeding. Rash. Cough. Signs of URTI, tonsillitis, inflamed tympanic membrane. Examine head and neck thoroughly for sites of primary lesion (infective or neoplastic). Check for lymphadenopathy elsewhere. Check for hepatosplenomegaly.

Investigations • Hb • FBC • ESR • U&Es • LFTs • TFTs (goitre) • Paul Bunnell • Toxoplasmosis screen • Mantoux • CXR • USS of lump • CT: lump, spread.

Treatment This is of the underlying disorder.

21

Organ and tissue transplantation

Transplantation has developed from an experimental procedure of 30 years ago to an established therapeutic option for most types of end-stage organ failure. For kidney, heart and liver transplantation a 1-year graft survival in excess of 80% can be expected.

CLASSIFICATION

This depends on the relationship between donor and recipient.

Autograft Tissue is transferred from one area of the body to another in the same individual, e.g. skin grafts.

Isografts Tissue is transferred between genetically identical individuals (e.g. monozygotic twins).

Allografts Tissue is transferred between genetically dissimilar individuals of the same species (e.g. cadaver renal transplants).

Xenografts Tissue is transferred between species. The only clinically applicable xenografts at the present time are temporary porcine skin grafts in human burns victims.

ORGAN AND TISSUE DONORS

LIVE RELATED DONORS

This type of organ donation relates chiefly to renal transplantation although it is now possible to transplant segments of pancreas, lobes of liver, and lobes of lung from living donors. In the past only 5% of kidney transplants in the UK have taken place from living donors although these numbers are increasing owing to the shortage of cadaver donors.

There are three potential histocompatibility matches:

- 'Perfect match' (2 haplotype match): all antigens match. There is a 25% chance of this occurring.
- 'Half match' (1 haplotype mismatch): half the antigens match. There is a 50% chance of this occurring.
- 'No match': no antigens match. There is a 25% chance of this occurring. In the past it was rare to use such a donor but it is now clear that the results from a 'no-matched' live related donor are almost as good as those from a well-matched cadaver donor.

The procedure of live-related donor transplantation and all its potential complications should be explained to the donor preferably with the next of kin present. Live related kidney donors must have a full medical and psychiatric assessment prior to donation.

Blood is taken initially for blood grouping and tissue typing. If this is compatible then a series of blood tests (i.e. Hb, FBC, ESR, U&Es, creatinine, LFTs, glucose) is carried out. Blood is also taken for hepatitis B, hepatitis C and HIV screening. A CXR and ECG are carried out. A crossmatch between donor lymphocytes and recipient's serum is also carried out. This test relates to the host lymphocyte immune response towards donor cellular antigens in vitro. If the reaction is positive then the transplant should not go ahead. If all the tests are satisfactory then the patient is admitted for arteriography. This is to assess that both kidneys are normal and that at least one of them has a single artery which is necessary for the anastomosis to the recipient's artery. Kidneys with multiple arteries may be used in cadaveric transplantation as they can be removed in these circumstances with a patch of aorta. However this clearly is not the case with a live donor. The IVU phase of the arteriogram checks for any abnormality in the excretory system.

LIVER UNRELATED DONORS

Recent experience has shown that transplants from non-blood relatives can often be as successful as those from blood relatives. At the present time, anyone with a close personal relationship, such as husbands, wives, partners or very close friends may be considered as possible donors. Live unrelated organ donation is strictly controlled by the Unrelated Live Transplant Regulatory Authority (ULTRA). Basically the procedures for organ donation with live unrelated donors are exactly the same as those for live related donors as outlined above. It is, however, important to ensure that no financial or other pressure is being put on the donor to donate. The last point is very important. To ensure that the donor's freedom is not abused, the law requires ULTRA to consider all proposed transplants between living people who are not close blood relatives. In addition to a full medical examination and explanation of the risks, an independent assessment has to be carried out. Both donor and recipient will be asked to see an independent assessor who is neither responsible for the recipient nor a member of the team who will do the transplant. The assessor has to make sure that the donor understands what is involved and to be sure about the reasons for wanting to donate and check that the donor is not under any form of pressure. The assessor also interviews the potential recipient. The assessor will send a report to ULTRA so they can check that there is no possible exploitation of the donor.

ULTRA need to be aware of the following:

- That the donor has not been paid to donate and has not been subjected to any other pressure. However, it is possible for the donor to be reimbursed legitimate expenses such as loss of earnings.
- That the doctor who asks for approval from ULTRA is acting on behalf of the donor.
- That both the donor and the recipient have been seen by the Independent Assessor and have been fully informed by the doctors responsible for both donor and recipient, that:
  a. the donor fully understands the nature and risks involved in donating an organ
  b. consent has been fully and freely given
  c. the donor is entitled to withdraw consent at any time before the operation.

CADAVER DONORS

General and specific criteria (→ Tables 21.1 and 21.2)

Selection of liver and heart and heart/lung donors depends on size match with the recipient. Also no attempt is made to match other than on blood group compatibility with these organs. HLA typing and crossmatching are not currently undertaken.

Obtaining permission for cadaver organ donation

1. A potential donor should be identified by the consultant in charge of the patient.

Table 21.1
General criteria for cadaver donors

Brainstem dead with intact circulation

Cause of death:
- cerebral trauma
- cerebral haemorrhage
- suicide
- primary cerebral tumour (histologically proven)
- cardiac arrest with brain death

Exclusions:
- malignancy
- HIV infection
- hepatitis B infection
- hepatitis C infection
- Creutzfeldt–Jakob disease (CJD)

Table 21.2
Specific criteria

Kidney	2–75 years with normal renal function
Heart	0–55 years with no cardiac disease
Heart/lung	0–55 years, non-smokers, no pulmonary disease including pulmonary oedema, acceptable blood gas levels
Liver	0–65 years, no liver disease or drug addiction
Pancreas	12–55 years, no history of diabetes, normal blood sugar
Corneas	No age limit, up to 24 hours after circulatory arrest, no history of corneal disease, no history of untreated viral infection at time of death, no history of neurological disease of unknown aetiology (e.g. multiple sclerosis, Alzheimer's disease or Creutzfeld–Jakob syndrome), few other contraindications (malignancy is not necessarily a contraindication)
Heart valves	0–65 years, no history of valve disease, can be removed up to 72 hours after circulatory arrest
Bone	18–60 years, no relevant medical history
Skin	0–70 years

2. Contact may be made with a transplant team prior to establishment of brainstem death to assess if the donor is suitable for organ donation.
3. The first set of brainstem death criteria are carried out. If they are satisfied the question of organ donation may be raised with the relatives. Consent should not be obtained until two sets of brainstem death criteria have been obtained.
4. If the relatives wish to know more about what is involved in transplantation, the Transplant Coordinators will speak to them and explain the details.
5. Blood is taken for tissue typing, blood group, HIV and hepatitis B and C screening.
6. Confidentiality must always be maintained.
7. Bereavement counselling and follow-up support should be arranged for the family; the Transplant Coordinators can help with this.

Tissue matching

ABO compatibility This must be present. Group O is a universal donor.

Human leukocyte antigen (HLA) matching HLA-A, B, C, D are on the short arm of chromosome 6. Attempts are made to match these antigens. They are important in live-related donor transplants, a perfect match giving a 1-year survival in excess of 95%. In cadaver transplantation the results are variable. In this context DR locus matching is important. A perfect match on the DR locus is associated with improved graft survival in cadaver transplants.

A cytotoxic crossmatch It must be negative. The recipient's blood is tested for cytotoxic antibodies against antigens on donor T lymphocytes. If such antibodies are present they would attach to and destroy the transplanted kidney, and therefore the donor is unacceptable.

ORGAN PRESERVATION

Organs are perfused with a balanced salt solution, e.g. hyperosmolar citrate at 4°C, and are stored surrounded by the same solution in sterile bags which in turn are surrounded by crushed ice.

Warm ischaemic time This is the time from cessation of circulation until perfusion with cold preservative. In heart-beating donors this time is theoretically zero.

Cold ischaemic time This is the time from perfusion with ice-cold preservative until circulation is re-established in the recipient. Table 21.3 shows appropriate times for warm and cold ischaemic time for different organs.

Table 21.3
Warm and cold ischaemic times

Organ	Warm	Cold
Kidney	30 min	Up to 48 h
Heart	0	Up to 4 h
Heart/lung	0	Up to 4 h
Lung	0	Up to 4 h
Liver	0	Up to 18 h
Small bowel	0	As soon as possible
Pancreas	0	Up to 12 h

SITING OF THE TRANSPLANT

Orthotopic The organ is situated in the place where the diseased organ had been, e.g. heart and liver transplantation.

Heterotopic The new organ is placed in a different site from the native organ, e.g. renal transplantation – the kidney is placed in the iliac fossa.

Paratopic The organ is placed alongside the native organ, e.g. pancreatic transplantation when the donor organ is placed in the lesser sac alongside the native pancreas.

REJECTION

There are four types of rejection.

Hyperacute This occurs with ABO incompatibility or preformed cytotoxic antibodies. It occurs on the operating table and in the case of the kidney it is seen to be flaccid, cyanotic and eventually thromboses. Nephrectomy is required, often at the time of transplantation or within 24 hours.

Accelerated acute rejection Rapid onset within a week of transplant. The success rate is poor.

Acute rejection This is the most common form of rejection and occurs within 3 months of transplantation. The kidney is infiltrated with T lymphocytes. This may be treated with methylprednisolone, ALG, ATG, or the monoclonal antibody OKT3.

Chronic rejection This is heralded by slow decline of renal function. Vascular intimal thickening occurs. The condition is untreatable.

IMMUNOSUPPRESSION

All transplant patients require immunosuppression for life. Large doses are given in the perioperative period but these are gradually scaled down to maintenance dose over a few months post-transplant. Drugs used include corticosteroids, antiproliferative drugs, e.g. azathioprine and mycophenolate mofetil, and calcineurin antagonists, e.g. cyclosporin and tacrolimus. Rejection episodes are treated with pulsed doses of methylprednisolone, ALG, ATG or monoclonal antibody. ALG, ATG or monoclonal antibodies may also be used prophylactically in high-risk or highly sensitized patients.

Corticosteroids *Prednisolone* is usually used in combination with cyclosporin or azathioprine. Prednisolone has multiple anti-inflammatory effects as well as immunosuppressive effects, the latter mainly the result of inhibition of cytokine production. Non-specific effect on cell-mediated and humoral immunity. Prednisolone is commonly given during transplantation and continued for at least the first few weeks. The dose is then gradually decreased or withdrawn to reduce the incidence of side-effects. Pulse doses of methylprednisolone are effective treatment for acute rejection episodes. The side-effects of corticosteroid include cushingoid features, hypertension, peptic ulceration, poor wound healing, osteoporosis, myopathy, cataracts, stunted growth, pancreatitis, avascular necrosis of bone, hyperglycaemia and diabetes, acne.

Antiproliferative drugs These include azathioprine which was the first widely used immunosuppressive drug and the newer drug, mycophenolate mofetil. Azathioprine is metabolized to 6-mercaptopurine by the liver and this in turn inhibits DNA and RNA synthesis by interfering with purine metabolism. In so doing it inhibits proliferation of lymphocytes in response to antigenic stimulation and impairs antibody production. Side-effects include nausea and vomiting, rashes, agranulocytosis, leukopenia, hepatic dysfunction, malignancy (especially skin malignancies and lymphoid tumours). Mycophenolate mofetil inhibits T and B cells by inhibiting an enzyme in the pathway of purine synthesis. It also prevents smooth muscle proliferation, which might have additional benefits for acute and chronic rejection. Its use is associated with a lower incidence of acute rejection episodes but the long-term results of this drug are unknown. The main side-effects of mycophenolate mofetil include haematological effects and gastrointestinal effects, particularly abdominal pain, diarrhoea and in some cases gastrointestinal haemorrhage.

Calcineurin antagonists These include cyclosporin and tacrolimus. Cyclosporin is a fungal metabolite that prevents the proliferation and clonal expansion of T lymphocytes by the inhibition of interleukin-2. It has considerably improved the results of organ transplantation since its introduction in 1983. The dose is titred to blood levels. Side-effects include nephrotoxicity, hypertension, hirsutism, tremor, gingival hyperplasia, hepatotoxicity. Tacrolimus has a similar mechanism to cyclosporin A but is considered more powerful. It is widely used in liver transplantation in which its greater water solubility and less dependence on bile salts absorption results in improved bioavailability. The side-effects of tacrolimus are similar to those of cyclosporin except that there is a lower incidence of hypertension, hirsutism, and gingival hyperplasia with tacrolimus.

Antilymphocyte globulin (ALG) and antithymocyte globulin (ATG) These are both prepared by immunizing animals with lymphocytes. Thymocytes are used to produce ATG. Antibody is collected and purified. The dose is monitored by T lymphocyte count in the peripheral blood. Complications include anaphylaxis and a high incidence of viral infection especially cytomegalovirus. ALG and ATG are used to treat acute rejection, or may be used prophylactically in highly sensitized patients.

Monoclonal antibody There are a large number of monoclonal antibodies directed against T cells and antigen-presenting cells. OKT3 is the most commonly used. It is specifically directed against T3 (CD3) antigen. It is used either as prophylaxis against rejection or for the treatment of acute rejection, especially when the patient is resistant to steroid. It is associated with pulmonary oedema if the patient is fluid overloaded. There is a higher incidence of herpes virus reactivation, opportunistic infections (cytomegalovirus and fungi), and Epstein–Barr-associated lymphoproliferative disorders and B cell lymphomas.

SPECIFIC ORGANS

KIDNEY TRANSPLANT

Recipient Almost any kidney disease is suitable for transplantation. Some diseases may recur in the transplant kidney, e.g. diabetic nephropathy, and membranoproliferative glomerulonephritis. If malignancy was the cause of renal failure, e.g. bilateral nephrectomy for Wilms' tumour or renal carcinoma, a period of time should be allowed for recurrence to occur. If it does not occur within that time period, then the patient is reassessed for transplantation.

Donor HLA typing is essential. Crossmatching should be negative. Kidneys can be safely kept for 36 hours, and occasionally up to 48 hours.

Operation This is heterotopic, the kidney being placed extraperitoneally in either the RIF or the LIF. The renal vein is anastomosed to the external iliac vein. The renal artery is anastomosed either end-to-end to the internal iliac artery or end-to-side to the external iliac artery. The ureter is anastomosed to the dome of the bladder. 70% of kidneys function immediately. 30% show delayed function due to ATN and require dialysis until the kidney begins to function.

Diagnosis of rejection

- Clinical general malaise, increased weight, decreased urine output.

- Laboratory: increased serum creatinine, decreased creatinine clearance.
- Radioisotope scan: DTPA shows reduced perfusion.
- Tru-cut needle biopsy.
- FNAC (in experienced hands).

Complications ATN, rejection, renal infarction due to renal artery or renal vein thrombosis, renal artery stenosis, urinary fistulae, ureteric obstruction. Lymphocele (a collection of lymph around the kidney which may compress the ureter causing ureteric obstruction).

Results

- 85–90% 1-year graft survival.
- 75% 5-year graft survival.

LIVER TRANSPLANT

Recipient Those with primary biliary cirrhosis, sclerosing cholangitis, chronic hepatitis, alcoholic cirrhosis, metabolic disease, biliary atresia in children. Hepatic resection where possible is preferred for malignant disease owing to the high recurrence rate post-transplant. Fulminant hepatic failure following hepatitis or drug overdose may be treated by liver transplantation.

Donor Blood group match. No HLA or cytotoxic crossmatch currently undertaken. Size compatibility required. Preservation can be undertaken for up to 20 hours using University of Wisconsin solution. Liver reduction techniques have been developed based on segmental anatomy of the liver such that parts of adult livers may be used in paediatric patients. Living related liver transplantation may also be undertaken usually using the left lateral segment.

Operation This is an orthotopic operation. The recipient's liver is removed. The donor vena cava is anastomosed to the recipient vena cava above and below the liver. The portal veins are anastomosed end-to-end. The donor hepatic artery on a patch of aorta is anastomosed to the common hepatic artery. End-to-end biliary tract anastomosis across a T tube is carried out.

Diagnosis of rejection Reduced bile output of poor quality down the T tube. Deteriorating LFTs. Biopsy.

Complications Early complications include acute rejection, vascular thrombosis, haemorrhage, biliary leaks and sepsis. Late complications include biliary infection, chronic rejection (vanishing bile duct syndrome) and recurrent disease.

Results

- 1-year graft survival depends upon the underlying liver disease. For chronic liver disease the 1-year graft survival is in excess of 80% but for fulminant hepatic failure is around 50%.
- 5-year graft survival. This is around 70% for chronic liver disease but only around 45–50% for fulminant hepatic failure.

Some individuals have lived for more than 25 years after liver transplantation. Late graft loss is less common than other forms of solid organ transplantation. About 20% of liver transplants at 5 years post-transplant appear to accept their liver grafts without the need for continuing immunosuppression. However, there are no criteria for defining this group prospectively.

HEART AND HEART/LUNG TRANSPLANT

Recipient End-stage heart disease with survival of 1 year unlikely, e.g. viral myocarditis, cardiomyopathies, severe IHD. Heart/lung transplants are usually carried out for cardiac problems associated with pulmonary vascular hypertension. The four possible lung transplant operations are heart/lung, double lung, sequential single lung, or single lung transplantation. The procedure used depends upon the lung condition. The commonest causes for lung transplantation in general are cystic fibrosis, bronchiectasis, primary pulmonary hypertension, emphysema, and idiopathic pulmonary fibrosis.

Donor Blood group match. No HLA or cytotoxic crossmatch. Size compatibility important. A safe time limit for cold ischaemia for the heart is 4–6 hours. The lungs are less tolerant of ischaemia than the heart. The lungs are usually ventilated with 80% oxygen and kept semi-inflated during storage.

Operation

Heart This is an orthotopic operation, the recipient's heart being removed. The recipient pulmonary veins are anastomosed to the left atrium and the recipient right atrium to the donor right atrium. The aorta and pulmonary arteries are anastomosed end-to-end to the corresponding recipient vessels. The operation is carried out on cardiopulmonary bypass.

Lung The technique depends upon whether it is a double lung transplant, sequential single lung transplant, or single lung transplant. A single lung transplant offers the advantage of maximum use of donor organs and relative technical simplicity. Cardiopulmonary bypass is not required. The main disadvantage of the single lung transplant is that there is only a limited amount of lung tissue and complications may result from the remaining diseased lung. The operation is therefore unsuitable for infective lung conditions such as bronchiectasis or cystic fibrosis.

Diagnosis of rejection

Heart Cardiac arrhythmias. Regular endomyocardial biopsies via forceps inserted via the external jugular vein and guided to the endocardium under radiographic control.

Complications

Heart Cardiac arrhythmias and death. Sepsis. Chronic rejection with small vessel disease and recurrent angina.

Lung Obliterative bronchiolitis

Results

Heart, heart/lung

- 85% 1-year graft survival
- 73% 5-year graft survival.

Lung

- 70% 1-year graft survival
- 50% 5-year graft survival

PANCREATIC TRANSPLANTATION

Recipient These are juvenile-onset diabetics who have concomitant renal failure and require kidney transplantation in addition. The aim is to prevent the development of other microangiopathic complications. The kidney and pancreas from the same donor are usually transplanted simultaneously, one organ into the RIF, the other into the LIF. The use of pancreatic transplantation alone to attempt to prevent the complications of diabetes is increasing.

Donor Blood group match. No history of diabetes. No family history of diabetes. Normal blood sugar.

Operation This is usually a hetertopic transplant, the pancreas being placed in either the right or the left iliac fossa. The majority of pancreatic transplants are whole pancreatic transplants with bladder exocrine drainage. The pancreas is removed with a duodenal segment, the latter being anastomosed to the bladder. The vascular anastomoses are based on the splenic artery and portal vein. These are anastomosed to the iliac vessels

Diagnosis of rejection Isotope scans. Reduction in urinary amylase where the pancreas is drained into the bladder. Biopsy.

Complications Graft thrombosis, fibrosis, pancreatic fistulae, rejection.

Results According to the expertise of the centre where the transplant is carried out there is a 50–80% 1-year graft survival. In centres with considerable experience of pancreatic transplantation, where the pancreas and kidneys are transplanted simultaneously the 1-year graft survival is 80% with a 5-year graft survival of 65%. Where pancreas transplantation alone is carried out, the 1-year graft survival is only around 50%.

The poor results and complications have encouraged an attempt to transplant isolated islets of Langerhans. These are injected via the portal vein into the liver. At the present time, the results are poor.

SMALL BOWEL TRANSPLANTATION

This remains an experimental procedure. The problems have not been solved and the operation is complicated by both technical problems and GVH disease.

GENERAL COMPLICATIONS

These include infection and malignancy.

Infection

Infection post-transplant may be dangerous and life-threatening and is related to use of immunosuppression. Infections may be bacterial, viral, fungal or protozoal. These include:

- *bacterial*, e.g. coliform urinary tract infections, septicaemia, chest infections, e.g. *Staph. pneumoniae*, tuberculosis
- *viral*, e.g. herpes simplex (cold sores on lips), herpes zoster, CMV, the latter giving rise to pneumonia, encephalitis and deterioration of graft function
- *fungal*, e.g. oral or vaginal candidiasis, aspergillosis
- *protozoal*, e.g. *Pneumocystis carinii*.

Management of infection When a transplant patient develops a fever and rejection has been excluded, aggressive investigation should be undertaken to elucidate the cause. Investigations include swabs of wound discharge, urine cultures, sputum cultures, blood cultures, viral studies, CXR, USS, CT scan, bronchoscopy, bronchial washings, lung biopsy. Treatment may have to be started on a 'best guess' basis. Appropriate therapy should be started as soon as laboratory confirmation of the diagnosis has been obtained. In severely ill patients with overwhelming infection, immunosuppressive drugs should be reduced or stopped until the infection is under control.

Malignancy

The incidence of malignancy is increased in all immunosuppressed transplant patients and therefore long-term follow-up is mandatory. Primary cancers develop in 5% of all recipients. There is a 100-fold increase compared with age match controls. Altered immunity with depressed tumour surveillance is an aetiological factor.

Skin cancers are the most common followed by non-Hodgkin's lymphomas. In cyclosporin-treated patients, non-Hodgkin's lymphoma occurs earlier in the post-transplant patient than with steroid and azathioprine therapy. Other cancers occur more commonly in transplant patients than in the general population.

Malignancy in transplant patients should be treated by standard methods. A decision to withdraw immunosuppression as part of the treatment of cancer is difficult. In general, patients with localized disease should be continued on immunosuppressive therapy, while the development of metastases is an indication for withdrawal of immunosuppression. However, decisions must depend on a careful consideration of the individual case.

Long-term follow-up of transplant patients Any patient who has had a transplant should be followed up long-term by the Transplant Unit. Patients remain on immunosuppression for life and long-term complications may develop. Surveillance for development of malignancies is important. Other important factors involve prompt and appropriate treatment of infection; advice on vaccination procedures (live vaccine should never be given to immunosuppressed patients); contact with infectious disease; travel abroad; pregnancy.

A

C

D

E

F

G

H

M

N

O

P

S

T

V